OSCEs at a Glance

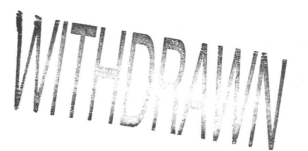

Contributors

Musculoskeletal
James Langdon   MB BS, BSc(Hons), MRCS(Eng)
Specialist Registrar in Trauma and Orthopaedics
Royal National Orthopaedic Hospital
Stanmore, Middlesex, UK

Psychiatry
Katherine Telford   BM BS, DM, MRCPCH, MRCPsych
Specialist Registrar in Child and Adolescent Psychiatry
Nottinghamshire Healthcare NHS Trust, Nottingham, UK

Stuart Whan   MB ChB, MRCPsych
Specialist Registrar in General Adult Psychiatry
Nottinghamshire Healthcare NHS Trust, Nottingham, UK

Radiology
Paula McParland   MB ChB, MRCP, FRCR
Specialist Registrar in Radiology
Southampton University Hospital NHS Trust, Southampton, UK

Surgery
Edward Fitzgerald   BA, BM, BCh(Oxon), MRCS(Eng)
Specialty Trainee; Research and Teaching Fellow
Department of Gastrointestinal Surgery
Nottingham University Hospital NHS Trust, Nottingham, UK

Photography
Amir Burney   FRCS, MSc
Teaching/Research Fellow (Surgery)
Sherwood Forest Hospitals NHS Foundation Trust
Mansfield, UK

OSCEs at a Glance

Adrian Blundell

BMedSci, BMBS, MRCP, MMed Sci (Clin Ed)
Specialist Registrar in Health Care of the Older Person and General Medicine
Sherwood Forest Hospitals NHS Trust
King's Mill Hospital
Sutton-in-Ashfield
Nottinghamshire
UK

Richard Harrison

BMedSci, BMBS, MRCS, MRCGP, MD, MBA
General Practitioner
Windsor
UK

WILEY-BLACKWELL

A John Wiley & Sons, Ltd., Publication

Library of Congress Cataloging-in-Publication Data

Blundell, Adrian.
  OSCEs at a glance / Adrian Blundell, Richard Harrison.
    p. ; cm.
  Includes bibliographical references and indexes.
  ISBN 978-1-4051-3057-8
  1. Diagnosis—Examinations, questions, etc. 2. Medical history taking—Examinations, questions, etc.
3. Clinical competence—Examinations, questions, etc . I. Harrison, Richard. II. Title.
  [DNLM: 1. Physical Examination—methods—Examination Questions. 2. Clinical Competence—Examination Questions. 3. Diagnosis—Examination Questions. 4. Medical History Taking—methods—Examination Questions. WB 18.2 B6587o 2009]
  RC71.B63 2009
  616.07′5—dc22

                                                                2008026358

ISBN: 978-1405-1-3057-8

A catalogue record for this book is available from the British Library.

Set in 9/11.5pt Times by Graphicraft Limited, Hong Kong
Printed and bound in Singapore by Fabulous Printers Pte Ltd

1   2009

Contents

Preface

Clinical examinations put fear into the hearts of many medical students. During a written exam, the mistakes can be 'private' whereas for clinical assessments there is always the danger of the hypothetical 'hole' being dug by the nervous student. Knowledge itself is only one requisite for becoming a competent doctor and, although important for clinical examinations, it is also essential to demonstrate the adequate skills and attitudes appropriate for a future doctor. There is still a tendency for students to focus too much of their work in the library rather than utilising the plethora of clinical signs and medical histories available on the wards. Facts alone will not permit success in clinical examinations and there is no substitute for perfecting your communication, history, examination and practical skills with a wide range of patients.

There are multiple OSCE books available but many substitute 'written' questions for true OSCE clinical stations. The other potential drawback is that many of them only cover one subject. This text presents potential OSCE stations from all the clinical subjects taught at medical school. We have used a case by case approach with the idea that the student should try to picture him/herself as they enter the station and are presented with the instruction and introduced to the patient or task. Each station consists of an example instruction with appropriate history or examination hints relevant to the case. Examiner questions are incorporated as discussion points. Where possible the answers to these viva topics have been given but, as a revision aid, this text needs to be used in combination with more comprehensive texts in each of the subjects. In addition to standard text books, useful information can be found on the websites of the National Institute for Health and Clinical Excellence and also the Royal College websites where multiple guidelines are written for use in clinical practice.

After our own personal experience of sitting OSCE style assessments, preparing students for them, and also as examiners, we feel this book uses a realistic approach to the OSCE exam and will help prepare students for the clinical exams throughout their medical school life.

Good luck.

Adrian Blundell
Richard Harrison

Acknowledgements

Many people have assisted in the development of this book. We are extremely grateful that they found time during their busy schedules to read various sections at various stages in order to make suggestions and corrections. While we have attempted to acknowledge those individuals as listed, there is one large group that also deserves a special mention – all the medical students and junior doctors in Nottingham, Oxford, London and Sydney that we have had the pleasure of teaching over the last few years and whose enthusiasm and ideas have helped form this revision guide.

We would also like to thank the following individuals: Naomi Bullen, Ashleigh Chalder and Asheeta Patel for their assistance with the setting up of the photographs; Pete Thurley for supplying some of the radiology images; Nicola Sherrington for the development of some of the mnemonics; and to the various development and production editors at Wiley-Blackwell for their support throughout the project – Vicki Noyes, Fiona Goodgame, Martin Sugden, Karen Moore and Helen Harvey.

Our final thanks go to our friends and family for their support and encouragement and in particular to Emma and Ruth who despite being author widows have agreed to marry us in the same year the book is to be published.

Section reviewers

We are indebted to the medical students and specialists who reviewed material during the early stages of the development of this book. We are also extremely grateful to the specialists listed below who have reviewed the manuscript at varying stages and have given valuable advice and feedback: Jonathon Bhargava, Consultant Ophthalmologist, Countess of Chester Hospital, Chester; Julian Boullin, Specialist Registrar in Cardiology, Kings College Hospital, London; Nick Clifton, Specialist Registrar in Otolaryngology, Queen's Medical Centre, Nottingham; Patrick Davies, Consultant Paediatrician, Paediatric Intensive Care Unit, Queen's Medical Centre, Nottingham; Chris Gilmore, Specialist Registrar in Neurology, Queen's Medical Centre, Nottingham; Adam Lawson, Consultant Hepatologist, Royal Derby Hospital, Derby; Hisham Maksood, Consultant Endocrinologist, Sherwood Forest Hospitals NHS Foundation Trust, Mansfield; Jane Partington, General Practitioner, Nottingham; Zudin Puthucheary, Senior Research Fellow & SpR Respiratory and ITU Medicine, Department of Health and Human Performance, University College, London; Emma Sawyer, GP Registrar, Nottingham; Ben Turney, Clinical Lecturer in Urology, University of Oxford.

Figures

Some figures in this book are taken from: Bull, P. & Clarke, R. (2007) *Lecture Notes: Diseases of the Ear, Nose and Throat*, 10th edition; Davey, P. (2006) *Medicine at a Glance*, 2nd edition; Grace, P & Borley, N. (2006) *Surgery at a Glance*, 3rd edition; Graham-Brown, R. & Burns, T. (2006) *Lecture Notes: Dermatology*, 9th edition; Impey, L. (2004) *Obstetrics and Gynaecology*, 2nd edition; James, B. *et al.* (2007) *Lecture Notes: Ophthalmology*, 10th edition; Miall, L., Rudolf, M. & Levene, M. (2007) *Paediatrics at a Glance*, 2; Norwitz, E. & Schorge, J. (2006) *Obstetrics and Gynaecology at a Glance*, 2nd edition; Olver, J. & Cassidy, L. (2005) *Ophthalmology at a Glance*; Ryder, R.E.J. *et al.* (2003) *An Aid to the MRCP Paces*, 3rd edition; Ward, J.P.T. *et al.* (2006) *The Respiratory System at a Glance*, 2nd edition; Weller, R. (2008) *Clinical Dermatology*, 4th edition; all Blackwell Publishing, Oxford and Buxton, P.K. (2003) *ABC of Dermatology*, 3rd edition. BMJ Publishing Group, London. Figure 11: Advanced life support algorithm is reproduced by permission of the Resuscitation Council UK. Figure 12: Hypertension: management of hypertension in adults in primary care is reproduced with permission by National Institute for Health and Clinical Excellence (NICE) (2006) CG034 London: NICE. Available from www.nice.org.uk/GG034. Figure 80: Screening timeline is reproduced by permission of the National Screening Committee.

Selected list of abbreviations

AAA	abdominal aortic aneurysm		FSH	follicle-stimulating hormone
ABG	arterial blood gas		FTT	failure to thrive
ACE	angiotensin-converting enzyme		FVC	force vital capacity
ACL	anterior cruciate ligament		GALS	gait, arms, legs and spine
ACTH	adrenocorticotrophic hormone		GCS	Glasgow Coma Scale
ADL	activity of daily living		GH	growth hormone
A&E	accident and emergency		GI	gastrointestinal
AF	atrial fibrillation		Glc	glucose
AIDS	acquired immune deficiency syndrome		GMC	General Medical Council
ANA	antinuclear antibody		GP	general practitioner
AP	anteroposterior		G&S	group and save
ASA	acetylsalicylic acid		Hb	haemoglobin
AV	atrioventricular		HDU	high dependency unit
AXR	abdominal X-ray		HIV	human immunodeficiency virus
BCG	bacillus Calmette–Guérin		HPC	history of presenting complaint
β-HCG	beta-human chorionic gonadotrophin		HR	heart rate
BMI	body mass index		HRT	hormone replacement therapy
BNF	*British National Formulary*		IBD	inflammatory bowel disease
BP	blood pressure		IBS	irritable bowel syndrome
BPH	benign prostatic hypertrophy		IM	intramuscular
BSL	blood sugar level		INR	international normalised ratio
Ca	calcium		ITU	intensive therapy unit
CCU	cardiac care unit		IUCD	intrauterine contraceptive device
CK	creatine kinase		IUGR	intrauterine growth retardation
CMV	cytomegalovirus		IV	intravenous
CNS	central nervous system		IVF	in vitro fertilisation
CO_2	carbon dioxide		Ix	investigation/s
COPD	chronic obstructive pulmonary disease		JVP	jugular venous pressure
CPR	cardiopulmonary resuscitation		LBBB	left bundle branch block
CRP	C-reactive protein		LDH	lactate dehydrogenase
CSF	cerebrospinal fluid		LFT	liver function test
CT	computerised tomography		LIF	left iliac fossa
CVA	cerebrovascular accident		LH	luteinising hormone
CVP	central venous pressure		LMN	lower motor neurone
CVS	cardiovascular system		LMP	last menstrual period
CXR	chest X-ray		LUQ	left upper quadrant
Δ	diagnosis		LV	left ventricle
D&C	dilation and curettage		LVF	left ventricular failure
ΔΔ	differential diagnoses		MCP	metacarpophalangeal
DH	drug history		MC&S	microscopy, culture and sensitivity
DIP	distal interphalangeal		MDT	multidisciplinary team
DNAR	do not attempt resuscitation		Mg	magnesium
DOB	date of birth		MI	myocardial infarction
DRE	digital rectal examination		MMR	measles, mumps and rubella
DVLA	Driver and Vehicle Licensing Agency		MMSE	mini mental state examination
DVT	deep vein thrombosis		MRC	Medical Research Council
EBV	Epstein–Barr virus		MRCP	magnetic resonance cholangiopancreatography
ECG	electrocardiogram		MRI	magnetic resonance imaging
ENT	ear, nose and throat		MS	multiple sclerosis
ERCP	endoscopic retrograde cholangiopancreatography		MSK	musculoskeletal
ESR	erythrocyte sedimentation rate		MTP	metatarsophalangeal
ET	essential thrombocythaemia		Mx	management plan
FBC	full blood count		NBM	nil by mouth
FEV_1	forced expiratory volume in 1 second		NSAID	non-steroidal anti-inflammatory drug
FH	family history		O_2	oxygen

OA	osteoarthritis	**sats**	oxygen saturations
OCP	oral contraceptive pill	**SFJ**	saphenofemoral junction
OD	once daily	**SH**	social history
OGD	oesophagogastroduodenoscopy	**SLE**	systemic lupus erythematosus
OSCE	objective structured clinical examination	**SOB**	shortness of breath
OTC	over-the-counter	**SOL**	space occupying lesion
PA	posteroanterior	**SPECT**	single photon emission computed tomography
PC	presenting complaint	**SpR**	specialist registrar
PCOS	polycystic ovarian syndrome	**SR**	systems review
PET	positron emission tomography	**STD**	sexually transmitted disease
PID	pelvic inflammatory disease	**Sx**	symptoms/signs
PIP	proximal interphalangeal	**TB**	tuberculosis
PMH	past medical history	**TFT**	thyroid function test
PO	per oral	**TIA**	transient ischaemic attack
PR	per rectum	**TNF**	tumour necrosis factor
prn	as required	**TSH**	thyroid-stimulating hormone
PV	per vagina	**U&E**	urea and electrolytes
RA	rheumatoid arthritis	**UMN**	upper motor neurone
RF	risk factors	**URTI**	upper respiratory tract infection
RIF	right iliac fossa	**US**	ultrasound
ROM	range of motion	**UTI**	urinary tract infection
RR	respiratory rate	**UV**	ultraviolet
RUQ	right upper quadrant	**VF**	ventricular fibrillation
Rx	treatment	**VT**	ventricular tachycardia
SAH	subarachnoid haemorrhage	**WCC**	white cell count

Types of station

History taking
Communication skills
Patient examination
Practical skills/procedures
Data interpretation

ESSENTIALS CHECKLIST

- Dress appropriately (local hospital policy)
- Wear name badge (+ white coat if expected)
- Be polite and considerate
- Read/listen to instructions carefully
- Use alcohol hand rub/wash hands
- Introduce yourself to examiners and patients
- Explain intentions and gain consent
- Treat simulated patients as if they were actual patients
- Obtain correct positioning and exposure of patient
- Maintain dignity of patient
- Ask about the presence of pain/ensure patient comfort
- Develop a rapport/treat patient with respect
- Explain your actions to the patient while examining
- Look at the examiners when presenting
- Speak clearly and confidently
- Maintain a logical approach when answering questions
- Thank the patient and examiner on completion

> Essentials checklist mnemonic
> – WINCER
>
> W - Wash hands
> I - Introduce
> N - Notice (i.e. be observant)
> C - Consent
> E - Expose
> R - Reposition

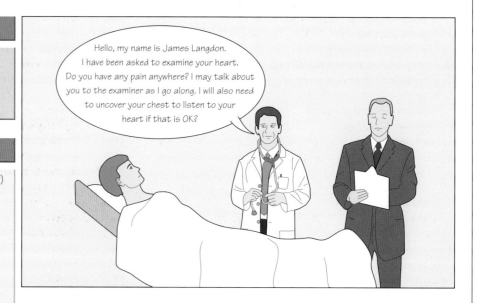

POTENTIAL PITFALLS

Forgetting elements of the ESSENTIALS CHECKLIST but in particular:

- Arriving late/dressing inappropriately
- Displaying inappropriate habits (e.g. sniffing, chewing gum, yawning)
- Forgetting about introductions and consent
- Forgetting about the importance of hand hygiene and (where appropriate) adequate sharps safety
- Not listening to or reading the instructions carefully and hence needing correction from the examiners
- Being rude, heavy handed or inconsiderate to the patient (or examiner!)
- Examining the patient from the left hand side of the bed
- Examining the patient in the wrong position
- Inadequately exposing the patient
- Looking at the patient while presenting rather than the examiner
- Fidgeting or fiddling with your hands while presenting
- Stating answers to questions without thinking adequately, and therefore not presenting answers in a logical order
- Looking like you have never performed a blood pressure measurement before (or other practical skill)
- Perfecting slick examination routines on 'normal' patients, but having seen few 'real' patients to then be able to pick up the abnormal signs
- Looking for clinical signs but not registering them
- Adequately covering 'textbook' revision but not examining enough patients or practising clinical skills

The OSCE has been increasingly used over the last 15 years, although one of the first descriptions was way back in 1979 by Harden and Gleeson [1]. This form of examination is now used extensively in medical schools in the UK. The main advantage is that it can be used to examine many different clinical skills with all students performing the same tasks, marked against explicit criteria by the same examiners.

Set up

An OSCE consists of a series of timed stations that each student rotates through. Each station involves a candidate carrying out a well-defined task. The time allocated for each station will vary with the required task, but in general each station lasts 5–10 minutes. The majority of stations have an examiner (or pair of examiners) who will assess the candidate's

performance using a structured marking sheet. If the station is purely data interpretation, then it is not always necessary to have an examiner present and the candidate will be required to complete a written task. Each station will have an accompanying instruction for the candidate to follow. The instructions can be presented in different ways:
• The examiner may ask the student to carry out a task
• The instructions may be posted at the station (e.g. on a poster near the patient)
• The candidate may receive the instructions prior to entering the station
• A rest station could be used to read through material relevant to the next station

OSCEs can be used at any stage during medical school. The exams in the earlier years concentrate on assessing the basic clinical skills and the emphasis is on the demonstration of correct technique, rather than interpreting the signs. This usually involves simulation-based cases rather than 'real' patient contact.

Types of station

The possibilities for individual OSCE stations are huge but generally they are divided into clinical, practical and data interpretation:

1 *Clinical stations*: These involve various aspects of communication or examination:
  • Obtaining and presenting medical histories
  • Performing a physical examination
  • Communication skills
These usually involve interaction with a patient who may be real or simulated (e.g. a student/actor/the examiner). The simulated patients rarely have abnormal clinical signs.

2 *Practical stations*:
  • Clinical skills (e.g. resuscitation, blood pressure measurement)
  • Procedural skills (e.g. cannula insertion, urethral catheterisation)
Mannequins or anatomical models are often substituted for the patient. The student may be required to explain and perform the procedure, gain consent or act on a result.

3 *Data interpretation stations*: These involve written or verbal discussion of a variety of results:
  • Examiner-led structured viva (e.g. discussion of laboratory results, interpretation of radiographs or electrocardiograms (ECGs))
  • Written station (e.g. 'Please interpret the following full blood count and answer the attached questions')
With the advent of improved information technology facilities, this type of knowledge can be adequately assessed during written exams, although some medical schools still include them in OSCEs.

The instructions

• Written or verbal instructions will be given to each candidate at the beginning of the station
• The patient, where necessary, will have had a chance to study written instructions summarising their condition (this is essential for simulated patients but real patients may just give their own history)
• Examiners will have instructions outlining the purpose of the station and the task to be carried out
• The examiners will also have read the student and patient instructions

The marks

Marking sheets will vary depending on the type of station and skill being assessed, but each task will be marked against explicit criteria. This will be in the format of a checklist of actions the student needs to perform. Patients may be asked their opinion of the candidate and it would be taken very seriously if the patient felt the student was rude or rough. Students may be examined by an individual or pair of examiners (who should mark independently). Once the station is completed an individual mark can be scored following agreement by the examiners and a statement as to the student's global performance is often included.

Preparation

There is increasing emphasis from the General Medical Council (GMC) that the clinical competence of medical students needs to be assessed and recorded. OSCE-type stations, using either 'real' or simulated patients, are ideal for this purpose. Clinical competence is a combination of three domains – knowledge, skills and attitudes. The GMC's document *Tomorrow's Doctors* clearly states that the attitudes and behaviour expected of future doctors needs to be developed during university along with clinical competence [2]. Students often underestimate the need to practise their clinical skills and bury their heads in the books until nearing the practical assessment, when there is a mad rush to the clinical skills laboratory to run through examination routines and a mad dash to the wards to see as many patients as possible. This behaviour remains common despite repeatedly reminding students of the practical nature of being a doctor and one of the main recommendations of *Tomorrow's Doctors* stating 'factual information must be kept to the essential minimum that students need at this stage of medical education' [2]. Start practising your clinical skills as early as possible, preferably with an 'OSCE buddy' or even 'OSCE group'. The skills tested in the OSCE and also 'real' life skills are best learnt in the clinical environment and not the library.

Technique

Technique does play a part in passing an OSCE. It is obvious which candidates have not practised their clinical skills sufficiently or who may have rehearsed routines on friends but have seen few abnormal physical signs. Emphasis is also on appropriate communication skills, which are necessary in all OSCE stations, not just the history and communication ones. This can be especially difficult if English is not a candidate's first language. The key to improving your presentation skills is practice. Once the presentation is perfected, the next skill is to become proficient at presenting discussion in a logical manner. The next few chapters cover in detail how best to use this book and deal with the skills of presenting in a logical order.

[1] Harden RM, Gleeson FA. *Assessment of Medical Competence. Using an objective structured clinical examination (OSCE).* ASME Medical Education Booklet No. 8. Association for the Study of Medical Education (ASME), Edinburgh, 1979.
[2] General Medical Council. *Tomorrow's Doctors.* General Medical Council, London, 2003. Available at www.gmc-uk.org.

How to use this book: work in groups of 2 or 3 and rotate the roles

History and communication stations	Use the information given for each character (student, patient or examiner) Role play the scenario with the examiner marking off points raised in the hints and tips checklist
Examination routines	The examiner should choose an example instruction to give to the candidate and then mark off the points raised in the hints and tips checklists. Real or simulated patients can be used
Cases	With real patients, the examiner should choose an instruction to give to the candidate and observe their performance If no patient is available, the examiner should ask the candidate to present the expected findings in an 'imaginary' patient with the condition, e.g. 'you have just seen a patient with mitral regurgitation, please present the possible findings' Ask relevant questions from the case as suggested
Data interpretation	The examiner can show the relevant information to the student and ask questions
Practical procedures	The examiner can ask the student to perform the various tasks and assess them using the checklist provided

OSCE presentation skills: hints and tips

Maintain eye contact with the examiner; avoid staring at the patient when presenting
Clasp hands behind your back to prevent fiddling
Speak clearly
Try to prepare your opening sentence in your head so as to start in a confident manner – first impressions are important
e.g. History station: 'Mrs X is a 56-year-old married woman who works as a receptionist ...'
e.g. Examination station: 'On examination Mr X is comfortable with no signs in the hands of cardiovascular disease, his pulse is ...'
e.g. Cases: 'The causes of a pleural effusion can be classified into transudates and exudates ...'
          'The causes of mitral regurgitation include ...'
Structure your findings logically; do not waffle
Present positive findings and relevant negative ones (e.g. no weight loss would be an important negative finding in a patient with dysphagia)
Try to present your differential diagnosis and problem list as a continuation of your findings, rather than waiting to be prompted
Although in common usage, try and avoid abbreviations
Do not be afraid of silences to collect your thoughts – it is better to think through an answer before rushing to the wrong conclusions
If you begin to start digging a hole, try and stop, apologise and ask to collect your thoughts and start again (if allowed)
Never use the terms cancer or malignancy when discussing differential diagnoses in the presence of patients

REMEMBER THE ELEMENTS OF THE ESSENTIALS CHECKLIST (CHAPTER 1) FOR *ALL* OSCE STATIONS. MISSING THESE WILL LEAD TO LOSS OF EASY MARKS.

This book can be used alone or equally well (if not better) with two or three friends. Take it in turns being the candidate, the patient and the examiner. Example student instructions for each station have been given and where possible the patient information has also been included, although for some stations improvisation will be necessary. Part of the skill is to realise the importance of inspection and piecing together the information obtained to come to a diagnosis. The diagnosis is often apparent from the end of the bed. The chapters in this book will act as aide memoirs. Remember to consider the patient 'as a whole' rather than focusing on one system or organ.

Communication skills are essential for *all* the stations. Make sure that you have plenty of practice in 'presenting patients' before the exam day so you are used to hearing your own voice. When asked questions, try and present the answers in a logical order rather than blurting out the first (and often the most obscure) answer. Try to avoid suggesting senior help immediately – the examiners want to know you are a safe clinician but you should be able to initially offer some sensible discussion. This book will introduce methods of being logical when presenting and answering questions. Remember the more you are talking the less time the examiners will have to ask tricky questions; you must, however, be talking sensibly!

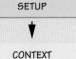

Communication hints

Communication skills: hints and tips

SETUP
- Gather the required facts (patient's notes, available letters) and personnel (e.g. patient's nurse or relative)
- Choose a suitable environment

CONTEXT
- Introduce, check identity and gain consent
- Ascertain the patient's (or relative's) prior knowledge of the situation in detail (one of the most important steps), e.g. 'your mother was admitted yesterday, can you tell me what you have been told up to now?'

CONTENT

Information gathering
- Use open and closed questions to collect appropriate information; be an active listener
- Avoid jargon and medical terminology but do not patronise
- Avoid confusing terms (e.g. shadows, growths, tumours) and use a term such as abnormality
- Use regular summaries and clarification, and check patient's understanding
- Explore the patient's ideas, concerns and expectations (ICE)
- Determine the impact, changes made and effects of the problem on the patient's life
- Do not be afraid of silences, especially after poignant phrases
  e.g. 'we have the results of your recent biopsy and I am sorry to say that I have some bad news (pause)'. Give this time to sink in before continuing, the patient may well respond during this pause and admit to what they were most worried about
- Apologise and acknowledge a person's feelings if necessary, but never blame colleagues about events that you are not responsible for
  e.g. a relative is angry about the GP not recognising that his wife had meningitis when seen 2 days earlier with flu-like symptoms. You cannot comment about the actions of the GP

Developing rapport
- Be empathic and sensitive, responding appropriately to the patients' emotions, encouraging them to express their feelings
- Be honest – if you are unsure about certain facts then state you will check with an appropriate person
- Use verbal and non-verbal communication and appropriate use of body language

CLOSURE
- Summarise and check the patient's understanding
- Agree a clear plan including adequate follow-up and support
- Arrange for further information to be given if necessary (leaflets, arrange appointments with other members of the health care team ± specialists ± support groups)
- Answer any questions or address concerns and offer contact details, e.g. bleep number

Ethical principles: hints and tips

Autonomy	Respect for the individual and their ability to make decisions with regard to their own health
Beneficience	Benefit the patient or others
Non-maleficence	Do no harm to the patient or others
Justice	Being fair or just to the wider community in terms of the consequences of an action

Answering ethical issues
- Present the case using the ethical principles listed above
- Acknowledge difficulties and be sensitive
- Present a balanced argument as there is often no completely correct answer
- Do not cause offence
- Display maturity and insight
- Be concise
- Close with summary
- Be aware of certain aspects of the law, e.g. confidentiality, criminality, DVLA rules
- Review the GMC website and documents such as 0–18 years and *Good Medical Practice*

OSCEs at a Glance. By A. Blundell and R. Harrison. Published 2009 Blackwell Publishing. ISBN: 978-1-4051-3057-8

4 History and examination hints

History stations: hints and tips

Background
Summarise serious medical conditions in the opening sentence

| Name, age, occupation |

Presenting complaint
The problem in the patient's own words

Systems review
Systemic symptoms
Cardiovascular
Respiratory
Gastrointestinal
Neurological
Genitourinary
Musculoskeletal
Consider more specialist histories if relevant, e.g. obstetric

| Relevant medical background (BKG) |

| Presenting complaint (PC) |

| History of presenting complaint (HPC) |

| Systems review (SR) |

History of presenting complaint
Mnemonic for symptom questions (particularly for pain): SOCRATES
Site
Onset
Character
Radiation/Relieving factors
Associated symptoms
Timing
Exacerbating factors
Severity

Risk factors
Summarise important risk factors as a separate section

| Risk factors (RF) |

Drug history
Prescription medication
Pills/inhalers/injections
Over-the-counter drugs
Homeopathic medicines
Allergy and adverse reactions
Compliance
Does the patient know what the drugs are for?

| Past medical history (PMH) |

| Drug history (DH) |

Past medical history (screening questions)
Previous medical problems
Previous operations/anaesthetics
Hospital admissions
Ask about: Heart problems, ↑BP, stroke,
rheumatic fever, asthma, COPD
TB, diabetes mellitus, jaundice,
epilepsy, kidney problems

Family history
Ask about parents' illnesses and ages
Ask about children
Family history of diseases

| Family history (FH) |

| Social history (SH) |

Social history
Impact of the illness on the patient and their relatives
Functional enquiry
Patient's mood and outlook
Smoking/alcohol/recreational drugs

Examination stations: hints and tips

Generic examination

Essentials checklist: WINCER
General inspection/observation
± screening test
System-specific inspection
Palpation
Percussion
Auscultation
Completion

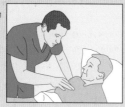

Generic neurological examination

Essentials checklist: WINCER
General inspection/observation
± screening test
System-specific inspection
Tone
Power
Reflexes
Coordination
Sensation
Completion

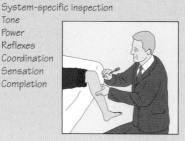

Generic musculoskeletal examination

Essentials checklist: WINCER
General inspection/observation
± screening test (function)
System-specific inspection (look)
Palpation (feel)
Move – active and passive
Measure
Special tests
Completion

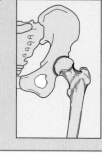

History stations

The general system for a *medical* history is outlined opposite. The other specialties use histories based around this structure but require more system-specific questions to be asked; these are summarised in the relevant chapters.

Taking a comprehensive history in an OSCE can only be expected if the station is of sufficient duration. A candidate would not be expected to do this in 5 minutes. In the shorter stations it is essential to listen carefully to the instruction, which will often guide a student towards appropriate questioning. Remain focused on the facts and relevant issues. A logical approach is essential, as is the skill of realising the pertinent questions to ask given a particular history, e.g. the importance of occupational history in someone with haemoptysis.

Each history station in this book has a list of hints and tips suggesting the information a candidate should be gathering. In general terms:
- *Remember the essentials checklist* (see Ch. 1)
- Ask some demographics, i.e. patient's name, age, occupation and marital status
- Determine the reason for the consultation, i.e. ascertain the patient's prior knowledge (e.g. if they have seen a doctor before, what information has already been given)
- If possible it is useful to ask a patient early in the consultation to list their serious medical or surgical conditions. In this way you already have a feel for their co-morbidities (i.e. background medical problems)
- Presenting complaint (PC) and history of presenting complaint (HPC): determine the symptomatology and associated features (i.e. SOCRATES)
- Systems review (SR): enquire about symptoms from other organ systems not already noted in the HPC
- Past medical history (PMH): include all serious medical and surgical problems in chronological order. Ask some disease screening questions as summarised opposite
- Further information should be obtained for major medical problems (e.g. stating that a patient has asthma means little on its own). Consider:
  - date of diagnosis
  - who made the diagnosis, e.g. GP, hospital doctor
  - why the diagnosis was made, i.e. what symptoms did they have at the time
  - how the diagnosis was made, e.g. biopsy, scan, laboratory test
  - what treatments the patient has had
  - frequency of hospital admissions
  - monitoring, e.g. investigations, hospital outpatients, GP visits
  - effect on life
- Drug history (DH) including allergies *and* adverse reactions:
  - compare the DH to the PMH; does the list make sense bearing in mind the PMH?
  - ask about over-the-counter (OTC) preparations
- Family history (FH):
  - ask about first-degree relatives (parents, children, siblings): are parents alive? If not what was their age and cause of death? Are there any diseases that run in the family?
  - ask about second-degree relatives (grandparents, uncles, etc.)
- Social history (SH): get a feel for the impact of the illness on the patient's and relatives' lives
- Consider summarising risk factors (e.g. cardiovascular) if appropriate
- Elicit and address any concerns the patient may have (e.g. 'do you have any other information that might be helpful, that we have not covered yet?')
- Verify what is concerning the patient the most

NB. This scheme is to be used as a guide and further avenues of questioning may need to be pursued depending on the individual patient, e.g. sexual, drug, travel and occupational histories.

Examination stations

- *Remember the essentials checklist* (see Ch. 1)
- Start in a confident manner (even if you are not) – first impressions are important
- Listen carefully to the instruction, e.g. 'please examine this man's praecordium' does not mean start by examining his hands
- Avoid having name badges and other objects dangling around your neck
- Hold your stethoscope or place it in your white coat pocket between stations. Do not have it placed around your neck!
- Examine from the right-hand side of the bed
- Take a physical step back and *inspect* from the end of the bed, observing the patient and surroundings
- Ask the patient to perform a *screening* movement if appropriate (e.g. take a deep breath for respiratory examination)
- Only talk through your routine if asked to, but make sure you guide the patient through each step (imagine they have never been examined before and so do not know what to expect) and be conscientious of their comfort at all times
- Treat the exam in a similar way to your driving test, i.e. make it clear to the examiners what you are looking for
- If you forget part of the routine, do not emphasise the fact by telling the examiners but fit it in at the next appropriate moment
- Follow the standard traditional routines shown opposite and summarised in more detail in each relevant chapter
- When you are looking for signs *actually look for them* and remember to comment on them when presenting
- State to the examiner what else you would like to examine in order to *complete* your assessment, e.g. blood pressure (BP) in a patient who you have found on neurological examination to have had a stroke
- Present exact facts rather than sitting on the fence, e.g. 'the conjunctiva are pale' rather than 'the eyes were possibly a little pale'
- Present accurate findings and summaries, e.g. 'these findings would be consistent with a right-sided pleural effusion' rather than just 'the patient probably has an effusion' or 'there is no evidence of scars on the anterior abdominal wall' rather than 'the patient has no scars' (the patient may have had a hip replacement!)
- Present positive findings and try and avoid too many negatives
- Try and summarise negative findings, e.g. 'there are no signs of chronic liver disease' rather than listing individually
- Present your findings in a logical order, i.e. the order you performed the examination, mentioning general observations and vital signs first
- Look at the examiner rather than the patient when presenting
- Avoid using potentially rude or distressing terminology, e.g. use the term mitotic lesion or neoplasia rather than cancer or malignancy and use the term increased BMI rather than fat
- After presenting the findings try and piece the information together into a diagnosis and, if possible, start suggesting investigations as part of a management plan

In essence *practise your routines until they are second nature* so you develop a confident, slick approach and develop an understanding of normal before abnormal.

Logical approach for a stable patient

History
Examination
Summary
Differential diagnoses
Problem list
Management plan

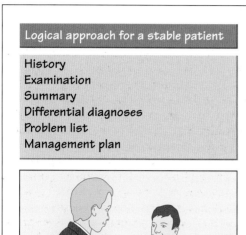

Management plan

Investigations
See algorithm below

Treatment

Medical   Surgical

Procedures

Cannula
Fluid aspirate
Lumbar puncture
Urinary catheter
Drain insertion

Location
Intensive care
Coronary care
General ward
Specialist ward
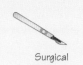

Monitoring
Chasing results
Reviewing the patient
Frequency of observations
Invasive monitoring, e.g. CVP

Multidisciplinary team
Physiotherapy
Occupational health
Dietician/speech therapy
Social work

Specialist review
Specialist opinion
 (doctor or nurse)
Further investigation
 or procedure

Patient education
Patient leaflets
Specialist opinions
Clear explanations
Support groups

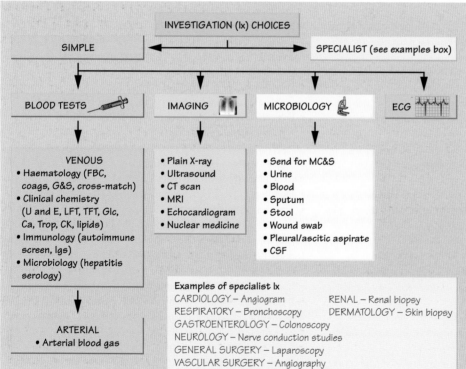

INVESTIGATION (Ix) CHOICES

SIMPLE ←——————————→ SPECIALIST (see examples box)

BLOOD TESTS   IMAGING   MICROBIOLOGY   ECG

VENOUS
• Haematology (FBC, coags, G&S, cross-match)
• Clinical chemistry (U and E, LFT, TFT, Glc, Ca, Trop, CK, lipids)
• Immunology (autoimmune screen, Igs)
• Microbiology (hepatitis serology)

ARTERIAL
• Arterial blood gas

• Plain X-ray
• Ultrasound
• CT scan
• MRI
• Echocardiogram
• Nuclear medicine

• Send for MC&S
• Urine
• Blood
• Sputum
• Stool
• Wound swab
• Pleural/ascitic aspirate
• CSF

Examples of specialist Ix
CARDIOLOGY – Angiogram   RENAL – Renal biopsy
RESPIRATORY – Bronchoscopy   DERMATOLOGY – Skin biopsy
GASTROENTEROLOGY – Colonoscopy
NEUROLOGY – Nerve conduction studies
GENERAL SURGERY – Laparoscopy
VASCULAR SURGERY – Angiography

Surgical sieve

Vascular
Inflammatory/infective
Traumatic
Autoimmune/allergic
Metabolic
Idiopathic/iatrogenic
Neoplastic
Substance abuse

Congenital
Dysplastic
Endocrine
Functional
Genetic
Hysterical

Patients seen in medical student exams are not acutely unwell and so can be assessed in a logical manner in order to determine a diagnosis and management plan. The approach is summarised opposite. This system helps a clinician make a diagnosis no matter what the presenting problem might be. This approach is also utilised in real life on the wards, although the process is dynamic, and the different areas can overlap, for example practical procedures can be performed while taking parts of the history.

History and examination: hints and tips
See Chapter 4.

Differential diagnoses, problem lists and management plans: hints and tips
When assessing a patient, try and formulate a list of differential diagnoses (ΔΔ). Next organise your thoughts into a problem list, taking into account other aspects of the history and examination rather than just the presenting complaint (e.g. non-urgent referrals, possible future investigations, impact of the illness on the patient and relatives, social problems, patient education). From the problem list it will be possible to determine a management plan (Mx). The main aspects of a management plan are described opposite.

For example, a 72-year-old female patient (weight 48 kg) with a known history of COPD is admitted to hospital with increasing SOB and a productive cough. Her blood tests have shown a ↑ white cell count and her chest radiograph shows consolidation in the right lower lobe. She has been on long-term steroids which cannot be weaned. She has had six admissions in the last 4 months but continues to smoke five cigarettes a day. She has rheumatoid arthritis which in addition to her COPD means she is limited in performing her activities of daily living. Her husband is fit and can help her but is due to be admitted for a hip replacement in 2 weeks' time. On previous admissions the doctors have felt that she might benefit from home oxygen therapy.

A possible problem list for this example would include:
• Infective exacerbation of chronic obstructive pulmonary disease (COPD) – needs treatment and monitoring
• Frequent admissions to hospital with exacerbations of COPD – optimise her treatment including a COPD nurse review in the community
• On long-term steroids – need to assess for side effects and consider osteoporosis prophylaxis
• Continues to smoke – offer smoking cessation advice as she cannot have home oxygen until she stops
• Discharge planning – husband due to be admitted to hospital in 2 weeks – will she be able to manage at home?
• Review inhalers and check technique – may have problems using some inhalers due to rheumatoid arthritis affecting her hands
• Currently on more than five medications = *polypharmacy*; admission is a perfect chance to carry out a full medication review
• Her weight is only 48 kg – consider nutritional assessment

Hints for problem lists
• Optimise medical conditions by considering further investigations or treatment
• Optimise risk factors
• Consider nutrition
• Show awareness of the complications of diseases and medications and look out for and treat these complications, e.g. osteoporosis prophylaxis for a patient on long-term steroids

• Involve other health care professionals, e.g. GPs, hospital specialists, nurse specialists, occupational therapists, physiotherapists, etc.
• Arrange adequate follow-up and monitoring of conditions
• Patient education
• Medication review

Investigation choices: hints and tips
Examiners will frequently ask about investigation (Ix) choices. Choose the simple ones first (unless asked for a definitive investigation), e.g. a patient who is admitted to hospital with a bleeding gastric ulcer may well need a gastroscopy at some point, but this is not the first test that would be carried out. Put yourself in your future shoes as the FY1 doctor and think what investigations you will be requesting. Remember the examiners are assessing your ability to become a safe foundation doctor; they are not assessing your ability to become a consultant.

An algorithm for investigation choices is summarised opposite. The heading 'imaging' is used instead of radiology to avoid missing out procedures carried out in other departments, e.g. echocardiogram.

State your investigations in the actual order you would request them, e.g. blood tests would nearly always come before imaging. It is also essential to understand the difference between an investigation and a routine part of the examination, e.g. think of blood pressure measurement as part of the cardiovascular examination, peak flow measurement part of the respiratory examination and urinalysis as part of the abdominal examination.

The only time not to start with the simple investigations is if the examiner asks for the definitive investigation, e.g. to confirm a patient has had a stroke, they need a computerised tomography (CT) scan of the head.

Possible viva questions
Many of the OSCE stations will involve some form of discussion around the problem presented. Most of the types of question will be centred on the following checklist:
• Aetiology
• Pathophysiology
• Symptoms
• Signs
• Common investigations
• Specialist investigations
• Poor prognostic features
• Treatment options
• Management
• Complications

Answering technique: hints and tips
Keep to a logical structure. Start broad and become more specific (e.g. 'the causes of a pleural effusion can be initially divided into exudates and transudates; exudates include . . .'). Use some form of *classification* in your answer, for example:
• The causes of *x* can be classified into cardiovascular, respiratory, endocrine . . .
• The causes of *y* can be classified into vascular, infective, neoplastic . . .
• Treatment can be divided into medical, surgical or multidisciplinary
• Treatment can be divided into acute, subacute or chronic (or early vs late)
• Postoperative complications can be divided into early and late
Remember to give examples in each category.

If unsure of the aetiology of a diagnosis then remember the mnemonic VITAMINS CDEFGH (see opposite).

Practical skills: hints and tips

Performing procedural skills competently is not just about the manual dexterity required

These stations test all three domains of learning (knowledge, skills and attitudes)

Types of station might include performing a procedure ...
- on an anatomical model or mannequin, e.g. cannula insertion (explanations given to the examiner)
- on a simulated or real patient, e.g. ECG recording
- on an anatomical model or mannequin but in the presence of a simulated patient, in order to explain the procedure and gain consent, e.g. diagnostic pleural aspiration

Remember:
- the importance of explaining the procedure to the patient and gaining consent (communication, attitude)
- the importance of knowing the indications, relevant anatomy and complications (knowledge)
- the ability to interpret results from performing the procedure, e.g. blood tests, peak flow rate (knowledge)
- the dexterity to perform the procedure (skill, knowledge)

The examiner can ask the student to perform the various tasks and assess them using the checklist provided

Station 1: Venepuncture

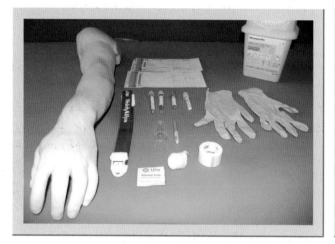

Station 2: Blood culture collection

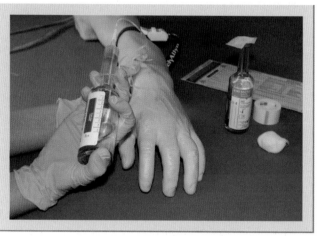

Station 3: Cannula insertion

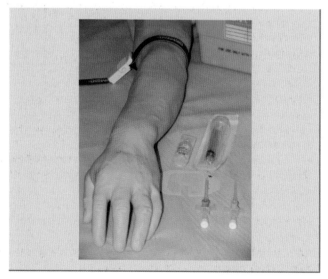

Station 4: Administering an IV injection

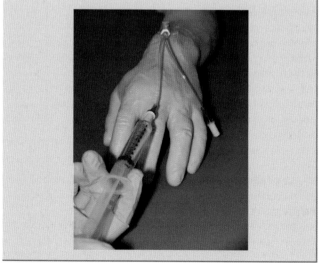

Station 1: Venepuncture

• *Mrs BP is attending a pre-op clinic prior to a right hemi-colectomy. Please take FBC, U&E, clotting and G&S blood samples using the mannequin's arm and prepare the samples for the lab*

Hints and tips

• Introduction/check correct patient/gain consent
• Explanation of procedure and reason for carrying it out
• Collect equipment (see opposite)
• Wash hands/wear gloves/apply tourniquet
• Select an appropriate vein by visualising and palpating
• Clean antecubital fossa (or alternate site) with alcohol wipe (allow this to evaporate)
• Attach needle to Vacutainer® holder
• Warn patient they will feel a sharp scratch
• Insert needle into the vein using an appropriate technique
• Once the needle has entered the vein, attach the Vacutainer® tubes one at a time – do not let the needle move once in the vein
• After removing the last of the tubes, release the tourniquet and then remove the needle
• Press with cotton wool over the puncture site (could ask patient to do this), keeping the arm straight to minimise bruising
• Dispose of sharps safely
• Tape cotton wool in place or use plaster (if no allergies)
• Label tubes, complete appropriate forms (including clinical information)
• Document which bloods have been taken
• Answer any questions the patient may have

Discussion points

• Please explain which blood bottles are used for each of the samples you have taken
• Do you know what additives are in the bottles and therefore which order they should be filled?

Station 2: Blood culture collection

• *Mr TG has a temperature of 38.2°C. You are his FY1 doctor and need to take blood cultures. Please explain this procedure to him and then demonstrate the technique using the mannequin*

Hints and tips

• Introduction/check correct patient/gain consent
• Explanation of procedure and reason for carrying it out
• Collect equipment (butterfly needle and Vacutainer® holder – see opposite)
• Wash hands/wear gloves/apply tourniquet and select vein as above
• Clean site with alcohol wipe (let dry)
• Once the site is clean, do not palpate the vein
• Warn patient they will feel a sharp scratch
• Insert butterfly needle and watch for the flashback
• Insert blood culture bottles into the Vacutainer® holder
• Allow ≈ 6 ml blood into each bottle
• Release the tourniquet/dispose of sharps safely
• Press with cotton wool over the puncture site as above
• Label the bottles correctly
• Complete the request form with appropriate clinical information
• Document the procedure in the patient's notes

Discussion points

• How would you investigate a patient with suspected bacterial endocarditis?

Station 3: Cannula insertion

• *Mr OS is a 50-year-old male, a known alcoholic, who has been admitted with haematemesis. Please demonstrate intravenous cannulation using the mannequin's arm*

Hints and tips

• Introduction/check correct patient/gain consent
• Explanation of procedure and reason for carrying it out
• Collect equipment (see opposite) – choose large-bore cannula and explain the rationale for this
• Wash hands/wear gloves/apply tourniquet
• Select an appropriate vein by visualising and palpating
• Clean the site with alcohol wipes
• Warn patient they will feel a sharp scratch
• Insert cannula using an appropriate technique
• Release the tourniquet
• Place an appropriate bung on the cannula
• Place a clear dressing, e.g. Tegaderm®, over the cannula
• Flush the cannula using 10 ml of normal saline
• Dispose of sharps safely
NB. If unsuccessful, remove the tourniquet and withdraw the cannula. Take a new cannula and commence the procedure again.

Discussion points

• What potential complications can occur from cannula insertion?
• For fluid resuscitation, which is better, a large-bore cannula or central venous catheter (central line)?

Station 4: Administering an IV injection

• *Mr JB has a K^+ of 7.8 with associated ECG changes. He needs 10 ml of 10% calcium gluconate and the nurse has asked you to administer it. A cannula is in situ*

Hints and tips

• Introduction/check correct patient/consent
• Explain your intention
• Prescribe drug correctly on the drug card
• Check for allergies and interactions with other drugs the patient is taking
• If unfamiliar with this drug then refer to the *British National Formulary*
• Check vial for correct drug, dose and date of expiry
• Double check this information with colleague
• Flush the cannula with saline to check patency
• Attach needle to syringe
• Break the glass vial safely and draw up the drug
• Clean the injection portal
• Inject the calcium gluconate slowly
• Dispose of all needles and ampoules safely (*do not recap needles*)
• Document the time of administration on the drug card
NB. Some drugs need to be reconstituted using a correct volume of diluent. Some drugs need to be infused slowly. The BNF has all the necessary information.

Discussion points

• What are the causes of a raised potassium?
• If a patient had an anaphylactic reaction to a drug you had just administered, what management would you instigate?

Station 5: Arterial blood gas collection

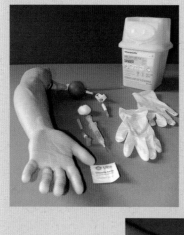

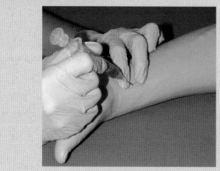

Station 6: Nasogastric tube insertion

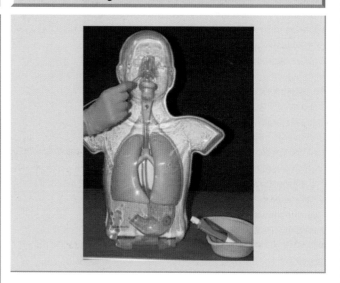

Station 8: Writing a prescription

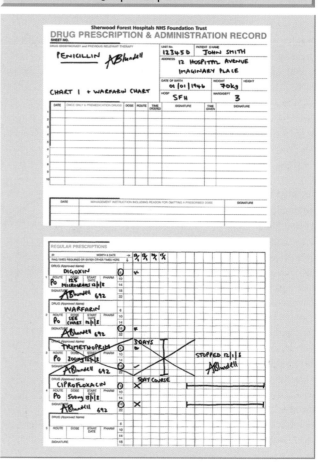

Station 7: Confirming and certifying death

Documenting confirmation of death
NAME, DATE, TIME and GRADE of DOCTOR as per all medical note entries
Asked to confirm death
Pupils fixed and dilated
No respiratory effort ⎫
No palpable pulse ⎬ for 1 minute
No heart sounds ⎭

Death confirmed at time and date
Rest in peace
Signature

Coroner referrals
Deaths within 24 hours of admission to hospital
Deaths where the deceased has not been seen by a medical practitioner
Unknown cause of death
Sudden, suspicious, unexpected or violent deaths
Deaths related to surgery or anaesthetic
Deaths due to alcohol or drugs
Deaths occurring in custody
Deaths related to industrial disease or accidents
Deaths occurring through neglect
Suicide

Station 5: Arterial blood gas collection

• *An 84-year-old male with known COPD has been admitted to hospital. Please take an arterial blood gas sample from his radial artery*

Hints and tips

• Introduction/check correct patient/consent
• Explanation of the procedure including the clinical reasons
• Preparation of equipment (see opposite)
• State to the examiner that you would perform Allen's test to ensure collateral blood supply via the ulnar artery
• Wash hands and put on gloves
• Attach needle to syringe and expel the heparin
• Position patient's arm with the wrist extended
• Locate the radial artery with the index and middle fingers of your left hand and clean the site with an alcohol swab
• Explain to patient that they will feel a sharp scratch
• Insert the needle (bevel upwards) at 60–90° to the skin towards the pulsation; advance slowly until arterial blood pulses into the syringe; collect approx. 2 ml
• Withdraw the needle and syringe and apply pressure for a few minutes over the puncture site with the swab
• Discard the needle in the sharps bin
• Expel air from the syringe, cap it and state you would take it to blood gas analyser, noting the FiO_2 and temperature of the patient

Discussion points

• You could also be asked to interpret an arterial blood gas result

Station 6: Nasogastric tube insertion

• *Mr H has been admitted following a stroke. He requires a fine-bore nasogastric tube for enteral feeding. Please discuss the procedure with Mr H and then demonstrate insertion of the tube*

Hints and tips

This station could be presented in several ways: as a pure skill, a pure communication or a combination.

You could be asked to insert a wide-bore (Ryles) tube or a fine-bore feeding tube. To confirm the position of the tube, measure the pH of the aspirate using pH indicator strips. (Radiography can be used to check fine-bore tube positioning.)

• Introduction/check correct patient/gain consent
• Explanation of reason for carrying out procedure including benefits versus risks and the fact that the procedure can be uncomfortable
• Collect equipment (see opposite) and place near the patient
• Wash hands and wear gloves
• Correct positioning of the patient (i.e. sat upright)
• Measure the proposed length necessary (ear lobe to nostril + nostril to just below xiphisternum)
• Lubricate the end of the tube with KY jelly
• The right nostril is used routinely, but check there is no obvious septal deviation or obstruction
• Pass the tube carefully into the nostril and pass along the floor of the nasal passage and into the nasopharynx
• Ask the patient to swallow when they feel the tube at the back of their throat (sipping water can help this process, although this would be unwise in a patient with an unsafe swallow)
• If the patient starts coughing then withdraw
• Continue passing the tube in to the appropriate length as calculated previously

• Inspect the patient's mouth to check the tube has not coiled
• Tape the tube in place and document the procedure in the notes
• Confirm the position using an appropriate method

Discussion points

• What are the complications of nasogastric (NG) tube insertion?
• How can one check the position of an NG tube?

Station 7: Confirming and certifying death

• *Mr ES, one of your patients, has died. He was admitted with pneumonia 3 days previously and also had a history of heart disease. Please demonstrate the procedure of confirming death using this mannequin and then complete the paperwork provided*

Hints and tips

• Confirm identity of patient with wrist band
• Shine a light in the pupils and check they are fixed and dilated
• Look, listen and feel for respiratory effort for 1 minute
• Palpate for a central pulse for 1 minute
• Listen for heart sounds for 1 minute
• Record the findings in the hospital notes
• Confirm with the staff that the relatives have been informed
• Complete a death certificate for your patient
• State to the examiner that you would verify that there were no indications for reporting the death to the coroner
• Complete the death certificate neatly and accurately, remembering that Ia must be the cause of death (i.e. pneumonia) and not the mode of death (e.g. respiratory failure)

Discussion points

• Which patients need referring to the coroner?

Station 8: Writing a prescription

• *Mrs TH has been in hospital for an elective procedure that she had 2 days ago. She has longstanding AF and is now complaining of some urinary symptoms. She has been started on trimethoprim but the microbiologist has just telephoned and asked you to change this to ciprofloxacin. Please complete her drug card. She is allergic to penicillin*

Hints and tips

In this station the examiner hands you the patient's drug chart but a simulated patient could also be in the room. (If unsure of drug doses or interactions, check in the BNF.) Each hospital will have their own prescription chart so please study these during your attachments.

• Check details on the front of the drug card match the patient and complete them if not already done so
• Ask about a history of allergies or adverse reactions
• Explain to Mrs TH that she has a urinary tract infection and you would like to treat this with antibiotics. Check that she is happy with this.
• Look through the current medication to check for any possible interactions with the new drug you would like to start
• Check to see if other treatment charts are in use and if so that this is noted (this patient is taking warfarin for her atrial fibrillation (AF) and has a separate warfarin treatment card)
• If safe to prescribe then complete the appropriate section of the drug card in *block capitals* using generic name and correct timing
• Document the indication if possible and both a start and stop date
• Sign and print name with bleep number

Station 9: Breaking bad news

Student info: You are the FY1 doctor in the breast surgery clinic. A 38-year-old lady with no previous medical history saw your SpR last week after noticing a right-sided breast lump. She has returned for the results of the biopsy which have shown invasive malignancy. She needs a right mastectomy ± radiotherapy. Your boss has asked you to organise the operation in the next 2 weeks. Please discuss this situation with the patient

Patient info: You are a 38-year-old high flying female executive and married with 2 children aged 14 and 10. You noticed a lump in your right breast 5 weeks ago and despite the fact your mother died of breast cancer, you were in denial. As it did not go away you consulted your GP who suggested referral to this breast clinic. A good friend had a similar lump which was found to be a fibroadenoma, which is what you are thinking this will turn out to be. Your mother died of metastatic breast cancer aged 52. You do not smoke or drink alcohol. You also have a busy 2 months coming up with work, having to prepare a presentation to give in San Francisco in 3 weeks time. An operation in the next 2 weeks would be extremely inconvenient

Station 10: Dealing with an angry relative

Student info: You are the FY1 doctor on the admissions ward and have just started your shift. An 84-year-old male patient admitted last night with non-specific symptoms has suddenly deteriorated with a reduced level of consciousness. It would appear that he has had a stroke. He is currently stable but requires an urgent head CT. The relatives have asked to speak to you for an update

Relative info: Your 84-year-old father has been unwell for several days and was admitted late last night with increasing confusion. The doctors overnight explained the problem was a urinary tract infection and dehydration and he would need antibiotics and fluids. The doctors put in a drip but your father only had 500 ml of fluid over a few hours. The bag has not been replaced and has now been empty for 5 hours. You are aware of the deterioration and are very angry about the lack of fluids despite overnight repeatedly asking the nurses to replace it. The explanation was that the doctor needed to write more fluids up. You feel this is clearly the reason he has gone downhill. If you are satisfied by the doctors' explanations then request to see your father at the end of the interview, if not then request to see a more senior member of the team and ask about making a complaint

Station 11: Dealing with an error

Student info: You are due to see Mr T, a 68-year-old male patient who has been called back to clinic because he was given the wrong results of a biopsy 3 weeks ago. There has been a mix up due to similar surnames. Having been told initially that the biopsy was OK, it turns out that it actually shows small cell lung cancer. Please discuss this with the patient who, following your consultation, will need to see the oncologists for consideration of chemotherapy. It is not operable

Patient info: You are Mr T, a 68-year-old smoker. You were found to have an abnormality on your chest X-ray 8 weeks ago and underwent a bronchoscopy. You were seen in clinic 3 weeks ago and told that the results of the tests had not shown any evidence of cancer. One of the doctors phoned you 2 days ago asking if you could attend the clinic today. They did not give a reason and you are now understandably concerned. The news 3 weeks ago had been a great relief to both you and your wife

Station 12: Dealing with consent

Student info: A 43-year-old lady was admitted with a severe headache. A CT scan is reported as normal and the consultant has asked for a lumbar puncture to be performed to exclude a subarachnoid haemorrhage. You are the FY1 doctor who will carry out the procedure under the supervision of your FY2. Please gain consent from the patient

Patient info: You are Mrs JB, a 43-year-old female. You developed a severe headache 13 hours ago. Your GP admitted you to hospital. The headache is still present although has improved following an injection and some tablets. You had a scan of your head 2 hours earlier and have been told that this is normal. The consultant came round a little while ago and muttered something about requiring a further test where they need to stick a needle in your back, which to be honest you think sounds painful. As your headache is a little better, you are not keen to have a further test. They did not say why you needed the test either. You have not heard of a lumbar puncture before and do not know what the procedure entails. You cannot understand why the scan of your head would not find a problem if one was there

Good communication is the crux to being a proficient clinician. Most of the complaints in the medical profession occur because of a breakdown in communication. Communication skills are necessary in some form at all OSCE stations, but some stations specifically assess the art of communication including attitudes and ethical issues.

Where is communication assessed?

- As part of history stations or specific communication stations
- When examining patients
- When presenting findings to an examiner
- In a written form at some stations
- When carrying out practical procedures or explaining them

Types of communication stations

- Explanation of procedures and treatments
- Gaining consent for procedures and treatments
- Breaking bad news
- Apologising for delays or errors in investigations and treatments

- Ethical issues, e.g. blood transfusion in a Jehovah's Witness
- Dealing with an angry patient/relative
- Discussing difficult topics
- Dealing with colleagues in difficulty
- Patient education

The emphasis on assessing medical students' communication, attitudes and ethical awareness has increased dramatically in recent years, and with good reason. These components are easily assessed in the OSCE environment, where the stations are run in various formats:

- An examiner guides the student through a structured viva, discussing a hypothetical situation that may involve ethical or attitudinal issues
- Aspects of communication are assessed using a simulated or real actor (occasionally the examiner may role play the part)

Sometimes information will need to be read prior to the station.

Remember the essentials checklist (see Ch. 1) and the hints in Chapter 3 for all the communication stations that follow.

Station 9: Breaking bad news

This is a difficult situation to tackle in 10 minutes, but is very realistic of life as a doctor. It is worth practising various aspects of breaking bad news: e.g. a diagnosis of cancer with available treatment options, a diagnosis of metastatic cancer with no treatment options, a diagnosis of a chronic disease (e.g. multiple sclerosis) and discussing resuscitation decisions with patients and relatives.

Hints and tips
- Introduce/check identity
- Verify reason for the patient attending and determine if anyone is with the patient
- Ascertain the patient's current knowledge of the situation
- Try to determine if the patient has any idea of what the diagnosis might be or if the previous doctor discussed the possibilities
- Present the diagnosis in an empathic, sensitive way
- Explore the patient's ideas, concerns and expectations
- Emphasise the importance of the diagnosis and treatment if necessary
- Offer time to think or contact her friends
- Use summaries and clarification where necessary
- Formulate a plan with the cooperation of the patient
- Offer further information through leaflets and arrange time to see specialist nurses
- Offer to arrange for the patient to see the consultant later in the clinic if necessary or if there are questions you cannot answer
- If, as is common, there is a lot of information for your patient to take on board, then a good way of assessing how much they have understood/retained is asking sensitively what they will be telling their spouse/friend
- At this point it is also worth remembering that it is often difficult to know how to break such dramatic news to the patient's children – she may wish for you to arrange help in discussing possible ways to do this

Station 10: Dealing with an angry relative
Hints and tips
- Introduce/check identity
- Ascertain the relative's knowledge of the situation, including diagnosis and management plans
- Acknowledge the relative's anger and give them time to express their views

- Apologise for the delay in prescribing fluids, offering a reason if you have one
- Present the updated information in an empathic and sensitive way and offer a reason for the deterioration
- Use summaries and clarification
- Formulate a definite plan that you will personally oversee
- Answer any further questions
- Offer an opportunity to discuss the situation with a more senior member of the team if necessary
- Stress the importance of sorting out the current situation, bearing in mind that if the relatives still wish to make a complaint later, then you can sort out the official channels, e.g. 'My only concern at the moment is to determine why your father has deteriorated and to try and improve his current condition with the antibiotics and fluids. If you still wish to make a more formal complaint, then I can arrange for you to speak to the correct personnel later today'
- Confirm your plan and check the family are in agreement with this, leaving them your contact details should they wish to speak to you again

Station 11: Dealing with an error
Hints and tips
- Introduce/check identity
- Ascertain the patient's current understanding of what the situation is (this will be more difficult in this case as you have asked him to attend and he may just be angry and want to know why)
- Explain the situation that has occurred, offering an appropriate apology
- Acknowledge the patient's anger
- Explain the steps that must now be taken in view of the change in diagnosis
- Formulate a definite plan including further investigations and referrals and offer to personally oversee this
- Use summaries and clarification
- Answer any further questions
- Offer an opportunity to discuss the situation with a more senior member of the team if necessary
- Offer leaflets and an opportunity to talk with the specialist nurses
- Confirm and agree a plan, including timing of follow-up

Station 12: Dealing with consent
Hints and tips
- Introduce/check identity
- Ascertain the patient's current understanding of the situation, including possible diagnosis, investigations up to now, what other doctors and nurses have said and what they expect to be happening next
- Summarise and clarify the results of the CT scan and the possible diagnosis
- Discuss the next step, i.e. the lumbar puncture, and ascertain if the patient has any knowledge of such a procedure
- Explain to the patient the procedure and the reason why it is necessary (i.e. a small number of subarachnoid haemorrhage (SAH) cases are not picked up on CT scan) including discussion of benefits versus risks and side effects
- Accept it is the patient's decision whether to have the procedure or not
- Offer some time to think about your discussion if necessary
- If the patient is happy to have the procedure then state the time you will be back to carry it out

Station 13: Explaining a procedure

Student info: You are the FY1 doctor on a medical ward. One of your patients, Keith Tomlinson, has a history of a change in their bowel habit. Your registrar has asked you to organise a barium enema for him. Please discuss this with the patient

Patient info: You are Mr Tomlinson, a 64-year-old male. You were admitted to hospital with some bleeding from your bottom but believe this is due to piles. It has resolved but you still seem to have rather stubborn bowels. This constipation has been for around 3 months. A doctor muttered about probably needing a further test because you have been found to be anaemic. You hope it is just some more blood tests that they wish to do as you do not really like hospitals and the thought of having more intimate investigations is rather alarming

Station 15: Requesting a post-mortem

Student info: You are the FY1 attached to the medical admissions unit. Last night a 76-year-old lady (Mrs Jolyson) was admitted with a presumed UTI. Her condition suddenly deteriorated late in the evening and the cause was not obvious. Despite active treatment of presumed septic shock, she arrested and died. You had briefly met her son during the original clerking and have arrived this morning to find him on the ward waiting to pick up the death certificate. He spoke to the doctor over night who had explained that she probably died of septicaemia due to her kidney infection. You feel that there were several confusing clinical findings which could not be explained by a UTI alone. You discuss the case with the coroner's officer, who is happy for the cause of death to be pyelonephritis. You still feel you are not completely sure what she died of and after discussing this with the consultant of the day, he suggests asking the relatives if a post-mortem can be carried out

Relative info: You are Mr Jolyson, the 48-year-old son of Mrs Jolyson. You came to the hospital when requested last night but your mother had died. This came as quite a big shock because you were under the impression that she had a urine infection. The doctors and nurses seemed to spend an awfully long time trying to get your mum better and in general you were impressed with the communication. One of the doctors explained that she had septicaemia due to the kidney infection and that is why she died. You have told your siblings this and have now come to pick up the death certificate. You see one of the doctors from the night before who asks if they can talk to you in more detail. You do not like the idea of a post-mortem but if the doctor communicates the reasons appropriately, you will consider a limited one, looking at the chest and abdominal organs, although you would not be happy if these were not returned to the body

Station 14: Resuscitation decisions

Student info: You are the FY1 doctor on the health care of the elderly ward. You have been looking after a 92-year-old man, Frank Spencer, who suffers with dementia (MMSE 13) and who has been admitted with aspiration pneumonia. This is his third admission in as many months. Over the last 3 days you have seen his wife and daughter on several occasions and have developed quite a good rapport, keeping them well informed of developments as they have happened. On the ward round yesterday, it was felt that if Mr Spencer deteriorated, resuscitation would not be in his best interests. You mentioned that you had got to know his family and would be happy to discuss this with them on their next visit

Relative info: You are 76-year-old Heather Spencer and have been married to Frank for 50 years. You have had a fantastic life but over the last 3 years he has been slowly deteriorating. This has been more marked since his 92nd birthday and although you are looking after him at home, you are not sure how long you will be able to manage even with the support services in place. You know he would not like to go into a nursing home, but you feel there may be no alternative. Each time he comes into hospital, it breaks your heart because although the hospital staff do their best and give him antibiotics to improve, he becomes weaker on each admission. You are not really sure how long he can last like this but you do feel he is suffering. The doctors have not previously spoken to you about resuscitation and although you do not want to make this decision on your own, you certainly do not want him to suffer

Station 16: Starting a treatment

Student info: You are the FY1 doctor on the cardiology ward. Vera Hunt, a 76-year-old lady has been diagnosed with atrial fibrillation. Your consultant has asked you to start her on warfarin and prepare her discharge. She will be seen in clinic in 6 weeks. You have met her a couple of times before

Patient info: You are Vera Hunt and are 76 years old. You have been admitted to hospital after having a funny turn. You collapsed after feeling your heart beat quickly. You live alone and are completely independent. You have had no falls apart from this admission and apart from high blood pressure, have no other medical history of note. The doctors have diagnosed an irregular heart beat and started you on a new tablet called digoxin. One of your friends has the same condition and they started her on rat poison but you have not been given that yet and to be honest you do not really fancy it, unless absolutely necessary. You do not smoke but you do like the odd glass of wine with dinner, possibly 6 or 7 a week. You are looking forward to going home

Station 13: Explaining a procedure

Although consenting patients for operations should be done by the doctor carrying out the procedure, there are several radiological tests that you will be required to know about and discuss with a patient. A barium enema is one such test that does not require formal written consent but should be clearly explained to the patient. The best way of knowing what is involved in such procedures is to go and watch them.

Hints and tips
• Introduce yourself and confirm your status/check identity of patient
• Ascertain the patient's current knowledge about the situation, i.e. why they think they were admitted and what they think is now going to happen
• Explain you would like to arrange a further test, called a barium enema, to determine if there is a reason for the constipation or anaemia

- Ascertain if the patient has any prior knowledge of this test
- Carefully explain the procedure
- Explain that it will be necessary for him to take a laxative substance in order to clear out his bowel prior to the procedure and on the morning will be allowed fluids only
- Stress that although the procedure is not painful it can be uncomfortable and is undignified
- He will be required to lie on a table in the radiology department and a tube will be placed per rectum through which barium can be inserted (as well as air); pictures of the bowel will be taken from various angles which will require the table to be moved around; the procedure will take around 20 minutes
- Check the patient's understanding of the procedure including the clinical indication and any risks
- Confirm that the patient is happy to proceed and check if he has any further questions
- Complete the appropriate request card, including clinical information and prescribe the bowel prep on the chart (if unsure of the bowel prep, state you would discuss with the radiology department)

Station 14: Resuscitation decisions
Hints and tips
- Explain to the examiner that you would arrange a meeting in a quiet room and be accompanied by Mr FS's nurse. Arrange for a colleague to hold your bleep
- Greet Mr FS's wife and daughter
- Ascertain their knowledge of the situation, including diagnosis and management plans
- Ask them how they are and how they think Frank is doing? (They may open up and say they do not feel he is doing very well at all)
- Clarify the current situation, i.e. diagnosis and treatment. Explain that although he is responding to the antibiotics, as this is his third admission in as many months, this could happen again
- Show sensitivity and caring while discussing the fact that, on future occasions, his response might not be so positive – have the family thought about the future?
- Admit that you need to discuss a difficult topic with them and broach the subject of needing to establish a plan of action if Mr FS were to deteriorate to the extent that his heart stopped. Had the family thought about it or indeed do they have any idea of how Mr FS felt about resuscitation?
- Clarify that this would not change his medical management in any way, but could prevent inappropriate actions in the event his heart stopped
- It is necessary to deal with emotions in such a situation, so do not rush and if necessary allow the family more time to think and talk amongst themselves
- At this point it may be fine to leave the family with the nurse but before leaving be clear as to the current plan and how they can contact you if they would like to talk further, giving details of the consultant if necessary
- Document the discussion carefully and if the family agreed with the DNAR, then complete the correct documentation (which will need to be signed by a senior doctor)

Station 15: Requesting a post-mortem
This is another consultation that should be handled by senior members of the team, although the early time following a patient's death is vital if requesting a post-mortem (PM) and junior doctors should be sensitive about this. Each hospital will have its own policy and documentation for requesting a PM.

Hints and tips
- Introduce yourself again and confirm identity of relative if unsure
- Express your sadness at the death of his mother
- Ascertain his knowledge of the events of the evening and the outcome and what information has already been given
- Acknowledge that this is both a difficult and sad time
- Explain that the working diagnosis is septicaemia from a kidney infection but several features did not fit in with this and you are concerned there may have been an underlying lung or heart problem such as a clot. Knowing the definite diagnosis could be helpful to both medical staff and the family members, especially if there was evidence of cancer or heart disease
- Explain that there are several options available, e.g. a limited post-mortem which would only look at certain organs
- Explain that a PM will not delay the funeral arrangements and there will be no visible incisions – the body can be viewed again after the PM
- If abnormal tissue is found, then with the relatives' permission, small pieces of this may be taken to be examined under a microscope
- Let the son have time to think and answer any other further queries. Offer a quiet room where he can contact other members of the family
- If in agreement, explain that the consent form is lengthy and that you will complete this with him and clarify any confusing areas
- State to the examiner that you would document the conversation in the notes and complete a clinical details information form for the pathologist
- Confirm to the son that you will contact him with the result and offer him your contact details so he can get in touch directly

Station 16: Starting a treatment
Hints and tips
- Greet Mrs VH
- Ascertain her current understanding of the diagnosis, implications of atrial fibrillation (AF) and possible complications
- Discuss the treatment options and the fact that you would like to start warfarin, explaining why
- Present a balanced argument for the benefits versus the possible risks of taking warfarin (benefit – to prevent stroke; risk – bleeding)
- Ascertain a negative history for falls and that she has no contraindications for anticoagulation (check alcohol history)
- Explain the logistics of starting this new drug (dose, frequency, need for monitoring the INR)
- Explain that if she notices any bleeding, e.g. in her urine, she must seek medical advice
- Explain that this drug can interact with some antibiotics, so she should be sure to tell future health care professionals that she is on it
- She should also limit her alcohol intake
- Answer any questions and clarify the dosing if necessary
- Check that the patient wishes to go ahead and start this medication (informed consent)
- State to the examiner that you would document this conversation in the notes, including the benefits, risks and possible side effects and also complete the warfarin chart with a correct loading dose

Station 17: Telephone information

Student info: You are the FY1 doctor on the health care of the elderly ward. You have been looking after Kenneth Jones who is 82 and has been admitted with a chest infection. He is improving on appropriate therapy but the CXR taken on admission has just been reported as being suspicious for an underlying lung neoplasm. This has not yet been discussed with him. He lives alone, is usually independent and is not confused. You have not met any of his relatives. A nurse comes to tell you that Mr Jones' daughter is on the telephone at the nurses' station asking to speak to a doctor. Please role play this scenario (a telephone has been provided and you are sitting with your back to the simulated relative)

Relative info: You are Kenneth Jones' daughter. He is 82 and normally completely independent. You see him once a week. He was admitted 3 days ago and told you on the phone that he had been told he had the flu and would be home soon. You are concerned that he has been losing weight and really not looking well. You have not been able to get in to the hospital yet to visit because you yourself have been unwell with a vomiting bug. You are keen to find out exactly what is happening and so have phoned the ward to speak to his doctor. You are concerned he has cancer because of his recent deterioration and long history of smoking but you do not feel it would be appropriate for the doctors to tell him this sort of news because it would 'destroy him'. You would rather know such information in advance

Station 19: Public safety

Student info: You are the FY1 doctor on the neurology ward. Peter Blundell, a known epileptic patient is due to be discharged home today. He was admitted 2 days ago following a fit after having been stable and fit free for the preceding 8 years. Your registrar has just telephoned the ward to ask you to remind Mr Blundell that he must not drive and will be seen in clinic in 6 weeks. You have not met Mr Blundell yet due to on-call shifts

Patient info: You are Mr Blundell, a 29-year-old male. You had epilepsy diagnosed in your late teens but have been fit free for the last 8 years. It was your birthday earlier in the week and you had a large amount of alcohol to drink and then collapsed in one of the bars. Your friends described you as having a shaking episode and you bit your tongue. You vaguely remember being told that you could not drive when your epilepsy was diagnosed, although you did not have a license at that time. You passed your driving test 6 years ago and are currently working as a pharmaceutical rep. This involves a significant amount of driving; in fact you are concerned that you will lose your job if you are not able to drive. This fit was obviously caused by your binge drinking and you cannot see a reason why you should stop driving, especially if your job is at risk

Station 18: Third party confidentiality

Student info: You are a GP. A 29-year-old married patient, Helen Robinson, comes to see you, concerned that she may be pregnant. A test confirms this and she is devastated. She asks to be referred for a termination as she is not ready to start a family because of career commitments. She does not want to discuss the situation with her husband because she knows he will want to start a family now. A few days later you notice Helen's husband, Mark, has an appointment with you. He has just entered your consulting room

Relative info: You are Mark Robinson and are 32 years old. You have arranged to see your GP, knowing that your wife has the same GP and visited a few days ago. She has really not been herself since, although she merely stated the GP had told her she had a viral illness. She has seemed distracted and has also been having some sickness in the mornings. Your suspicion is that she is pregnant and is keeping this information from you. You are hoping the GP will explain what is going on

Station 20: Self-discharge

Student info: You are the FY1 doctor on call on a Sunday afternoon. You have been asked by the nurses to review a patient on the cardiology ward who wants to go home. Brian Johnson is a 29-year-old male admitted 4 weeks earlier with infective endocarditis. The microbiologists have advised a 6-week course of intravenous antibiotics. Mr Johnson is an IV drug abuser, heavy smoker and heavy drinker. The nurses state that he often wanders off the ward and seems to be getting increasingly frustrated by his admission

Patient info: You are Mr Brian Johnson, a 29-year-old IV drug abuser who smokes 25/day and drinks 40 units of alcohol a week. You have been previously well but were admitted 4 weeks ago with an infection on a heart valve that the doctors have said was caused by IV drug abuse. You have had treatment for 4 weeks now and feel completely well in yourself. You are, however, getting increasingly frustrated with being in hospital. Many of the nurses look down on you, probably because of your background. All the other patients on the ward are old and unwell. The nurses do not like you going off to smoke. You are not sleeping well due to the noise of the ward. You feel that you would do better at home, as your mum has offered to let you stay with her on discharge, as long as you stay off the drugs. The nurses have informed you that you cannot go home until the doctors say so, but you know your rights. You have agreed to talk to one of the on-call doctors

Station 17: Telephone information

This is a common scenario on the ward. This station makes it clear that you have not met the patient's relatives before.

Hints and tips

- Thank the nurse and ask her if it is possible to put the call through to the doctors' office (remember the easiest way of breaching confidentiality is when conversations take place on the busy ward environment)
- Introduce yourself
- Establish the caller's identity (if in any doubt a doctor should take the person's number and call them back, after checking in the medical records)
- Explain that it is not possible to give information over the telephone without the permission of the patient
- If the relative mentions that she does not want information relaying to her father first, then discuss the principle that it is his right to know and make decisions as he has the capacity to do so (respect his autonomy)
- Agree some form of plan: if Mr KJ is well enough to come to the phone, then invite him to speak to his daughter and with his permission information could then be given; if he is too unwell then state you will go and ask his permission and telephone her back, bearing in mind that you should only tell her what you have already discussed with him. The ideal is to realise that the telephone is not the best medium for communication and offer to arrange a time for her to come in and discuss the case
- Explain to the examiner that any conversations would be clearly documented in the patient's notes

Station 18: Third party confidentiality

Hints and tips

- Introduce yourself
- Ascertain the husband's reason for attending surgery
- Confirm that it is not possible for you to discuss the health problems of other patients, including his wife
- The husband may try different angles to wean information out of you but you must be very strict with confidentiality
- Encourage the husband to discuss his feelings with his wife
- Verify that the patient did not have another reason for attending today, related to his own health
- Apologise if necessary but under no circumstances discuss the health problems of his wife
- Document the consultation

This case is a relatively straightforward case of maintaining confidentiality. It could be developed in a viva to a discussion regarding opinions on abortion and maternal and paternal rights. Alternative stations could involve situations where confidentiality may be breached at the doctor's discretion, e.g. in cases of public safety (see Station 19) or, for example, where a 32-year-old male has been diagnosed with human immuno-deficiency virus (HIV), but does not wish his partner to be informed – his partner may be at risk.

Station 19: Public safety

Hints and tips

- Introduce and explain your position/check identity of patient
- Ascertain the patient's current understanding of the situation and the reason for his admission
- Confirm the diagnosis and check the patient understands this
- Ascertain an occupational history and realise the significance of a driving ban
- Discuss that Mr PB will need to inform the Driver and Vehicle Licensing Agency (DVLA) of the diagnosis and that he will not be able to drive for 12 months and that if he did drive his insurance policy would not be valid
- Acknowledge that this situation is difficult as he currently relies on driving for his occupation but reinforce that informing the DVLA is a legal requirement and stress that this decision is not only for his safety but also that of the general public
- Suggest that Mr PB talks to his employer and attempts to find a temporary new position
- If Mr PB refuses to accept your advice then arrange for one of your senior colleagues to see him
- This station could become confrontational if not handled with care, but if a patient continues to drive despite adequate effort to advise them against this, then a doctor has a duty to inform the DVLA – it would be better to avoid threats to the patient and use careful communication to convince them of the correct course of action
- Confirm the clinic appointment in 6 weeks time, when the matter can be discussed further
- Explain to the examiner that this conversation would be clearly documented in the notes

Station 20: Self-discharge

Hints and tips

- Introduce yourself and explain your position/check identity of patient
- Ascertain the patient's current understanding of the situation, including diagnosis, what it means and what other doctors and nurses have said
- Ascertain the reasons why the patient would like to self-discharge and appreciate these if necessary (although do not comment on other people's actions)
- Explain that you would recommend that the patient stays in hospital to complete the intravenous antibiotics and clarify that the patient understands the importance of completing the treatment and the possible consequences of not doing so
- If there are problems that you think could be resolved, then suggest these, e.g. you could offer to talk to the nursing staff to agree that he can leave the ward at set times
- Clarify that if the patient left the hospital, this would be against medical advice and he would be required to complete a self-discharge letter
- Advise that you could arrange for a member of his team to talk in more detail, but this might have to wait until Monday
- If he still insists on leaving, then complete the correct paperwork
- Consider an alternative course of action, e.g. a course of oral antibiotics, but speak to microbiology about this
- Speak to your senior on call if necessary
- Arrange follow-up and make a note for the team to contact the GP about the discharge
- State that you would contact the cardiology team on Monday morning to let them know about the events
- Document all discussions and agreed plans in the notes

Station 21: Basic life support

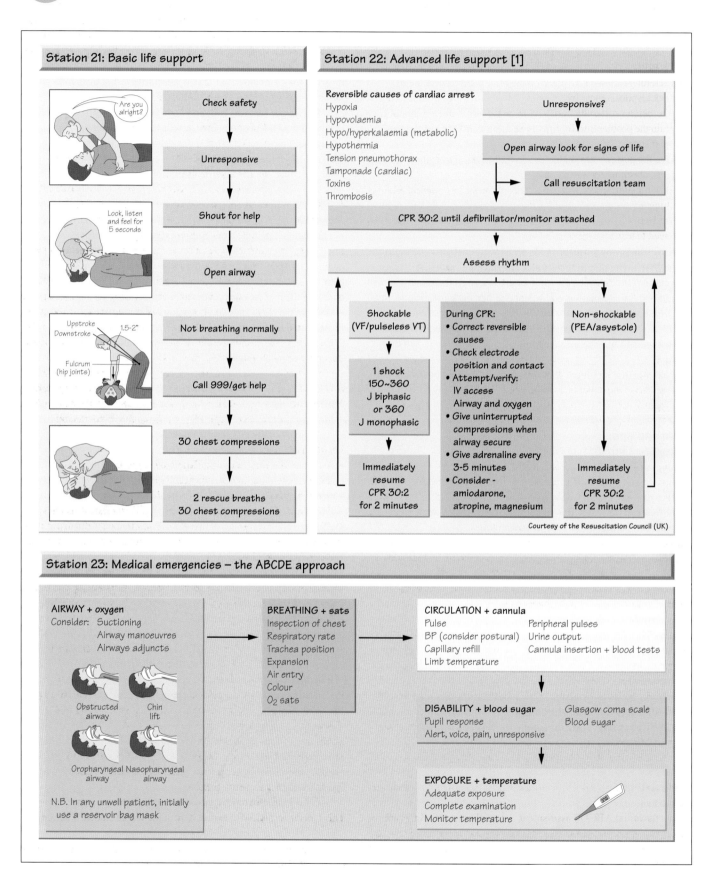

Check safety

↓

Unresponsive

↓

Shout for help

↓

Open airway

↓

Not breathing normally

↓

Call 999/get help

↓

30 chest compressions

↓

2 rescue breaths
30 chest compressions

Station 22: Advanced life support [1]

Reversible causes of cardiac arrest
Hypoxia
Hypovolaemia
Hypo/hyperkalaemia (metabolic)
Hypothermia
Tension pneumothorax
Tamponade (cardiac)
Toxins
Thrombosis

Unresponsive?

↓

Open airway look for signs of life

→ Call resuscitation team

↓

CPR 30:2 until defibrillator/monitor attached

↓

Assess rhythm

Shockable (VF/pulseless VT)

1 shock
150~360
J biphasic
or 360
J monophasic

↓

Immediately
resume
CPR 30:2
for 2 minutes

During CPR:
• Correct reversible causes
• Check electrode position and contact
• Attempt/verify: IV access Airway and oxygen
• Give uninterrupted compressions when airway secure
• Give adrenaline every 3-5 minutes
• Consider – amiodarone, atropine, magnesium

Non-shockable (PEA/asystole)

Immediately
resume
CPR 30:2
for 2 minutes

Courtesy of the Resuscitation Council (UK)

Station 23: Medical emergencies – the ABCDE approach

AIRWAY + oxygen
Consider: Suctioning
Airway manoeuvres
Airways adjuncts

Obstructed airway   Chin lift

Oropharyngeal   Nasopharyngeal
airway   airway

N.B. In any unwell patient, initially use a reservoir bag mask

→

BREATHING + sats
Inspection of chest
Respiratory rate
Trachea position
Expansion
Air entry
Colour
O_2 sats

→

CIRCULATION + cannula
Pulse   Peripheral pulses
BP (consider postural) Urine output
Capillary refill   Cannula insertion + blood tests
Limb temperature

↓

DISABILITY + blood sugar   Glasgow coma scale
Pupil response   Blood sugar
Alert, voice, pain, unresponsive

↓

EXPOSURE + temperature
Adequate exposure
Complete examination
Monitor temperature

Station 21: Basic life support

• *You are walking home one evening when you spot a person collapsed on the pavement. Please assess the person and take whatever action you see fit. You are alone (you have a mobile phone). There is no evidence of cervical spine trauma.*

Hints and tips

• Check for your own safety first
• Check responsiveness by shouting and giving the person a shake
• If the person responds, leave them in the same position and try to ascertain the problem, calling an ambulance if necessary
• If no response, shout for help
• Move the person onto their back and open the airway (head lift and chin tilt), checking for any foreign body
• Check for signs of breathing (look, listen and feel for 10 seconds) – if breathing, move into recovery position
• If no breathing, call 999 or physically go for help – remember you may need to leave the person
• Then 30 chest compressions (rate 100 per minute)
• Combine two rescue breaths with each set of compressions
• Stop to recheck only if there is respiratory effort
• Continue resuscitation until further help arrives, the person starts breathing or you become exhausted

Station 22: Advanced life support

Scenarios in an OSCE will range from patients already found collapsed to those that are initially medically unwell (see Station 23) who may arrest. The stations may assess airway management (using basic airway manoeuvres and adjuncts), safe defibrillation or leading an arrest scenario following the algorithms opposite.

Station 23: Medical emergencies

Student info: *You have been asked by the nurses to review Mr SP who is on the orthopaedic ward. He is 84 and underwent repair of a right fractured neck of femur yesterday. He has been quite well during the day but the nurses are now worried about him as he seems confused and is not feeling well. They have asked you to attend urgently*

Examiner info: *Initial observations are: patent airway, respiratory rate (RR) 30, crackles left base, saturations on room air 86%, heart rate (HR) 120, blood pressure (BP) 90/50, temperature 38°C. The patient has developed a hospital-acquired pneumonia. The observations can change depending on the action of the student*

Hints and tips

Follow the ABCDE protocol as discussed opposite.
• *Airway*: patent but the patient is unwell so apply oxygen using a reservoir mask
• *Breathing*: RR is high and there is evidence of crackles at the left lung base; measure oxygen (O_2) sats
• *Circulation*: tachycardia and hypotension; insert large-bore cannula and give IV fluids (500 ml normal saline). Send blood tests
• *Disability*: alert although confused, blood sugar level (BSL) 4.2, pupils equal
• *Exposure*: no obvious skin infections and, in particular, the wound site is clean

During the initial ABCDE assessment, act on abnormal findings appropriately and then reassess the response to your interventions. If the patient deteriorates at any time then return to the *airway*. Following this initial assessment it will be necessary to use a logical approach to determine the diagnosis (see Ch. 5). State to the examiners that you would review the patient's hospital notes, drug chart and observations.

The most likely diagnosis is a hospital-acquired pneumonia, but other sources of infection need to be considered as do other causes of hypoxia post-operatively. The reason for the confusion in this man is multifactorial and it is important for you to know the causes of delirium and how to assess this (see Station 78, Ch. 30).

Ix	*Bloods*	FBC, U&E, CRP, ABG,
	ECG	
	Imaging	CXR (portable if the patient is unwell)
	Micro	Blood cultures, urine for MC&S
Mx	*Rx*	Oxygen, IV fluids, IV antibiotics, thromboembolic prophylaxis, paracetamol
		Review medications, specific management of delirium
	Location	Consider transfer to medical ward or HDU
	Monitoring	Regular observation, strict fluid balance
	MDT	Consider chest physiotherapy
	Specialists	Senior medical doctor, liaise with orthopaedic surgeons

Student info: *You are the FY1 on the gastro team and the nurses have asked you to see a patient on your ward urgently. He was admitted overnight with melaena on a background of alcoholic liver disease. On admission he was clinically stable and he is awaiting a gastroscopy. He has passed more melaena and is not looking well. He is not on oxygen but does have a 20 gauge cannula in his left hand*

Examiner info: *Initial observations are patent airway, RR 24, clear lungs, saturations on room air 92%, HR 120, BP 80/50, temperature 36°C. On exposure the patient has had a large amount of melaena. The observations can change depending on the action of the student*

Hints and tips

Follow the ABCDE protocol as discussed opposite.
• *Airway*: patent, commence oxygen via a reservoir mask
• *Breathing*: RR 24, sats 92% on room air, chest clear
• *Circulation*: HR 120, cool peripheries, capillary return 4 seconds, BP 80/50. Insert two large-bore cannulae. Commence fluid resuscitation (500 ml IV normal saline stat). Take blood for routine tests and cross-match
• *Disability*: alert, BSL 5
• *Exposure*: large amount of melaena, nil other problems

The diagnosis is most likely an upper GI bleed due to oesophageal varices. This man needs resuscitation and stabilisation before transferring for endoscopy.

Ix	*Bloods*	FBC, clotting, U&E, LFT, Glc, cross-match 4 units, ABG (assess metabolic state)
	ECG	
Mx	*Rx*	O_2, IV fluids, blood transfusion, consider terlipressin, correct clotting abnormalities, consider vitamin K
	Procedures	Consider urinary catheter and central line
	Location	Gastro ward or HDU if necessary
	Monitoring	Regular observation, central venous pressure (CVP), strict fluid balance, regular blood tests, OGD
	Specialists	Senior medical help
		Inform on-call gastro doctor and arrange gastroscopy

This type of scenario will evolve depending on the student's actions.

[1] Resuscitation Council UK. *Adult advanced life support algorithm.* Resuscitation Council UK, 2005. Available at www.resus.org.uk.

Cardiovascular symptoms

Chest pain	Syncope	Breathlessness	Orthopnoea
Palpitations	PND	Dizziness	Peripheral oedema

Station 24: Palpitations

Causes of atrial fibrillation (THE ATRIAL FIBS)

Thyroid disease (hyperthyroidism)	Ischaemic heart disease
Hypertension / Hypothermia	Atrial dilatation / Atrial myxoma
Electrolyte imbalance (e.g. hypomagnesaemia)	Lone (i.e. idiopathic)
	Fever (e.g. endocarditis, chest infection)
Alcohol	Infarct / Ischaemia
Thromboembolic disease (PE)	Bad valves (e.g. mitral stenosis)
Rheumatic heart disease	Stimulants (e.g. cocaine)

Station 25: Chest pain

Management of acute MI

ABCDE	Morphine + antiemetic	R - Reassurance
High flow oxygen	Thrombolysis if indicated	O - Oxygen
Aspirin 300 mg	Consider angioplasty	M - Morphine
Clopidogrel 300 mg	Monitoring on CCU	A - Aspirin
GTN spray or infusion		N - Nitrates
		C - Clopidogrel
		E - Enoxaparin

Station 26: Hypertension

Classification of hypertension

Normal	Systolic < 120	and Diastolic < 80
Prehypertension	Systolic 120–139	or Diastolic 80–89
Stage 1 hypertension	Systolic 140–159	or Diastolic 90–99
Stage 2 hypertension	Systolic > 159	or Diastolic > 99

Causes of hypertension

Primary = essential > 90%
Secondary
- Renal (renal artery stenosis, polycystic kidneys, glomerulonephritis)
- Endocrine (Cushing's, Conn's, phaeochromocytoma)
- Drugs (steroids, OCP)
- CVS (coarctation of the aorta)
- Others (pre-eclampsia, 'white coat hypertension')

Treatment of hypertension
- Lifestyle factors (stop smoking, reduce alcohol, exercise, reduce weight, reduce salt intake, reduce stress)
- Address cardiovascular risk factors
- Drugs

Choosing drugs for patients newly diagnosed with hypertension

Younger than 55 years	55 years or older or black patients of any age
Step 1	
A	C or D
Step 2	
A + C or C + D	
Step 3	
A + C + D	
Step 4	

Add • Further diuretic therapy, or • Alpha-blocker, or • Beta-blocker
Consider seeking specialist advice

Abreviations
A = ACE inhibitor (consider angiotensin-II receptor antagonist if ACE intolerant)
C = calcium-channel blocker
D = thiazide-type diuretic
Black patients are those of African or Caribbean descent, and not mixed-race, Asian or Chinese patients

Risk factors for ischaemic heart disease

+ve PMH	↑ Cholesterol	↑ BP
Smoking	+ve FH	Diabetes

Secondary prevention post MI

Lifestyle	Physical activity
	Smoking cessation
	Dietary advice
	Increased omega 3 fatty acids (oily fish)
	Sensible alcohol intake
Optimise risk factors	
Cardiac rehabilitation	
Drugs	ACE/aspirin /b-blocker/statin
	Clopidogrel for up to 12 months
Consider need for coronary revascularisation	

Differential diagnosis of chest pain

Diagnosis	History hints	Examination hints
MI	Central crushing chest pain. Radiation to arms, jaw. Nausea, vomiting, sweating, unwell. Risk factors	Sweaty, cold, clammy. Tachycardia. Signs of shock or cardiac failure
Angina	Central chest pain ± radiation. Known precipitant. Alleviated by nitrates or rest	Tachycardia
Pulmonary-embolism (PE)	Sudden-onset SOB. Pleuritic chest pain. Haemoptysis. May just have increased SOB. Risk factors	Often none specific. Tachycardia. ↑ RR. Signs of shock. Pleural rub
Pleurisy	Sharp, pleuritic chest pain. Recent chest infection. Systemic symptoms	Fever, signs of consolidation, pleural rub
Pneumothorax	Sudden-onset SOB. Localised pleuritic chest pain. Risk factors	↓ Air entry. ↑ RR. Tracheal deviation (late sign). Signs of shock
Aortic dissection	Central 'tearing' chest pain. Radiation to back. Unwell. Nausea, vomiting, dizzyness. Risk factors	Unwell. BP variation in each arm. Radio, radial delay. Absent pulses. Signs of shock. Neurological deficits. Aortic regurgitation
Pericarditis	Central chest pain, sharp in nature. Often relieved by sitting forward. Systemic symptoms. Recent viral illness	Fever, tachycardia. Pericardial rub. Signs of vasculitic disease
Dyspepsia	Central chest, burning, epigastric pain. May radiate to back. Food associations. Exacerbated by lying flat	Epigastric tenderness
Musculo-skeletal	History of injury. Pain exacerbated by movement	Reproducible tenderness (not a specific sign for musculoskeletal pain)

Station 24: Palpitations

Student info: *Mrs MH is an 84-year-old female referred by her GP to the cardiology clinic with a history of palpitations. You are the cardiology FY1 doctor. Please take a history to present to your consultant*

Patient info: *You are Mrs MH and are 84 years old. PMH: TIA 2 years ago (1-hour history of right-hand weakness) and ↑BP. DH: aspirin, simvastatin, perindopril and bendrofluazide. You have had two episodes of palpitations over the last month while sitting down, each lasting 10 minutes. They felt regular and were associated with a central chest discomfort (no radiation, SOB, or nausea). You get intermittent dizziness on standing in the morning approximately 1 hour after taking your tablets. You live alone in your bungalow, are mobile with a stick, have had no falls, are a non-smoker and drink six cups of coffee a day and two sherries at night. You are concerned because your friend had a similar sounding episode to this and then was found collapsed at home having had a presumed heart attack*

Hints and tips
- Determine the patient's reason for coming to hospital and ascertain her current knowledge of the situation
- Determine symptomatology
- Need exact timing, onset and previous episodes of associated chest discomfort or SOB; ask the patient to tap out the rhythm
- Determine if any symptoms of hyperthyroidism
- Full DH; elicit details of the PMH, including events of the previous TIA and investigations performed at this time
- Full social history including details of alcohol, tobacco and caffeine intakes. Ask about mobility and falls
- Address any concerns the patient has, e.g. the recent death of her friend
- Summarise and agree a management plan

Discussion points
- How would you investigate this patient?
- What are (i) the causes of, (ii) treatment options for, and (iii) complications of atrial fibrillation?
- How would you manage a patient with a supraventricular tachycardia?

ΔΔ Paroxysmal AF or SVT; sinus tachycardia

Ix		
Bloods	FBC, U&E, Mg, thyroid function test (TFT), Glc
ECG	
Imaging	CXR, echocardiogram
Other	24-hour cardiac tape (or 7-day event)

Station 25: Chest pain

Student info: *Mr GS is a 62-year-old male who has been referred to hospital by his GP with chest pain. You are the medical FY1 doctor. Please take a full history which you then need to present to the consultant on the post take ward round*

Patient info: *You are Mr GS, 62 years old. PMH: GORD, no known ↑BP, ↑lipids or diabetes. You started having episodes of chest tightness 4 weeks ago on walking up the hill near your house. These episodes would resolve after 1–2 minutes of rest. There was associated SOB but no radiation or associated symptoms. Earlier this morning you had an episode of chest tightness of greater intensity walking around the house which only resolved after 30 minutes. There was associated nausea and SOB and you felt unwell. The pain has now gone. You live in a house with your wife who has multiple sclerosis and you are the main carer. You smoke 10 cigarettes a day, drink no alcohol and weigh 95 kg. Your father died of a myocardial infarction (MI) aged 68; your brother, who is 52, had a recent angiogram but the results are unknown*

Hints and tips
- Ascertain the patient's understanding of the reason the GP has referred him to hospital
- Elicit the salient points about the current chest pain and events over the last 4 weeks, determining current and previous exercise tolerance
- Elicit his risk factors for heart disease and in particular the details of his brother's recent investigations
- Determine impact of symptoms on quality of life and ability to look after his wife and if patient has an understanding of what the diagnosis might be
- Elicit any concerns the patient may have; summarise and agree a plan

Discussion points
- Can you discuss the management of MI and state how the management of ST elevation MI differs to non-ST elevation MI?

ΔΔ Acute coronary syndrome

Ix		
Bloods	FBC, U&E, lipids, Glc, cardiac enzymes (creatine kinase (CK), troponin at 12 hours)
ECG	
Imaging	CXR; consider echo if indicated
Other	Consider coronary angiography

Station 26: Hypertension

Student info: *Mr RH is 56 years old. His BP has been 200/110 on repeated measurements that his GP has taken and he has been referred to your clinic. Please take a full history and be prepared to discuss with the examiner the advice and management you would recommend*

Patient info: *You are Mr RH and are 56 years old. You are a self-employed window cleaner and weigh 105 kg, smoke 10 cigarettes a day and drink 30 units alcohol per week. You have high BP despite starting atenolol 6 weeks ago, but have no cardiovascular symptoms. You are married with no children but are having some marital difficulties which are not being helped by the fact that work is quiet and the atenolol has led to problems with impotence. Your mother died of a stroke aged 72 and your father (82 years) has ↑BP and angina following a MI at the age of 64. You feel well and wonder why your GP has sent you to hospital*

Hints and tips
- Ascertain the patient's understanding of the reason for referral to hospital
- Determine symptomatology
- Determine his risk factors for heart disease and elicit his other PMH
- Elicit full family history, drug and allergy history and the fact that compliance with the atenolol has been poor due to impotence
- Determine social history including marital and work problems
- Ascertain patient's understanding of high BP and possible complications associated with this
- Elicit any concerns the patient has
- Summarise and agree management

Discussion points
- How would you investigate this patient?
- What are (i) the causes of and (ii) complications of hypertension?

Ix		
Bloods	FBC, U&E, lipids, Glc
ECG	
Imaging	CXR; consider echocardiogram and renal US
Other	Consider 24-hour BP monitoring

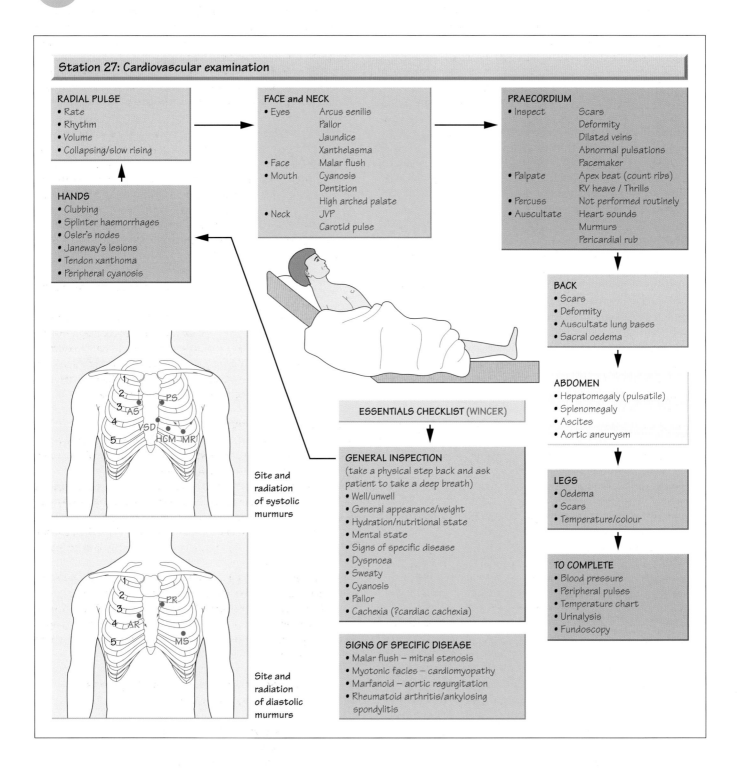

Station 27: Cardiovascular examination

RADIAL PULSE
- Rate
- Rhythm
- Volume
- Collapsing/slow rising

HANDS
- Clubbing
- Splinter haemorrhages
- Osler's nodes
- Janeway's lesions
- Tendon xanthoma
- Peripheral cyanosis

FACE and NECK
- Eyes   Arcus senilis
  Pallor
  Jaundice
  Xanthelasma
- Face   Malar flush
- Mouth   Cyanosis
  Dentition
  High arched palate
- Neck   JVP
  Carotid pulse

PRAECORDIUM
- Inspect   Scars
  Deformity
  Dilated veins
  Abnormal pulsations
  Pacemaker
- Palpate   Apex beat (count ribs)
  RV heave / Thrills
- Percuss   Not performed routinely
- Auscultate   Heart sounds
  Murmurs
  Pericardial rub

BACK
- Scars
- Deformity
- Auscultate lung bases
- Sacral oedema

ABDOMEN
- Hepatomegaly (pulsatile)
- Splenomegaly
- Ascites
- Aortic aneurysm

LEGS
- Oedema
- Scars
- Temperature/colour

TO COMPLETE
- Blood pressure
- Peripheral pulses
- Temperature chart
- Urinalysis
- Fundoscopy

Site and radiation of systolic murmurs

Site and radiation of diastolic murmurs

ESSENTIALS CHECKLIST (WINCER)

GENERAL INSPECTION
(take a physical step back and ask patient to take a deep breath)
- Well/unwell
- General appearance/weight
- Hydration/nutritional state
- Mental state
- Signs of specific disease
- Dyspnoea
- Sweaty
- Cyanosis
- Pallor
- Cachexia (?cardiac cachexia)

SIGNS OF SPECIFIC DISEASE
- Malar flush – mitral stenosis
- Myotonic facies – cardiomyopathy
- Marfanoid – aortic regurgitation
- Rheumatoid arthritis/ankylosing spondylitis

Station 27: Cardiovascular examination

- *This 55-year-old female presents with exertional dyspnoea and orthopnoea. Please examine her cardiovascular system*
- *This 65-year-old female has been referred by her GP with a newly diagnosed heart murmur. Please examine her praecordium*
- *Please examine this patient's peripheral pulses*

Examination routine

- Introduction/consent/ask about pain
- *Exposure*: adequate exposure of the upper body and neck is required but respect dignity by covering female breasts with a blanket while examining the peripheries. The legs and feet should also be exposed at least up to the knees so as to avoid missing any scars or peripheral oedema

- *Position*: lying at 45°
- *General inspection*:
  - take a physical step back and observe the patient and surroundings
  - assess whether the patient is well/unwell, comfortable lying at rest or dyspnoeic, in any pain, cachetic, jaundiced or pale
- *Screening test*: ask the patient to take a deep breath in
- *System-specific inspection*:
  - look for clues around the bedside, e.g. nitrate spray
  - observe the general appearance to see if there is any evidence of specific diseases or syndromes, e.g. Marfan's or Down's syndrome, ankylosing spondylitis, COPD
- *Hands*:
  - note the temperature and look carefully for finger clubbing, cyanosis and peripheral stigmata of infective endocarditis (splinter haemorrhages, Osler's nodes, Janeway lesions)
  - palpate the right radial pulse and examine for rate and rhythm. Check for a collapsing pulse (aortic regurgitation) by raising the patient's arm above their head (check they do not have shoulder pain first) while feeling the brachial pulse with your left hand and placing your right fingertips over the radial artery
  - check for differences in the radial pulses and also state that you would like to check for radiofemoral delay (coarctation of the aorta)
  - state that you would like to check the blood pressure
- *Head and neck*:
  - look for any sign of a malar flush (red cheeks that can be a sign of pulmonary hypertension due to mitral stenosis)
  - check the sclera for signs of pallor or jaundice and note any arcus senilis or xanthalasma
  - examine the lips, mouth and tongue for central cyanosis
  - check the state of dentition and look for evidence of a high arched palate
  - feel a carotid pulse for rate, volume and character (better assessed with a central pulse)
  - examine the JVP (see Station 36, Ch. 16). Decide if the JVP is raised or not and look for any changes with inspiration
- *Praecordium inspection*: check for scars, deformities, dilated veins or evidence of a pacemaker
- *Praecordium palpation*:
  - palpate for the apex beat (usually fifth intercostal space in the midclavicular line), demonstrating the position by counting the rib spaces. The apex beat can be difficult to feel, so if necessary ask the patient to move onto their left side. Assess the character; tapping = palpable first heart sound (e.g. mitral stenosis), forceful and sustained = increased pressure (e.g. hypertension or aortic stenosis), forceful but not sustained = increased volume (e.g. aortic or mitral regurgitation)
  - feel for a right ventricular heave (left parasternal heave) by placing the heel of your hand over the left lower sternal edge (right ventricular hypertrophy or left atrial enlargement) and finally move your hand over the pulmonary area to feel for a palpable second heart sound (pulmonary hypertension) and the aortic area for a thrill (i.e. palpable murmur)
- *Praecordium auscultation*:
  - commence with the diaphragm of your stethoscope over the apex (mitral area). Listen and distinguish the first and second heart sounds and determine if they are of the normal intensity and if there is any splitting
  - determine if there are any added sounds, prosthetic sounds or murmurs
  - if a murmur is heard in this position, listen at the axilla for radiation

- repeat this routine at the left lower sternal edge (tricuspid), the puLmonary area (**L**eft sternal edge in the second intercostal space) and the ao**R**tic area (**R**ight sternal edge in the second intercostal space)
- remember to be seen timing the cardiac cycle with the carotid pulse while listening (systole corresponds to the carotid pulse, S1 occurs just before systole and S2 just after)
- change to the bell and listen over the carotid artery on each side for any evidence of radiation of murmurs (aortic stenosis) or carotid bruits
- position the patient in the left lateral position to listen for mitral stenosis (bell)
- ask the patient to sit forward and listen (diaphragm) over the left lower sternal edge for the murmur of aortic regurgitation (the patient needs to be in full expiration while you are listening, i.e. 'please breathe in deeply, breathe out and now hold your breath'). In general if a murmur is heard it would look proficient if you try to demonstrate a change in the murmur with respiration (see below)
- While the patient is sitting forward listen to the lung bases (if any evidence of crackles or decreased air entry then complete a quick respiratory examination on the back)
- Assess for sacral oedema
- Check the legs and feet looking for signs of scars, peripheral oedema or peripheral vascular disease
- *Completion*: state to the examiners that you would like to complete your examination by checking the peripheral pulses, performing urinalysis (haematuria in endocarditis, proteinuria in hypertension), performing fundoscopy (hypertensive changes, Roth's spots of endocarditis) and looking at the temperature chart. Depending on your findings you may also wish to perform a respiratory or abdominal examination

A note on heart sounds

Diagnosing the wrong murmur in an exam is unlikely to cause a fail, especially if a student has demonstrated a competent examination routine and has talked about the findings sensibly.
- *S1*: marks beginning of systole (feel carotid pulsation); comprises mitral and tricuspid valve closure; closing of mitral valve slightly precedes the tricuspid (pressure is higher in left ventricle)
- *S2*: occurs just after systole; comprises aortic (A2) and pulmonary (P2) valve closure; aortic valve closes slightly before pulmonary (pressure is higher in aorta)
- *Inspiration*: this causes increased negative intrathoracic pressure, which causes increased blood return to the right side of the heart, therefore right-sided heart murmurs are louder on inspiration. The increased blood in the right ventricle causes the pulmonary valve to stay open slightly longer and so a physiological splitting of the second heart sound can occur on inspiration

Summary of common cardiology investigations

Bloods	FBC (anaemia, raised white cell count (WCC))
	CRP (endocarditis)
	Cardiac enzymes (CK, troponin)
	Glc (diabetes)
	Lipid profile (hyperlipidaemia)
	U&E (renal impairment)
ECG	
Imaging	CXR, transthoracic echocardiogram, TOE
Micro	Blood cultures (endocarditis)
Other	24-hour cardiac memo tape (24-hour tape)
	Exercise tolerance testing (ETT) (treadmill test)
	Coronary angiography

Station 28: Mitral stenosis

History hints

SOB ↓ ET
Cough Fatigue
Palpitations
PMH: rheumatic fever (RF),
embolic event (e.g. TIA)

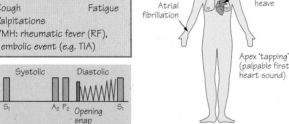

Examination hints

Female > male
Malar flush/low volume pulse/atrial fibrillation
Scars (thoracoplasty/thoracotomy/sternotomy)
Tapping apex/loud S1
Mid-diastolic rumbling murmur – low pitched (left lateral position at
  apex with bell) + opening snap
Murmur increases with exercise
Signs of chronic heart failure
Signs of pulmonary hypertension
Signs of endocarditis
Signs of embolic complications

Station 29: Mitral regurgitation

History hints

SOB ↓ ET
Orthopnoea/PND Angina
Fatigue
PMH: ischaemic heart disease,
RF, connective tissue disease

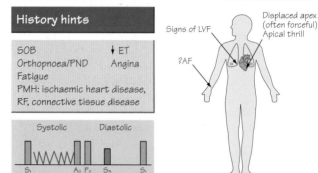

Examination hints

Scars – previous valvotomy
Possible atrial fibrillation
Displaced apex (often forceful)
Apical thrill
Soft S1
S3 if rapid ventricular filling
Pansystolic murmur at apex radiating to axilla
Signs of cardiac failure
Signs of endocarditis
Signs of embolic complications
Signs of connective tissue disease

Station 30: Aortic stenosis

History hints

SOB (Sx on exertion)
Chest pain
Syncope
Dizziness
PMH: RF

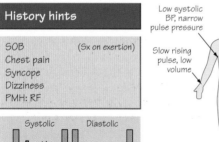
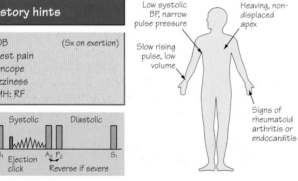

Examination hints

Low volume, slow rising pulse
Low systolic blood pressure
Narrow pulse pressure
Heaving non-displaced apex
Ejection systolic murmur over aortic area radiating to carotids
Soft or absent S2
Signs of left ventricular dysfunction (late sign)

Station 31: Aortic regurgitation

History hints

SOB Orthopnoea
↓ ET Palpitations
PMH: RF, connective tissue
disease
FH: aortic dissection

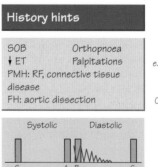
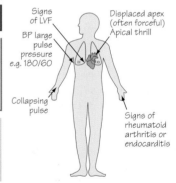

Examination hints

Large volume, collapsing pulse
Wide pulse pressure
Displaced apex (often forceful)
Early diastolic murmur (aortic area to LLSE)
Eponymous signs (Corrigan's, De Musset's, Quincke's, Muller's)
Signs of cardiac faliure
Signs of endocarditis
Signs of embolic complications
Signs of connective tissue disease

- *Examine this patient's praecordium*
- *This patient suffered with rheumatic fever when 7 years old. Please listen to their heart*
- *This patient has been presenting with episodes of syncope, please examine their cardiovascular system*

Hints and tips
- If examining the whole cardiovascular system try and decide what the murmur may be before auscultation, using the hints opposite
- If more than one murmur is heard, determine which is predominant
- If unsure whether there are different murmurs or just one radiating throughout the praecordium, move your stethoscope small distances across the chest wall from the mitral to aortic area, listening closely for a change in character
- The instructions may wish a full cardiovascular examination to be carried out but often you will be directed to a specific part

Approach to murmurs
- Inspect for peripheral signs
- Timing (i.e. systolic, diastolic)
- Loudest area
- Radiation
- Volume and pitch
- Added sounds (e.g. opening snap)
- Effect of dynamic manoeuvres (e.g. respiration)

Station 28: Mitral stenosis

Causes	Rheumatic heart disease	
	Congenital	
	Systemic lupus erythematosus (SLE)/rheumatoid	
	Carcinoid	
ΔΔ	Left atrial myxoma	
Ix	*ECG*	
	Imaging	CXR (enlarged left atrium); Echo
Rx	*Medical*	Treat AF and heart failure
		Antibiotic prophylaxis
	Surgical	Valvotomy/valvuloplasty
		Mitral valve replacement

Discussion points
- Do you know any diagnostic criteria for rheumatic fever?
- Can you describe any symptoms or signs of rheumatic fever?

Station 29: Mitral regurgitation

Causes	Ischaemic heart disease	
	Rheumatic heart disease	
	Mitral valve prolapse	
	Infective endocarditis	
	Connective tissue disease	
Ix	*ECG*	
	Imaging	CXR; Echo
Rx	*Medical*	Treat heart failure
		Diuretics/ACE inhibitor
		Antibiotic prophylaxis
	Surgical	Mitral valve repair/replacement

Discussion points
- What are the possible ECG findings in mitral regurgitation?

- Would you recommend antibiotic prophylaxis, and if so for which procedures?
- What are the indications for surgery?

Station 30: Aortic stenosis

Causes	Degenerative	
	Congenital bicuspid valve	
	Rheumatic heart disease	
Ix	*ECG*	(?left ventricular hypertrophy)
	Imaging	CXR; Echo
	Other	Coronary angiography (only as part of pre-op Ix)
Rx	*Medical*	Monitoring
		Antibiotic prophylaxis
	Surgical	Valvuloplasty or replacement

Discussion points
- How can you differentiate between aortic sclerosis and aortic stenosis?
- In mixed aortic valve disease, how can you determine which is the dominant lesion?
- What are the indications for surgery in aortic stenosis?

Station 31: Aortic regurgitation

Causes	Infective endocarditis	
	Rheumatic heart disease	
	Connective tissue disease	
	Rheumatoid arthritis	
	Ankylosing spondylitis	
	Aortic dissection	
	Prosthetic valve leak	
Ix	*ECG*	
	Imaging	CXR; Echo
	Other	Consider CT aortogram
		Coronary angiography
		Specific tests depending on the likely cause, e.g. vasculitic screen, septic screen
Rx	*Medical*	Diuretics/ACE inhibitor
		Antibiotic prophylaxis
	Surgical	Aortic valve replacement

A note on pulmonary hypertension
Raised pressure in the pulmonary arteries for whatever reason can cause pulmonary hypertension and lead to right heart strain and failure.

- *Please discuss some causes of pulmonary hypertension and describe the sequence of signs that may develop*

Signs	Loud P2	Tricuspid regurgitation
	Diastolic murmur of	Raised JVP
	pulmonary regurgitation	Pulsatile hepatomegaly
	Right ventricular heave	Peripheral oedema

Causes

Related to pulmonary venous hypertension, e.g. chronic left ventricular failure (LVF), ventricular septal defect, atrial septal defect, mitral stenosis/regurgitation
Related to arterial obstruction, e.g. thromboembolic disease, vasculitis
Related to hypoxia, e.g. living at high altitude, restrictive lung conditions, sleep apnoea, COPD

Station 32: Tricuspid regurgitation

History hints

SOB
Oedema
Abdominal swelling
PMH: COPD,
  mitral stenosis
IV drug user

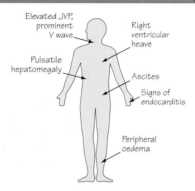

Elevated JVP, prominent V wave
Right ventricular heave
Pulsatile hepatomegaly
Ascites
Signs of endocarditis
Peripheral oedema

Examination hints

Raised JVP with
  prominent V waves
Right parasternal heave
Pansystolic murmur
  LLSE
Pulsatile hepatomegaly
Ascites
Peripheral oedema
Peripheral signs of
  endocarditis
Fever

Summary of common murmur timings

Timing	Abnormality
Pansystolic	MR, TR, VSD
Midsystolic (ejection)	AS, HOCM
Late systolic	Mitral valve prolapse
Early diastolic	AR
Mid diastolic	MS

Station 33: Prosthetic heart valves

Examination hints

Mitral valve
• Midline sternotomy scar
• Metallic S1 click (closing of the prosthesis) followed by metallic opening snap
• Normal S2
• May be systolic murmur
Aortic valve
• Midline sternotomy scar
• S1 normal
• Ejection click (opening of valve)
• Ejection systolic murmur and S2 click (closure)

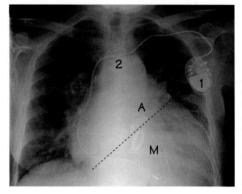

A chest radiograph showing evidence of both mitral (M) and aortic (A) valve replacements. Note the sternotomy wires (2), cardiomegaly and pacemaker (1)

Station 34: Cardiomyopathy

History hints

Exertional SOB, chest
  pain or dizziness
Recent viral illness
High alcohol intake
FH: sudden death or
  known cardiomyopathy
PMH: connective tissue
  disease

Examination hints

Pulse - ?AF, ?jerky character
Prominent a wave in the JVP
Forceful apex, double impulse
Midsystolic murmur (LLSE) – can be
  increased by valsalva or exercise
Pansystolic murmur of mitral regurgitation
Signs of chronic liver disease
Signs of connective tissue disease

Station 35: Infective endocarditis

History and examination hints - four phenomena

Infective	Fever, malaise, nights sweats, rigors
Heart damage	Murmurs, heart failure
Vascular	Major arterial emboli, septic pulmonary infarcts, mycotic aneurysm, intracranial haemorrhage, conjunctival haemorrhages, and Janeway's lesions
Immunological	Glomerulonephritis, Osler's nodes, Roth spots, rash and rheumatoid factor

Classification of non-ischaemic cardiomyopathy

DILATED CARDIOMYOPATHY
Absence of coronary artery disease
Global systolic dysfunction
Normal LV wall thickness
Causes:
Idiopathic
Genetic (e.g. myotonic dystrophy)
Infective (e.g. post viral)
Infiltrative (e.g. haemachromatosis)
Toxins (e.g. alcohol)
Endocrine (e.g.hypothyroidism)
Connective tissue disease (e.g. SLE)

HYPERTROPHIC CARDIOMYOPATHY
Hypertrophy of the
  myocardium
Usually asymmetrical
  hypertrophy of the
  septum
Can cause outflow
  tract obstruction
Diastolic dysfunction
Causes:
Genetic

Outflow tract obstruction
Aorta
LA
Mitral valve
Aortic valve
Asymmetrical septal hypertrophy
LV

RESTRICTIVE CARDIOMYOPATHY
Rarest form
Stiff myocardium
Congestive cardiac failure
Diastolic dysfunction
Rare
Similar signs to constrictive pericarditis
Causes:
Idiopathic
Infiltrative (e.g. amyloid)
Granulomatous (e.g. sarcoid)
Endomyocardial Fibrosis

Station 32: Tricuspid regurgitation

• *Please examine this patient's praecordium and describe the murmur*
• *This patient has a heart murmur, please perform a structured examination to demonstrate how you would determine the valve lesion*

Discussion points

• What are the causes of tricuspid regurgitation (TR)?
• How might you approach the management of a patient with TR?

Causes

Primary causes	Rheumatic heart disease
	Infective endocarditis
	Carcinoid syndrome
	Trauma (steering wheel)
	Congenital
Secondary causes	More common and due to dilatation of the right ventricle, e.g. COPD, mitral stenosis, cor pulmonale
Rx *Medical*	Diuretics/vasodilators
	Treat underlying cause, e.g. lung disease
Surgical	Annuloplasty; valve replacement (rare)

Station 33: Prosthetic heart valves

• *This patient suffered with rheumatic fever when they were a child, please auscultate their praecordium*

Hints and tips

• Listen carefully from the end of the bed for a clicking noise if a metallic valve
• Remember there could be a murmur as well as a prosthetic sound
• Remember that more than one valve may have been replaced

Discussion points

• What are the complications of valve replacement?
• What types of valve are you aware of?

Complications	Thromboembolic events
	Infective endocarditis
	Leakage
	Haemolysis
	Haemorrhage due to anticoagulation

Station 34: Cardiomyopathy

• *This 45-year-old male has been complaining of exertional breathlessness. He has a background of chronic alcohol use. Please examine his cardiovascular system*

Discussion points

• What are the causes and management of cardiomyopathy?
• Describe ECG changes associated with each of the cardiomyopathies

Ix	*ECG*	
	Imaging	Echo, CXR
	Other	Targeted at the specific cause (e.g. ferritin levels for haemochromatosis)

Dilated cardiomyopathy

ECG findings	Left bundle branch block (LBBB)
	Bifid, wide p waves (left atrial enlargement)
	Anteroseptal Q waves
	Left ventricular hypertrophy (LVH)
	Arrhythmias (e.g. AF, VT)
Rx *Lifestyle*	Smoking cessation; reduce alcohol
Medical	Treat specific underlying cause if present
	Control heart failure and AF (anticoagulation)
Surgery	Consider cardiac transplant

Hypertrophic cardiomyopathy

ECG findings	LVH
	Bifid, wide P waves
	Q waves (inferior, anterior)
	Axis deviation
	Conduction abnormalities
Rx *Lifestyle*	Smoking cessation; reduce alcohol
	Avoid strenuous exercise
Medical	β-blocker (e.g. metoprolol)
	Consider antiarrhythmic (e.g. amiodarone)
	Endocarditis prophylaxis
Surgery	Implantable defibrillator/pacemaker
	Myomectomy

Restrictive cardiomyopathy

ECG findings	Low voltage complexes
	Conduction abnormalities
Rx *Medical*	Treat underlying cause, e.g. steroids for sarcoid
	Symptomatic treatment, e.g. diuretics
Surgery	Cardiac transplant

Station 35: Infective endocarditis

• *This patient has had a swinging fever, please examine the cardiovascular system*

Hints and tips

Although unusual to find a patient with endocarditis in an OSCE, many of them are stable and remain in hospital for prolonged courses of antibiotics so could be utilised as part of a history or examination station.
• Look for the presence of a peripherally inserted long line in the antecubital fossa – this could suggest a prolonged course of treatment

Discussion points

• Discuss the treatment of infective endocarditis
• How can the response to treatment be monitored?
• What organisms are responsible?
• Can you explain the difference between acute and subacute bacterial endocarditis?
• Do you know of any clinical criteria for diagnosing infective endocarditis?

Risk factors	Valve disease, especially rheumatic
	Prosthetic valves; IV drug abuser
Ix *Bloods*	FBC, CRP, erythrocyte sedimentation rate (ESR), U&E
ECG	
Imaging	CXR; transthoracic echocardiogram; TOE
Micro	Multiple blood cultures; urinalysis + MC&S

---

[1] Durack DT, Lukes AS, Bright DK. New criteria for diagnosis of infective endocarditis: utilization of specific echocardiographic findings. Dukes Endocarditis Service. *Am J Med* 1994;**96**(3):200–9.

Station 36: Jugular venous pressure

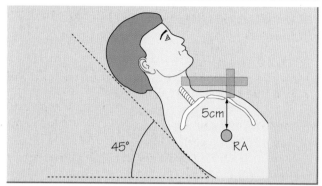

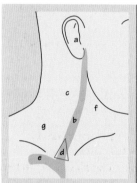

a, intertragic notch
b, internal jugular vein (IJV)
c, sternocleido-mastoid (SCM)
d, IJV between two heads of SCM
e, subclavian vein
f, anterior triangle
g, posterior triangle

Causes of a raised JVP

Congestive heart failure	Right ventricular failure
Tricuspid regurgitation	Pericardial tamponade
Constrictive pericarditis	Hyperdynamic circulation
Superior vena caval obstruction	Fluid overload

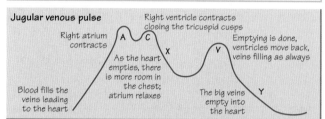

Abnormal JVP waveforms

Dominant a wave
Pulmonary hypertension
Hypertrophic cardiomyopathy
Tricuspid stenosis

Cannon waves
Complete heart block
Atrial flutter
Ventricular tachycardia

y descent
Rapid descent - severe TR, constrictive pericarditis

Absent a wave
Atrial fibrillation

Dominant v wave
Tricuspid regurgitation

Kussmaul's sign
Paradoxical rise on inspiration
Causes: constrictive pericarditis
cardiac tamponade

Station 37: Cardiac failure

History hints

RVF	LVF
Swelling of the ankles	SOB
Abdominal distension	Orthopnoea/PND
Nausea	↓ET
Fatigue	Cough
SOB	Cardiac RF
PMH: chronic lung disease, known heart disease (as per LVF)	PMH: ischaemic heart disease, BP, cardiomyopathy, renal disease

NYHA classification

Class I
No symptoms

Class II
Symptoms with moderate exertion

Class III
Symptoms with minimal exertion

Class IV
Symptoms at rest

CXR changes with LVF

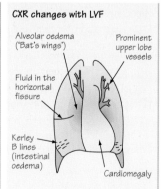

Alveolar oedema ('Bat's wings')
Prominent upper lobe vessels
Fluid in the horizontal fissure
Kerley B lines (intestinal oedema)
Cardiomegaly

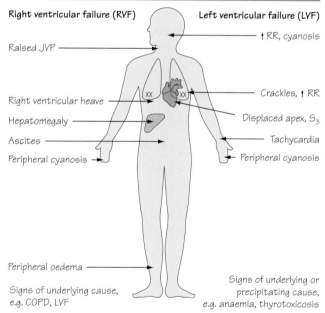

Right ventricular failure (RVF)

Raised JVP
Right ventricular heave
Hepatomegaly
Ascites
Peripheral cyanosis
Peripheral oedema
Signs of underlying cause, e.g. COPD, LVF

Left ventricular failure (LVF)

↑ RR, cyanosis
Crackles, ↑ RR
Displaced apex, S₃
Tachycardia
Peripheral cyanosis
Signs of underlying or precipitating cause, e.g. anaemia, thyrotoxicosis

Generalised cardiac cachexia if chronic heart failure

Station 36: Jugular venous pressure

- *Please examine this patient's JVP*
- *Please draw the waveform of the normal JVP using the paper provided*
- *This patient is known to have a heart murmur, please examine the JVP and describe your findings, stating possible diagnoses*

Hints and tips

- Check there is adequate lighting
- Be able to demonstrate surface anatomy (clavicle, two heads of sternomastoid, manubrium, angle of Louis) and show the path of the right internal jugular vein
- Look in the area between the two heads of the sternomastoid (red triangle on figure opposite) and then follow a path towards the angle of the jaw
- Ask the patient to breathe deeply while observing
- If noted, demonstrate the ways to differentiate it from the carotid pulse:
  - not palpable
  - occludable (apply pressure at the base of the neck)
  - complex waveform with double impulse
  - moves with respiration (decreases with inspiration)
  - abdominojugular reflex
- Draw the waveform if requested

Discussion points

- What are the causes of a raised JVP?
- How can the JVP be differentiated from the carotid artery?

Station 37: Cardiac failure

- *This patient has been complaining of orthopnea, please examine the cardiovascular system*
- *Please examine this woman's fluid balance status*

Hints and tips

Patients in the OSCE will not be acutely unwell, so a patient that might appear will have stable chronic heart failure. Such a patient could be utilised in an examination station or equally well as part of history taking or communicating a new diagnosis. Alternatively the treatment of acute left ventricular failure (LVF) could be discussed as part of a viva, or assessed in an emergency station with the use of a mannequin.

Discussion points

- What are the causes of heart failure?
- What are the management priorities in acute LVF?
- Discuss the management of heart failure
- Do you know any classifications of cardiac failure?
- How would you investigate a patient with suspected LVF?

Causes of left ventricular failure

- Myocardial disease: ischaemic heart disease, cardiomyopathy
- Increased preload (i.e. volume overload): mitral regurgitation, aortic regurgitation
- Increased afterload (i.e. pressure overload): hypertension, aortic stenosis

- Restrictive left ventricular filling: constrictive pericarditis, cardiac tamponade, mitral stenosis

Precipitating causes

Cardiac	Arrhythmias
Endocrine	Hyperthyroidism
Haematology	Anaemia
Infectious	Endocarditis
Drugs	Non-steroidal anti-inflammatory drugs (NSAIDs)
Iatrogenic	Excess IV fluids

Causes of right ventricular failure

- LVF: any cause of LVF (chronic LVF → raised pulmonary pressure → secondary right ventricular failure)
- Increased preload (i.e. volume overload): atrial septal defect
- Increased afterload (i.e. pressure overload): pulmonary hypertension (see Ch. 14), pulmonary stenosis
- Myocardial disease: right ventricular myocardial infarction

Ix of cardiac failure

Bloods	FBC, U&E, LFT, TFT, cardiac enzymes (CEs)
	ABG
ECG	ischaemic changes, left ventricular hypertrophy, arrhythmias
Imaging	CXR (see opposite)
	Echo

Mx of acute LVF

ABCDE (see Ch. 11)

Rx	Oxygen, diuretics, morphine, metoclopramide
	Nitrates if systolic BP > 90
	Need to ascertain the underlying cause and treat this as appropriate
Procedures	Urinary catheter, consider central and arterial lines
Location	Coronary care unit (CCU) or HDU
Monitoring	Continuous observation, strict fluid balance including daily weights
Specialists	Senior medical doctor
	Cardiologist
	Consider intensive therapy unit (ITU)/anaesthetic opinion
	Patient may need ventilatory support ± inotropic support if in cardiogenic shock

General Mx of heart failure

Rx	Treat underlying cause
	Optimise cardiovascular risk factors
	Diuretics
	ACE inhibitor/AII receptor antagonist
	Cardioselective β-blocker – once the patient is stable
Monitoring	Fluid balance, weight, routine bloods
	Consider spironolactone
Specialists	Heart failure specialist nurse
	Cardiologist
Education	Fluid balance

Station 38: ECG recording – explanation

Introduction
Explain purpose of the appointment
Ascertain whether the patient has had an ECG before
Explain what an ECG is
Explain what the ECG can show
Describe the process of performing an ECG:
• upper body needs to be exposed
• electrodes and leads will be attached
• need to lie still
• safe, no chance of electric shock
Answer all patient's questions
Reassure patient

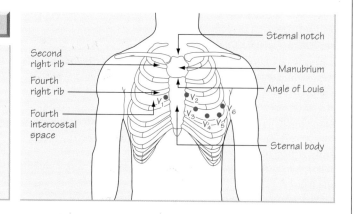

Station 39: ECG recording – procedure

Introduction
Explain purpose of the appointment
Ascertain if the patient has had an ECG done before
Perform the procedure adequately communicating to the patient each
 of the steps as follows:
• prepare machine and electrodes
• expose the patient's chest
• apply the electrodes to the limbs and praecordium
• ask the patient to lie still while you take the recording
If happy with the trace, remove the electrodes and ask the patient to
 redress

Station 40: ECG interpretation – summary

Remember to interpret the ECG in combination with the patient's
clinical findings and then use the following routine

1. Rate
2. Rhythm
3. Axis
  → a. Regular or irregular?
  → b. Tachycardic, bradycardic or normal?
  → c. Narrow QRS or broad QRS?
  → d. P waves present?
  → e. Relationship between P wave and QRS complex?

4. Waveforms
  → a. P wave and PR interval
  → b. QRS complex
  → c. ST segment
  → d. T wave & QT interval

Station 41: Blood pressure measurement

Examination hints

General observation, e.g. Cushingoid
Complete CVS examination
Peripheral pulses/abdominal bruits
Fundoscopy
Urine dipstick
Consider measuring BP in both arms and postural

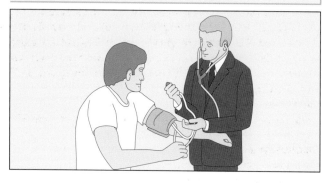

Station 41: Overview
Introduction
Explain purpose of the appointment
Patient to be seated, arm exposed on support
Ensure suitably sized cuff
Wrap the cuff around the upper arm and centre the bladder over the
 brachial artery
Warn the patient that the cuff will inflate and become tight on the arm
 which may be uncomfortable
Estimate the BP by palpation
Auscultate over the brachial artery while inflating and then deflating
 the cuff
Record systolic and diastolic BP on the paper provided
Answer patient's questions and give reassurance
State to examiner that under certain clinical scenarios it would be
 necessary to check the BP in both arms and also with the patient
 lying and standing

Station 42: Postural BP measurement

Patient should be lying down for 10 minutes
Measure BP with patient lying
Stand patient up (or sit up, if not able to stand)
Measure BP at 0, 1 and 3 minutes
Note any symptoms
Document the BP on a chart with the timings clearly recorded

Station 38: ECG recording – explanation

Student info: *Mrs PM is a 79-year-old female who is being admitted for a hysterectomy in 1 week and is attending her pre-operative assessment where she needs an ECG to be performed. Please explain the process of recording the ECG to her, answering any questions she may have and then indicate on the graphic where you would place the electrodes on the praecordium*

Patient info: *You are Mrs PM and are 79 years old. You have never had an ECG before and are very worried about the procedure. Your father died of a heart attack aged 45 years. You are worried about what the ECG might show and the consequences of this*

Hints and tips

This station is testing your communication skills rather than the actual skill of recording an ECG.

- Determine the patient's reason for coming to hospital
- Explain the reason for needing an ECG
- Ascertain the patient's prior understanding of the procedure
- Explain the procedure, making clear that it is completely painless
- Explain that the ECG is performed to measure the electrical activity of the heart
- Emphasise that it will be necessary to expose the patient to apply the sticky pads for the electrodes
- Emphasise that she will need to lie still during the procedure
- Explain that the ECG can tell us information about the rate and rhythm of the heart and also if there has been any previous damage or strain
- Reassure Mrs PM that this is part of the routine process of preparing a patient for an operation and as she has had no symptoms the ECG is unlikely to show any abnormalities, but if there were any abnormal changes you would explain these to her
- Address any concerns the patient has

Station 39: ECG recording – procedure

Student info: *Mr RH is a 36-year-old male who has been admitted following an episode of chest pain the day before. He is clinically well and your registrar has reviewed the initial ECG but has asked if you can perform a second one*

Patient info: *You are Mr RH, a 36-year-old male. You had an episode of short-lasting left-sided chest pain yesterday. The pain has now gone following some analgesia. You feel it is related to weight lifting. The doctors feel it is a musculoskeletal injury and will let you home if the ECG recording is normal. You had an ECG taken when you first arrived at the hospital*

Hints and tips

This station is testing your ability to carry out the skill of recording an ECG. Some of the explanations from Station 38 will need to be used while carrying out the procedure.

- Determine the patient's reason for coming to hospital
- Explain the reason for needing an ECG
- Ascertain if the patient has had an ECG done before
- Explain your actions as you are carrying them out
- Prepare the ECG machine and expose the patient adequately
- Place the limb and chest electrodes in the correct position
- Ask the patient to lie still and record the ECG
- If the trace is technically adequate, remove the electrodes and ask the patient to get redressed
- Answer any questions the patient may have

Station 40: ECG interpretation – summary

A full ECG interpretation is outside the remit of this book. ECGs could be included in an OSCE as a data interpretation station or as part of a cardiovascular station. In general, ECG knowledge will be tested in a written exam. The key is to follow a logical routine (see opposite).

- Check patient details and check calibration
- Look at the rhythm strip first
- Calculate rate
- Determine rhythm by deciding where the impulse starts (sinoatrial node, atria, around the atrioventricular node or ventricle) and how it is conducted (normal, slow, fast)
- Determine axis
- Look at each waveform individually
- If there are areas of ischaemia, try and determine the territory involved
- State any causes or management if asked

Station 41: Blood pressure measurement

Student info: *Mr FM is 45 and has attended your surgery for a routine 'well man' check up. Please measure his blood pressure*

Patient info: *You have attended your GP for a routine 'well man' check up. Your main concern is that your brother, who was 5 years older than you, has recently died following a brain haemorrhage. You have been told that this happened because of his high blood pressure*

Hints and tips

This station tests communication skills, practical skills and also understanding. A variation on the theme would be to ask a student to measure a postural BP (see Station 42 opposite).

- Determine the patient's reason for coming to the surgery
- Explain the reason for checking BP
- Explain the procedure. Has the patient had their BP checked before?
- Ask the patient to expose their arm while you check your equipment
- Choose the right size of cuff (a standard cuff in an obese patient will lead to a falsely raised reading)
- Place the cuff around the upper arm with the bladder over the brachial artery and warn the patient that the cuff will inflate and become tight which could cause some discomfort
- The arm needs to be supported and horizontal at the level of the heart
- Check the systolic pressure by palpation – inflate the cuff while palpating the radial artery and note when it disappears, inflate a further 20 mmHg and then deflate slowly until the pulse can be felt again
- Inflate the cuff to the same level as before but this time auscultate over the brachial artery and determine the systolic and diastolic BP. As deflation occurs five different sounds are heard (Korotkoff sounds). Phase 1 is the first sound and indicates systolic BP. The sound eventually becomes muffled (phase 4) and then disappears (phase 5). Use phase 5 as the diastolic
- Record the measurements on the chart provided
- State to the examiners that you would like to check a postural BP

Discussion points

- What are the causes of hypertension?
- How do you investigate hypertension?
- What are the causes of postural hypotension?
- What happens to BP on inspiration?
- What do you understand by the term pulsus paradoxus?
- Discuss some management principles of hypertension (see Ch. 12)

Respiratory symptoms

Breathlessness	Fever
Haemoptysis	Apnoea attacks
Post nasal drip	Weight loss
Daytime somnolence	Snoring
Reflux symptoms	Cough
Chest pain	Voice disturbance

Specific respiratory history points

Exercise tolerance	Occupation
Atopy	Diurnal variation
Pets	Asbestos/dust exposure
Previous respiratory problems	Smoking history
Previous intubation	Peak flow when well

NB. Nocturnal symptoms are important, e.g. cough, inhaler use

Station 43: Asthma

Features of severe asthma attack

PEF 33–50% predicted or best
Inability to complete sentence in
 1 breath
RR > 25 breaths/min
Pulse > 110 beats/min

Features of life-threatening asthma attack

PEF < 33% predicted or best
Cyanosis/silent chest/poor
 respiratory effort
$SpO_2 < 92\%$
Hypotension
Bradycardia/arrhythmias
Exhaustion/confusion/coma
Normal $PaCO_2$

Management of acute severe asthma

ABCDE
Oxygen driven nebulised high dose salbutamol
PO or IV steroids
Antibiotics if pneumonia
Close monitoring of sats + ABGs
Early referral to ITU if deterioration
CXR – to exclude pneumothorax
High flow oxygen
Nebulised ipratropium
Consider IV magnesium

British Thoracic Society, Scottish Intercollegiate Guidelines Network. *British Guideline on the Management of Asthma. Thorax 2008;***63** (Suppl IV). Available at www.brit-thoracic.org.uk.

Clinical features to differentiate COPD from asthma

	COPD	Asthma
Smoker or ex-smoker	Nearly all	Possibly
Symptoms under age 35	Rare	Often
Chronic productive cough	Common	Uncommon
Breathlessness	Persistent and progressive	Variable
Night time waking with breathlessness and/or wheeze	Uncommon	Common
Significant diurnal or day to day variability of symptoms	Uncommon	Common

Station 44: Lung malignancy

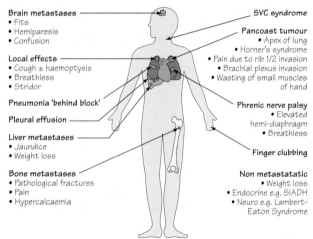

Brain metastases
• Fits
• Hemiparesis
• Confusion

Local effects
• Cough ± haemoptysis
• Breathless
• Stridor

Pneumonia 'behind block'

Pleural effusion

Liver metastases
• Jaundice
• Weight loss

Bone metastases
• Pathological fractures
• Pain
• Hypercalcaemia

SVC syndrome

Pancoast tumour
• Apex of lung
• Horner's syndrome
• Pain due to rib 1/2 invasion
• Brachial plexus invasion
• Wasting of small muscles
 of hand

Phrenic nerve palsy
• Elevated
 hemi-diaphragm
• Breathless

Finger clubbing

Non metastatatic
• Weight loss
• Endocrine e.g. SIADH
• Neuro e.g. Lambert-
 Eaton Syndrome

Cellular types of lung cancer		% cases
Small cell lung cancer		15–20
Non-small cell lung cancer	Squamous	25–30
	Adenocarcinoma	40–60
	Large cell	10–15

Station 45: Pneumothorax

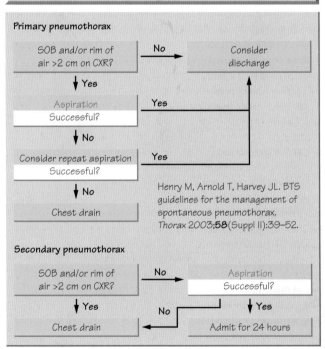

Primary pneumothorax

SOB and/or rim of air >2 cm on CXR? — No → Consider discharge

↓ Yes

Aspiration Successful? — Yes →

↓ No

Consider repeat aspiration Successful? — Yes →

↓ No

Chest drain

Henry M, Arnold T, Harvey JL. BTS guidelines for the management of spontaneous pneumothorax. *Thorax* 2003;**58**(Suppl II):39–52.

Secondary pneumothorax

SOB and/or rim of air >2 cm on CXR? — No → Aspiration Successful?

↓ Yes ↓ No ↓ Yes

Chest drain ← Admit for 24 hours

Station 43: Asthma

Student info: *Mr BS is a 22-year-old male with a history of an annoying cough which is persisting despite a course of antibiotics. Take a history and be prepared to discuss the management with your examiner*

Patient info: *You are Mr BS aged 22 years. You had eczema in childhood and suffer with hay fever. You have had a dry cough for a few weeks, which is worse in the early morning, and have noticed some mild SOB when exercising which you put down to smoking. You smoke 15/day and work as a bar man. There is no family history of note and no regular medications. You have a cat*

Hints and tips

• Determine the patient's reason for visiting the GP and ascertain knowledge of the current situation
• Determine symptomatology
• Full respiratory history with specific points (see opposite)
• Ask specifically about nocturnal wakening and early morning cough
• Establish the history of atopy
• Realise the importance of occupational history
• Establish smoking history
• Assess impact of the symptoms on the patient's life
• Address any concerns the patient has
• Discuss management and agree a plan

Discussion points

• How would you investigate a patient with suspected asthma?
• Discuss the management of asthma including educating the patient about keeping an 'asthma plan'
• Explain the stepwise management of asthma
• Discuss the severe and life-threatening signs of acute asthma
• Discuss the management of acute asthma

Station 44: Lung malignancy

Student info: *Mr AB is a 72-year-old male who has been referred with haemoptysis. You are the FY1 in clinic. Please take a full history in order to present the case to the consultant.*

Patient info: *You are Mr AB, a 72-year-old male who has had 3–4 episodes of haemoptysis over the preceding month, producing fresh blood, approximately half a spoonful, each time. COPD was diagnosed 8 years ago. DH: salbutamol nebs prn, tiotropium and symbicort inhalers. There have been three admissions with breathing problems over the last 5 years and six courses of steroids over the same time period. Until 4 months ago your exercise tolerance was 200 m but more recently has reduced to 50 m on the flat despite using increased doses of salbutamol. You have no chest pain but weight loss of 6 kg. You smoke 15 cigarettes a day, worked in the navy and were exposed to asbestos. You live alone. You suspect you have lung cancer*

Hints and tips

• Ascertain the patient's current knowledge and understanding of the reason the GP has referred him to hospital
• Elicit the salient points about the recent haemoptysis
• Demonstrate awareness of the previous diagnosis of COPD and the impact of this illness
• Establish the deterioration in respiratory function and exercise tolerance
• Elicit the weight loss and any other associated symptoms
• Determine impact of symptoms on quality of life
• Elicit any concerns the patient may have
• Demonstrate awareness of the impact of this diagnosis on the patient

Discussion points

• What is your differential diagnosis?
• Discuss the different types of lung cancer
• Explain the clinical features associated with lung cancer

△△ Exacerbation of COPD; lung malignancy
    Chest infection; pulmonary embolus

Ix *Bloods* FBC, U&E, LFT, calcium (Ca)
      ECG
      Imaging CXR, consider CT of the thorax
      Micro Sputum culture (+ send for cytology)
      Other Bronchoscopy ± bronchial washings and biopsy if lesion is visualised

Station 45: Pneumothorax

Student info: *Mr GF is 20 and has attended A&E complaining of some left-sided chest pain. Please take a full history, formulate a differential diagnosis and suggest appropriate investigations*

Patient info: *You are Mr GF, a 20-year-old male, 6ft 5in tall with no previous medical problems. You experienced sudden-onset left-sided chest pain last night; there was no relief with paracetamol. You made a recent trip to Australia for diving and are also due to fly to Malaysia in 10 days time. You smoke 20/day. There is no SOB at rest but you did notice a little SOB when climbing the stairs. There is no FH of note*

Hints and tips

• Determine the patient's reason for coming to hospital
• Determine symptomatology and elicit change in exercise tolerance
• Elicit full risk factors for possible thromboembolic disease
• Appreciate the significance of the recent flight and diving trip
• Address any concerns the patient has regarding future flying and diving
• Educate the patient about the importance of smoking cessation (the future risk of a further pneumothorax is greater in smokers)

Discussion points

• How would you investigate this patient as the FY1 doctor in A&E?
• What signs would suggest a tension pneumothorax?
• What are the causes of a pneumothorax?
• Describe the treatment of a patient with a pneumothorax

Causes

Spontaneous
  Primary   No known underlying lung disease
             Thought to be due to rupture of small bleb (small air-filled sac)
             Usually young tall men
             Cigarettes and positive family history are associated
  Secondary Underlying lung disease, e.g. COPD, TB, cystic fibrosis, asthma
Traumatic e.g. knife wound
Iatrogenic e.g. central venous catheter insertion

Ix *Bloods* FBC, D-dimer (if PE is suspected)
      ECG
      Imaging CXR
             Consider CT pulmonary angiogram (or ventilation perfusion scan if normal CXR) if pulmonary embolism (PE) is suspected

△△ Left-sided pneumothorax; pulmonary embolus; pleurisy

Station 46: Respiratory examination

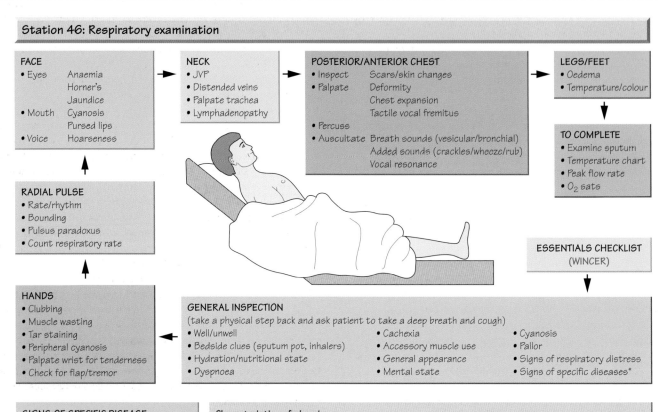

FACE
- Eyes — Anaemia
  - Horner's
  - Jaundice
- Mouth — Cyanosis
  - Pursed lips
- Voice — Hoarseness

NECK
- JVP
- Distended veins
- Palpate trachea
- Lymphadenopathy

POSTERIOR/ANTERIOR CHEST
- Inspect — Scars/skin changes
- Palpate — Deformity
  - Chest expansion
  - Tactile vocal fremitus
- Percuss
- Auscultate — Breath sounds (vesicular/bronchial)
  - Added sounds (crackles/wheeze/rub)
  - Vocal resonance

LEGS/FEET
- Oedema
- Temperature/colour

TO COMPLETE
- Examine sputum
- Temperature chart
- Peak flow rate
- O_2 sats

RADIAL PULSE
- Rate/rhythm
- Bounding
- Pulsus paradoxus
- Count respiratory rate

ESSENTIALS CHECKLIST
(WINCER)

HANDS
- Clubbing
- Muscle wasting
- Tar staining
- Peripheral cyanosis
- Palpate wrist for tenderness
- Check for flap/tremor

GENERAL INSPECTION
(take a physical step back and ask patient to take a deep breath and cough)
- Well/unwell
- Bedside clues (sputum pot, inhalers)
- Hydration/nutritional state
- Dyspnoea
- Cachexia
- Accessory muscle use
- General appearance
- Mental state
- Cyanosis
- Pallor
- Signs of respiratory distress
- Signs of specific diseases*

SIGNS OF SPECIFIC DISEASE
- Sputum pot – bronchiectasis, pneumonia
- Rheumatoid arthritis – rheumatoid lung, fibrosis
- Ankylosing spondylitis – upper lobe fibrosis
- Cachexia – COPD, fibrotic lung disease, neoplasm, bronchiectasis
- Clubbing – bronchiectasis, fibrosis, neoplasm, lung abscess, empyema, cystic fibrosis

Timing of crackles
Early = large airways, e.g. infection, pulmonary oedema
Middle = medium airways, e.g. infection, bronchiectasis
Late = small airways, e.g. fibrosis

Character
Coarse e.g. pus (infection) fluid (oedema)
Fine e.g. fibrosis, fluid (oedema)

NB. Pulmonary oedema is the great mimic, so interpret the sign in the context of the case
NB. Two conditions can coexist

Characteristics of wheezing

Site and disease	Tone		Timing		Location	
	Monotonic	Polyphonic	Inspiration	Expiration	Trachea or mouth	Chest
Stridor, as in upper airway infections; laryngospasm; postsurgical or postintubation damage; extrathoracic tracheal stenosis; and endotracheal lesions	+		+		+	
Intrathoracic or lobar bronchial obstruction, such as by a foreign body; airway stenosis; intrathoracic tracheomalacia or bronchomalacia; and endobronchial	+			+	+	+
Diffuse obstruction of several large airways, as in asthma		+		+	+	+

Diagram showing the surface markings of the lobes and suggested areas for percussion

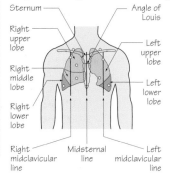

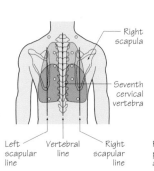

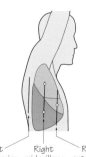

Sternum — Angle of Louis
Right upper lobe — Left upper lobe
Right middle lobe — Left lower lobe
Right lower lobe
Right midclavicular line — Midsternal line — Left midclavicular line

Right scapula
Seventh cervical vertebra
Left scapular line — Vertebral line — Right scapular line

Right posterior axillary line — Right midaxillary line — Right anterior axillary line

Station 46: Respiratory examination

- *This 55-year-old female presents with increasing SOB over the last 6 months. Please examine her respiratory system*
- *This 65-year-old smoker presents with SOB, weight loss and haemoptysis. Please examine*
- *Please demonstrate how you would examine this patient for signs of carbon dioxide retention*
- *Please demonstrate expansion, percussion and auscultation on this patient's praecordium*

Examination routine

- Introduction/consent/ask about pain
- *Exposure and position*: as per the cardiac examination (see Ch. 13)
- *General inspection*:
  - take a physical step back and observe the patient and surroundings. Asymmetry of chest expansion is best observed from the end of the bed, as is Horner's syndrome
  - assess whether the patient is well/unwell, comfortable lying at rest or dyspnoeic, in any pain, cachetic, jaundiced, cyanosed or pale
- *Screening test*: ask the patient to take a deep breath in and out, and then give a cough
- *System-specific inspection*:
  - look for clues around the bedside, e.g. nebuliser, sputum pot
  - observe the general appearance to see if there is any evidence of specific diseases or syndromes, e.g. chronic bronchitis, emphysema, rheumatoid arthritis, ankylosing spondylitis
  - note if there are any signs of respiratory distress (accessory muscle use, intercostal indrawing of the ribs or asymmetry) and listen to the patient's breathing (?stridor, audible wheeze)
- *Hands*:
  - look for finger clubbing, cyanosis, tar staining and wasting of the small muscles of the hand
  - squeeze the wrists for any tenderness (hypertrophic pulmonary osteoarthropathy (HPOA))
  - palpate the radial artery for any evidence of a bounding pulse and note the rate and rhythm
  - while assessing the pulse rate also count the respiratory rate
  - check for evidence of a carbon dioxide (CO_2) retention flap or tremor
- *Head and neck*:
  - look for signs of central cyanosis, pursed lip breathing or Horner's syndrome (ptosis, miosis – see Ch. 39)
  - examine the JVP for evidence of right heart failure due to chronic pulmonary disease (see Ch. 16)
  - palpate the position of the trachea
  - ask the patient to lean forward and examine for lymphadenopathy in the cervical and supraclavicular regions
- *Chest*: it is now time to assess the chest – as a suggestion, start with the back first (i) because the patient is already sitting forward, (ii) the signs are usually more obvious and (iii) large breasts can make examination more difficult anteriorly when a student is already feeling anxious. To examine the back, either ask the patient to sit forward or, if able, sit on the edge of the bed
- *Chest inspection*: note any scars, deformities (scoliosis or kyphosis, pectus excavatum), radiotherapy markings or obvious asymmetry while observing the chest wall movement
- *Chest palpation*:
  - examine chest expansion by gripping your fingers in the intercostal spaces on either side of the chest and holding your thumbs off the skin and parallel in the midline (ask the patient to fully expire first)
  - if you wish to carry out tactile vocal fremitus, this is the correct time. This gives the same information as vocal resonance and so both are not essential
- *Chest percussion*: percuss at the areas demonstrated opposite. To assess the apices it is acceptable to percuss directly onto the clavicles (but needs clear instructions to the patient). Always compare right with left when assessing percussion
- *Chest auscultation*:
  - with the diaphragm of your stethoscope, auscultate in the same areas that you percussed. Ask the patient to breathe in and out through their mouth (it is not necessary to get the patient to breathe as deeply as possible – this can be quite uncomfortable for the patient and is also often noisy!)
  - assess the breath sounds. Vesicular are normal whereas bronchial represent upper airway transmitted breath sounds through areas of consolidation (bronchial breath sounds are similar to the sounds heard when listening over the trachea). Next listen for the added sounds of crackles, wheezes and pleural rubs
  - finally, assess vocal resonance in the same areas
- Now move to the anterior chest and repeat the above steps
- Complete the examination by inspecting the feet and ankles for peripheral cyanosis or oedema
- *Completion*: state to the examiners that you would like to complete your examination by performing a peak flow rate, checking the temperature chart, oxygen saturations and sputum pot. If there is a suspicion of cor pulmonale or pulmonary hypertension it would also be necessary to perform a cardiovascular examination

Neat tricks

To demonstrate chronic airflow limitation, ask the patient to breathe in fully and then blow out as hard and as fast as possible. This is known as the forced expiratory time and if expiration is prolonged for more than 3 seconds, it suggests airflow limitation.

If crackles are heard, ask the patient to cough and see if the character changes (fibrotic crackles will not change in character).

Summary of common respiratory investigations

Bloods	FBC (anaemia, raised WCC)
	CRP (infection)
Imaging	CXR
	CT chest
	CT pulmonary angiogram (CTPA)
	Ventilation/perfusion scan (V/Q scan)
Micro	Sputum MC&S
	Pleural aspirate
Other	Bronchoscopy ± biopsy and washings
	Pulmonary function testing
	Thoracoscopy (pleural biopsy)

Station 47: Pleural effusion

History hints

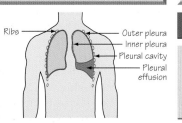

Ribs
Outer pleura
Inner pleura
Pleural cavity
Pleural effusion

SOB
Chest pain
Occasionally cough
Symptoms related to
    underlying cause

Examination hints

Examine the peripheries carefully for a possible cause, e.g. rheumatoid arthritis (RA)

Expansion	↓ if large
Percussion	Stony dull
Breath sounds	↓
Added sounds	None
Vocal resonance	↓
Other	? Mediastinal shift (away from side)

Causes

Transudate – Cardiac failure, nephrotic syndrome, hepatic cirrhosis, myxoedema, hypoalbuminaemia

Exudate – Infectious (para-pneumonic, TB, empyema)
    Neoplastic (bronchial cancer, mesothelioma, secondaries)
    Autoimmune (SLE, RA)   Gastro (pancreatitis)

Station 49: Bronchiectasis

History hints

SOB   Chronic productive cough
Ask about volume and colour of sputum
History of recurrent chest infections when younger

Examination hints

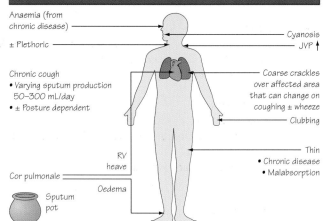

Anaemia (from
chronic disease)

± Plethoric

Chronic cough
• Varying sputum production
  50–300 mL/day
• ± Posture dependent

RV
heave

Cor pulmonale

Oedema

Sputum
pot

Cyanosis
JVP ↑

Coarse crackles
over affected area
that can change on
coughing ± wheeze

Clubbing

Thin
• Chronic disease
• Malabsorption

Station 48: Interstitial lung disease

History hints

Gradual onset of increasing SOB   PMH of autoimmune disease
Dry cough   DH, occupational history, pets
Asymptomatic   Other symptoms related to
History of exposure to allergens,   underlying cause
    e.g. extrinsic allergic alveolitis

Examination hints

Clubbing, cyanosis, crackles
Clubbing more common with cryptogenic
Crackles are classically fine end inspiratory
Other signs related to underlying cause (e.g. RA, SLE)
Signs of steroid effects
REMEMBER IF CRACKLES ARE HEARD ASK THE PATIENT TO COUGH

Station 50: COPD

History hints

SOB, wheeze, cough, sputum   History of smoking
Steroid usage   Usual exercise tolerance
Frequency of exacerbations   Frequency of hospital admissions

Examination hints

Look for inhalers, spacer, nebuliser, oxygen, sputum pot
Hyperexpanded chest
Paradoxical movement of lower ribs
Reduced cricosternal distance
Cyanosis, cachexia
CO_2 flap, bounding pulse, tar-stained fingers
Use of accessory muscles, pursed lips
Evidence of cor pulmonale (raised JVP, ankle oedema)
Wheeze, reduced air entry
NB. Some patients may have no abnormal physical signs

Assessment of severity of airflow obstruction according to FEV_1 as a % of the predicted value [1]

Severity	FEV_1
Mild airflow obstruction	50–80% predicted
Moderate airflow obstruction	30–49% predicted
Severe airflow obstruction	<30% predicted

MRC dyspnoea scale [1]

Grade	Degree of breathlessness related to activities
1	Not troubled by breathlessness except on strenuous exercise
2	Short of breath when hurrying or walking up a slight hill
3	Walks slower than contemparies on level ground because of breathlessness, or has to stop for breath when walking at own pace
4	Stops for breath after walking about 100 m or after a few minutes on level ground
5	Too breathless to leave the house, or breathless when dressing or undressing

Station 47: Pleural effusion

- *Please perform expansion, percussion and auscultation on the back of Mr AG who has been complaining of increasing SOB*
- *Mrs TH has no previous history of lung disease and has been getting increasingly SOB over the last month. Please examine her respiratory system and present your positive findings*

Hints and tips

- Examination as described in Chapter 19
- *Completion*: examine other relevant systems depending on the proposed cause, e.g. CVS if suspecting heart failure

Discussion points

- What are the causes of a pleural effusion?
- How would you manage a patient with a pleural effusion?
- What investigations do you send the pleural fluid off for when performing a diagnostic tap?

Ix		
Bloods	FBC, U&E, LFT, CRP, TFT, Albumin (rheumatoid factor/lactate dehydrogenase (LDH))	
	Consider ABG	
Imaging	CXR ± ultrasound (US) of the chest	
ECG		
Micro	Diagnostic aspirate for MC&S	
	Also send fluid for protein/glucose/LDH/pH and cytology	
Other	Consider CT chest	
	Consider echo	
	Medical thoracoscopy (or pleural biopsy)	

Criteria for diagnosing an exudate

- Protein > 30 g/dl

This is based on a serum albumin of 40 g/L so this figure needs to be corrected when the patient has hypoalbuminaemia. A more accurate measure is:

- Pleural/serum protein ratio > 0.5 *or*
- Pleural/serum LDH ratio > 0.6

NB. An aspirate with a pH of < 7.2 and a low glucose suggests an empyema which needs insertion of an intercostal drain. The pH is inaccurate as a marker for empyema in neoplastic processes.

Other causes of a dull lung base

- Raised hemidiaphragm
- Pleural thickening (normal vocal resonance)
- Lower lobe collapse (mediastinal shift towards side)
- Consolidation

Mx

ABCDE if necessary (see Ch. 11)

Rx	Aim treatment towards underlying cause
Procedures	Aspiration of fluid
	Insertion of intercostal drain (US guided)
	Consider pleurodesis
Monitoring	Regular O_2 sats ± ABG
Specialists	Respiratory physician and consideration for thoracoscopy

Station 48: Interstitial lung disease

- *Mrs VB has a history of rheumatoid arthritis. Please examine her respiratory system*

Hints and tips

- *Completion*: examine other relevant systems depending on the proposed cause, e.g. musculoskeletal if suspecting rheumatoid lung disease

Discussion points

- What are the causes of bilateral crackles and how can you differentiate them clinically?
- What are the causes or associations of interstitial lung disease?
- How would you investigate a patient with suspected interstitial lung disease?

Ix		
Bloods	Antinuclear antibody (ANA), rheumatoid factor, ESR	
	ABG – hypoxaemic respiratory failure	
Imaging	CXR – reticular nodular changes	
	High resolution CT chest	
Other	Pulmonary function tests (forced expiratory volume in 1 second (FEV_1)/forced vital capacity (FVC) > 0.8, i.e. restrictive)	
	Consider bronchoscopy and biopsy	

Causes

Idiopathic	Idiopathic pulmonary fibrosis (also known as cryptogenic fibrosing alveolitis)
Extrinsic allergic alveolitis	e.g. farmer's lung, bird fancier's lung
Drugs	e.g. amiodarone, methotrexate
Pneumoconioses	e.g. asbestosis, silicosis
Connective tissue disease	e.g. rheumatoid disease, scleroderma, ankylosing spondylitis
Granulomatous lung disease	e.g. sarcoidosis
Radiation	

Mx

ABCDE if necessary (see Ch. 11)

Rx	Oxygen
	Consider steroids or other immunosuppressive drugs, e.g. azathioprine
	Advise influenza vaccinations
Monitoring	Regular O_2 sats ± ABG
Specialists	Respiratory physician
Education	Avoidance of precipitants

Station 49: Bronchiectasis

- *Please examine the respiratory system of this patient who suffered with several episodes of pneumonia as a child*

Hints and tips

- *Completion*: following auscultation, ask the patient to cough and listen again to see if the crackles change in character
- Examine the sputum pot

Discussion points

- What are the causes of bronchiectasis?
- Discuss the management options for a patient with bronchiectasis

Ix		
Bloods	Consider immunoglobulins	
	Aspergillus precipitins	
	ABG	
Imaging	CXR – ring shadows	
	High resolution CT thorax	
Micro	Sputum MC&S	

Causes   Congenital – cystic fibrosis, primary ciliary dyskinesia
syndromes (e.g. Kartagener's)
Childhood infections, e.g. measles, TB
Post-obstructive
Allergic bronchopulmonary aspergillosis
Hypogammaglobulinaemia
Chronic aspiration
Recurrent pneumonia

Mx
ABCDE if necessary (see Ch. 11)
Rx   Antibiotics for exacerbations
Bronchodilators
Mucolytics
Advise influenza vaccination
MDT   Physiotherapist for postural drainage
Complications   Cor pulmonale
Massive haemoptysis
Metastatic infection, e.g. cerebral abscess

Station 50: COPD

• *Please demonstrate the examination of the respiratory system on this smoker*

Discussion points
• What diagnoses are collectively referred to as COPD?
• What are the causes of COPD?

Hints and tips [2]
Characterised by airflow limitation that is only partially reversible and usually progressive. Damage to the lungs is a combination of airway damage (obstructive bronchiolitis) and parenchymal damage (emphysema) – the contributions of each vary between individuals. The underlying mechanism is an inflammatory response usually to noxious substances (e.g. cigarette smoking).

Airflow obstruction is defined as a FEV_1 of < 80% predicted and a FEV_1/FVC ratio of < 0.7. There is often an overlap with chronic asthma although usually less reversibility.

Ix   *Bloods*   FBC (polycythaemia, anaemia)
α_1-antitrypsin (early onset, +ve FH, non-smoker)
ABG – ?hypercapnic respiratory failure

ECG
Imaging   CXR – hyperexpanded, bullae
Consider high resolution CT thorax
Consider echo
Micro   Sputum MC&S
Other   Spirometry: low FEV_1, FEV_1/FVC < 0.7
Transfer factor for carbon monoxide
Pulse oximetry
Causes   Smoking
Environmental
Occupational (dust)
α_1-antitrypsin
Untreated asthma

General management principles [2]
• Assess and monitor disease
• Optimise risk factors
• Manage stable disease
• Manage exacerbations
Consider the following:
• ABCDE if necessary (see Ch. 11)
• Bronchodilators
• Anticholinergics
• Steroids if responsive
• Antibiotics for infections
• Long-term oxygen therapy
• Patient education
• Regular exercise
• Smoking cessation
• Vaccinations
• Pulmonary rehabilitation
• Aminophylline
• Mucolytics

---

[1] National Institute for Health and Clinical Excellence. *Chronic Obstructive Pulmonary Disease*. Clinical Guideline No. 12. NICE: London, 2004. Available at www.nice.org.uk.

[2] GOLD. *Global Strategy for the Diagnosis, Management and Prevention of COPD*. Global Initiative for Chronic Obstructive Lung Disease (GOLD), 2007. Available at British Thoracic Society www.goldcopd.org.

Station 51: Previous TB

History hints

Cough	SOB	Haemoptysis
Weight loss	Night sweats	Nationality
Foreign travel	Contacts	PMH and FH
IV drug use	Immunosuppressed	Fever

Examination hints

Chest deformity
Scars – thoracotomy, thoracoplasty, supraclavicular (phrenic nerve crush)
Absent ribs
Tracheal deviation (towards side)
Crackles (apical), reduced expansion, pleural effusion

General
• Malaise
• Fever and weight loss
• Night sweats

Lymph node TB
• Painless lymph node enlargement

Respiratory TB
• Dyspnoea
• Cough/sputum
• Haemoptysis
• Crackles

Adrenal TB
• Addison's disease (commonest cause worldwide)

Renal TB
• Haematuria
• Sterile pyuria
• Chronic renal failure

Neurological TB
• Meningitis
• Cerebral abscess
• Nerve lesions

Cardiac TB
• Pericardial TB
• Calcification and tamponade

Spinal TB
• Vertebral collapse
• Paralysis

Skin TB
• Lupus vulgaris

Large joint TB

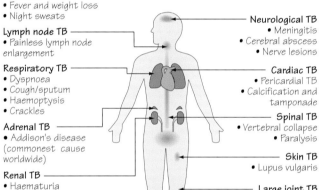

Station 53: Pneumonectomy/lobectomy

History hints

History of chronic lung condition with previous surgery

Examination hints

Expansion	↓
Percussion	Dull
Breath sounds	↓
Added sounds	None
Vocal resonance	↓
Other	? Mediastinal shift (towards side)

Chest radiograph
The most striking abnormality is the complete white-out of the left lung. There is associated volume loss on this side and deviation of the mediastinum to the left. This would be consistent with a diagnosis of left-sided pneumonectomy

Station 52: Obstructive sleep apnoea

History hints

Daytime somnolence	Cat napping
Morning headache	Snoring
Mood disturbance	Decreased libido
Decreased cognitive performance	Irritibility
Partner may describe apnoeic episodes	Poor sleep
History of falling asleep while driving	

Examination hints

Overweight	Large collar size
Hypertension	Micrognathia
Middle-aged man	Cyanosis
Septal deviation	Signs of cor pulmonale
CPAP equipment	

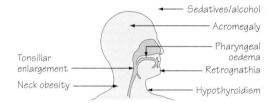

Station 54: Pneumonia

History hints	Examination hints	
SOB	Expansion	↓
Productive cough	Percussion	Dull
Travel	Breath sounds	Bronchial
Fever	Added sounds	Crackles
Malaise	Vocal resonance	↑
Confusion	Other: Tachypnoea, sputum pot, hypotension,	
Myalgia	fever, tachycardia	

Severity score for CAP [1]

Score 1 point for each of:
• Confusion (mental test score <8 or new disorientation)
• Urea >7mmol/L (i.e. includes use of laboratory tests)
• Respiratory rate >30/min
• Blood pressure (SBP<90 mmHg or DBP <60 mmHg)
• Age >65 years

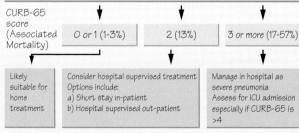

CURB-65 score (Associated Mortality): 0 or 1 (1–3%) | 2 (13%) | 3 or more (17–57%)

| Likely suitable for home treatment | Consider hospital supervised treatment. Options include: a) Short stay in-patient b) Hospital supervised out-patient | Manage in hospital as severe pneumonia Assess for ICU admission especially if CURB-65 is >4 |

Station 51: Previous TB

- *This 62-year-old female had a respiratory illness 40 years ago. Please examine her respiratory system*

Hints and tips

- Examination as described in Chapter 19
- Before the advent of chemotherapy, the aim of treatment was to cause lung hypoxia via different surgical procedures:
  - thoracoplasty = rib removal
  - plombage = insertion of polystyrene balls in the thoracic cavity
  - phrenic nerve crush – caused paralysis of the diaphragm

Discussion points

- What areas of the body can be affected by TB?
- What are the treatment options?
- How does one diagnose TB?

Ix	Bloods	FBC, U&E, LFT, CRP, ESR
		Consider ABG
	Imaging	CXR
	Micro	Sputum culture: Ziehl–Neelsen stain for acid-fast bacilli (AFB) – three early morning samples
		Urine for AFB if suspecting renal tract involvement
	Other	For extrapulmonary TB – send appropriate sample for culture or perform aspiration or biopsy of affected tissue, e.g. lymph node
		Mantoux test: +ve in post-primary pulmonary TB

Types of infection

1. *Primary pulmonary TB*:
   - Granuloma formation usually in the upper lobes (the Ghon focus)
   - 'Primary complex' = Ghon focus + hilar lymphadenopathy
   - Healing occurs with fibrosis and calcification
2. *Post primary pulmonary TB*:
   - Due to reactivation or failure of healing due to immunocompromised patient
   - Local and distant spread can occur (see opposite)
   - Miliary TB – haematogenous disseminated spread to several organs

High-risk groups

- Immunocompromised (HIV, diabetes mellitus)
- Ethnic minorities
- Young and old
- Health workers
- Contacts

Causes of apical fibrosis: STARE

- **S**arcoidosis
- **T**B
- **A**nkylosing spondylitis
- **R**adiation
- **E**xtrinsic allergic alveolitis

Station 52: Obstructive sleep apnoea

- *Mr DS has been investigated by the psychiatrists for a change in mood but no cause has been found. He has also been suffering with daytime tiredness. His GP has asked the respiratory team for an opinion. Please examine him and comment on any findings*

Hints and tips

- *Completion*: examine other relevant systems depending on your proposed cause, e.g. endocrine if suspecting acromegaly or hypothyroidism
- Offer to estimate the patient's BMI and measure their collar size

Discussion points

- What conditions predispose to obstructive sleep apnoea?
- How would you investigate a patient with suspected obstructive sleep apnoea and what are the management options?
- What are the associated complications of obstructive sleep apnoea?

Ix	Bloods	FBC (polycythaemia), ABG, TFT, Glc, lipids
	ECG	
	Imaging	CXR, consider echo
	Other	Overnight pulse oximetry
		Overnight video sleep studies
		Polysomnography
		Other investigations to rule out an obvious predisposing condition, e.g. acromegaly

Predisposing conditions	Obesity
	Large neck
	Tonsillar enlargement
	Hypothyroidism
	Acromegaly
	Craniofacial abnormalities
	Alcohol
Complications	Hypertension
	Type II respiratory failure
	Pulmonary hypertension

Mx		
Rx		Treat predisposing conditions
		Optimise BP control/diabetes/↑lipids?
		Continuous positive airways pressure (CPAP) overnight
Specialists		Consider ENT referral for tonsillectomy (in exceptional cases)
Education		Alcohol reduction, smoking cessation, weight loss

Station 53: Pneumonectomy/lobectomy

- *Mr Johnson has a history of lung cancer. Please examine his lungs*

Hints and tips

- Patients with previous lobectomy or pneumonectomy are often stable and can therefore be used in the OSCE exam
- Look carefully for scars and signs of mediastinal shift

Indications for lobectomy/pneumonectomy

- Neoplastic process
- Benign tumours
- Infective processes, e.g. TB
- Trauma

Station 54: Pneumonia

- *This patient has been unwell for 5 days with a productive cough. Please examine his lungs*

Discussion points

- What are the common pathogens implicated in community- and hospital-acquired pneumonia?

- What are the complications of pneumonia?
- How do you investigate a person with suspected pneumonia?

Classification
- Community-acquired pneumonia (CAP)
- Hospital-acquired pneumonia
- Aspiration
- Pneumonia in immunocompromised

Causes of CAP

Bacteria	*Streptococcus pneumoniae*
	Haemophilus influenzae
	Moraxella catarrhalis
	Pseudomonas (cystic fibrosis or bronchiectasis)
	Staphylococcus aureus (post viral)
Atypical organisms	*Mycoplasma, Legionella*
Viral	Influenza
Protozoal	*Pneumocystis carinii*
Ix *Bloods*	WCC/CRP
	Consider atypical respiratory serology
	Consider ABG
Imaging	CXR
Micro	Sputum culture
	Blood culture
	Urine for *Legionella* or pneumococcal antigen

Mx

ABCDE if necessary (see Ch. 11)

Treatment	Oxygen, IV fluids, antibiotics (assess severity to determine if IV or oral)
Location	Assess severity to determine admission or not
Monitoring	Regular observation including O_2 sats and RR, ABGs
MDT	Consider chest physiotherapy
Specialists	Consider ITU review if necessary and in particular if CURB65 score > 4
Complications	Pleural effusion
	Lung abscess
	Empyema
	Cavitation
	Septic shock and organ failure

Causes of cavitation on CXR
- Infective: *S. aureas*, *Mycobacterium* TB, *Klebsiella*, atypical mycobacteria
- Neoplastic: squamous cell carcinoma
- Inflammatory: lung abscess
- Autoimmune: Wegener's granulomatosis

[1] British Thoracic Society. *British Thoracic Society Guidelines for the Management of Community Acquired Pneumonia in Adults – 2004 update.* 2004. Available at www.brit-thoracic.org.uk.

Station 55: Peak flow measurement

Teaching a procedure to a patient – generic advice
Introduction/consent
Explanation of reason for carrying out procedure
Explanation of equipment
Explanation of procedure with demonstration if
 necessary
Observation of procedure with corrections if
 necessary
Check understanding
Ask if patient has any questions or queries

Station 56: Inhaler technique

Sit up straight or stand
Tilt head back a little
Remove cap and shake the inhaler
If first use or not been used for a few days then spray 1 puff into the air
Take a few deep breaths and then breathe out gently
Place the inhaler in your mouth (do not bite it!) and form a seal with
 your lips
Breathe in slowly and simultaneously press down on the canister to release the drug
Continue to full inspiration and hold your breath for 10 seconds (or as long as you can)
If a further dose is required, wait 30 seconds and repeat

Station 57: Oxygen therapy

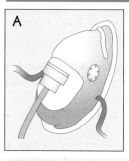
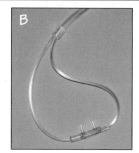
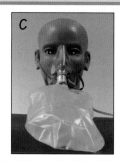
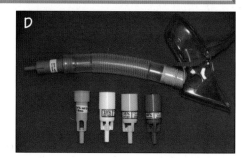

Oxygen therapy – revision points
Low-flow devices:
(A) Simple face mask (e.g. Hudson)   (max. FiO_2 30–50%)
(B) Nasal cannula   (max. FiO_2 30–60%)
(C) Reservoir bag   (max. FiO_2 60–80%)
• Low-flow devices give a variable amount of oxygen depending on the minute volume (MV)
 of the patient (MV = respiratory rate x tidal volume), i.e. the greater the ventilation, the
 lower the inspired oxygen for a given flow rate of supplemental oxygen
• Difficult to accurately measure the FiO_2 so not recommended for use with unwell COPD
 patients

High-flow devices:
(D) Venturi mask   (max. FiO_2 24–60%)
• High-flow devices give a precise concentration of oxygen depending on the valve used

Indications for oxygen therapy
Cardiac or respiratory arrest   Tachypnoea (RR > 24)
Hypoxaemia (SaO_2 < 90% or PaO_2 < 8 kPa)   Hypotension   Metabolic acidosis

Which mask?
REMEMBER HYPOXIA KILLS BEFORE HYPERCAPNIA
If in doubt use a reservoir bag and check an ABG
Monitor the patient closely and check an ABG if there
 is a change in oxygen concentration or any clinical
 deterioration

Nasal prongs: Stable patient
Reservoir mask: Acutely unwell patient
Simple face mask: Unwell patient but requiring
                        FiO_2 < 50%
Venturi mask: Patient requiring accurate FiO_2,
                        i.e. hypercapnic ventilatory failure

As a general rule aim SpO_2 > 94%
If a patient has hypercapnic ventilatory failure then aim
 for SpO_2 88–92%

Station 55: Peak flow measurement

• *Miss AP (22 years old, height 167 cm) has attended her GP with a history of intermittent wheeze. The GP has made a diagnosis of asthma and has asked you to measure the patient's peak flow rate. Please perform this task and record the measurement on the chart provided*

Hints and tips

This station is testing your ability to explain the procedure to the patient and then record the result. See opposite for general overview, but remember the following tips:
• Introduction/consent
• Explanation of reason for carrying out procedure and explanation of the equipment
• The indicator must be at the base of the numbered scale
• Patient should sit upright or stand up
• Hold the device horizontally without touching the scale
• Take in a deep breath
• Ask the patient to place the meter in her mouth and close lips tightly around the mouthpiece (do not put tongue in the hole)
• Ask the patient to blow out as hard and as fast as she can without obstructing the indicator
• Note the number obtained from the scale

• Patient should perform this procedure three times and note the highest number recorded on the chart
• Show the patient a predicted peak flow chart and explain what her predicted peak flow rate should be
• Ask the patient if they have any further questions
NB. With good communication skills and clear instructions it should not be necessary to demonstrate the skill to the patient first, unless the instruction specifically asks for this.

Discussion points

• What pattern would be demonstrated on the peak flow diary if your diagnosis of asthma was correct?
• What treatment would you prescribe initially and at follow-up if there was no improvement in symptoms?
• At what level of peak flow would you advise your patient to seek medical help?
• What are the important history points with a patient with asthma?

Station 56: Inhaler technique

• *Miss AP (from Station 55) has been given a salbutamol inhaler (pressurised metered dose). Please explain the correct procedure for administering this drug*

Hints and tips

See opposite for the actual inhaler technique and use the hints and tips from Station 55.

Station 57: Oxygen therapy

• *This station tests your ability to correctly administer oxygen therapy in various clinical situations. The examiner will explain a scenario and then you need to choose the most appropriate oxygen therapy from the samples available*
• *Please name each of the oxygen delivery systems displayed and tell the examiner what inspired oxygen concentrations can be achieved with each. Then discuss scenarios where you would use each device*

Hints and tips

• Hypoxaemia is defined as a reduction below normal levels of oxygen in arterial blood, i.e. PaO_2 of < 8.0 kPa or $SaO_2 < 90\%$
• Hypoxia is the reduction below normal levels of oxygen in the tissues, i.e. hypoxaemia can lead to hypoxia
• Low-flow devices give a variable amount of oxygen depending on the patient's breathing pattern but can still deliver high concentrations of oxygen (i.e. if the patient is breathing slowly)
• High-flow devices deliver a set concentration of oxygen depending on the valve and providing the correct flow rate is set (the flow rate is stated on the valve)
• High-flow devices can deliver low concentrations of oxygen
• Humidification should occur if prolonged high concentrations of oxygen are being used
• Reservoir bag masks deliver 70–80% oxygen when flow is set to 15 L/min. Note the reservoir needs to be filled with oxygen before the mask is placed on the patient
• A non-rebreathe valve separates the mask from the bag so the patient cannot exhale back into it
• Oxygen saturations are not always accurate – if in doubt then check an ABG

Predicting the PaO_2

• The PaO_2 for a patient needs to be interpreted taking into account the inspired oxygen concentration (FiO_2). Hence it is *essential* to document how much oxygen the patient is on
• The arterial oxygen concentration (PaO_2) should be approximately 8–10 kPa lower than the FiO_2, e.g. if the FiO_2 in room air is 21%, in a healthy person the PaO_2 should be 11–13 kPa; if the FiO_2 is 40%, the PaO_2 should be approx. 30–32 kPa

Example scenarios
Scenario 1
An 84-year-old female with known COPD has been admitted to your ward with increasing SOB and a productive cough. ABGs: pH 7.38, PaO_2 6.3, $PaCO_2$ 5.8 (on 2 L/min via nasal cannula), RR 30.
• *Please discuss the best oxygen therapy to use in this situation and your plan for monitoring progress*
Your patient is hypoxaemic and needs her inspired oxygen concentration increasing. Use a venturi mask at a concentration sufficient to reach SaO_2 of 88–92%. Her ABG should be repeated after 20–30 minutes or earlier if there is any clinical change.
• *What are the criteria necessary to consider non-invasive ventilation?*

Scenario 2
A 36-year-old male with no previous PMH is admitted to A&E with a pneumonia. ABGs: pH 7.4, PaO_2 8.8, $PaCO_2$ 3.7 (on 24% venturi), RR 28.
• *Would you change this man's oxygen therapy and if so what would you choose?*
Any acutely unwell patient should be given oxygen via a reservoir bag mask initially. Progress can be monitored by checking oxygen saturations or repeating a blood gas. A simple face mask could be used following the initial assessment if his SaO_2 remain > 92%.
• *What are the clinical indications for oxygen therapy?*

Scenario 3
A 64-year-old male has just returned to the ward following an inguinal hernia repair. He is previously fit and healthy and has no history of respiratory disease. Although a little drowsy, the rest of his observations are normal and clinically he looks well. The nurse has found his saturations to be 89% on room air. She has asked for your advice.
• *Please administer oxygen to the mannequin provided explaining your actions to the examiner*
• Introduction/consent
• Check correct patient
• Explain your actions to the patient
• Check the SaO_2 using pulse oximetry
• Comment that the sats are low and offer some reasons for this possibility
• State that you would like to check the arterial blood gas (ABG shows PaO_2 8.6, otherwise normal parameters)
• Suggest nasal prongs as the patient is post-op and has had no previous lung disease
• Apply the nasal cannula correctly to the patient and turn the oxygen to the correct flow rate
• State intention to review patient in 30 minutes or earlier if necessary
• Prescribe oxygen on the treatment chart

Station 58: Chest radiograph interpretation – normal chest

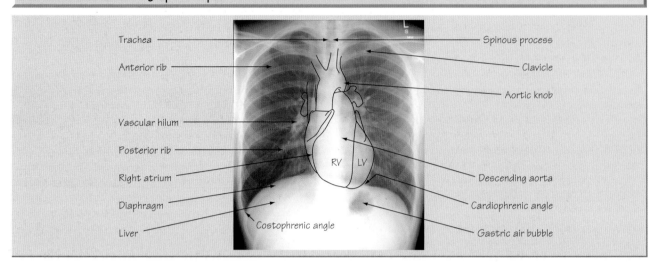

Trachea — Spinous process
Anterior rib — Clavicle
— Aortic knob
Vascular hilum —
Posterior rib —
Right atrium — Descending aorta
RV LV
Diaphragm — Cardiophrenic angle
Liver — Costophrenic angle — Gastric air bubble

The silhouette sign

A useful sign for determining which lobe is involved. Consolidation can cause loss of the solid-gas interface between the heart borders, diaphragms or mediastinum

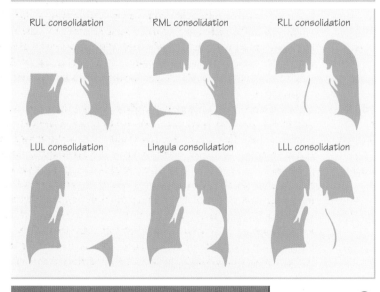

RUL consolidation   RML consolidation   RLL consolidation

LUL consolidation   Lingula consolidation   LLL consolidation

Technical hints – see text for detail

A - Date and name
B - AP/PA: Is it anteroposterior or posteroanterior?
C - Right diaphragm 2 cm higher than left
D - Check ribs for fractures and metastases
E - Soft tissues and breast shadows
F - Well positioned? Trachea should be midway between clavicles
G - Penetration: The disc spaces should just be visible through the cardiac shadow
H - Lung fields

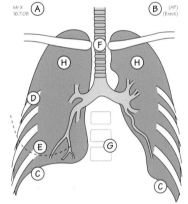

CT of the chest

1 - Oesophagus
2 - Right lung
3 - Right main bronchus
4 - Right pulmonary artery and branches
5 - Superior vena cava
6 - Ascending aorta
7 - Pulmonary trunk
8 - Mediastinum and heart
9 - Left pulmonary artery and branches
10 - Left main bronchus
11 - Left lung
12 - Descending aorta

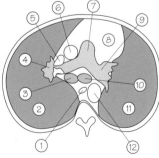

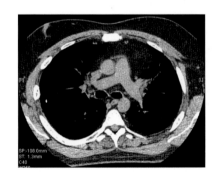

Station 58: Chest radiograph interpretation – normal chest

Technical hints (see opposite)

- Always interpret the radiograph in the light of the clinical findings
- Make sure it is the correct patient (A) and know the history and examination findings (this may not be available in your exam however!)
- Determine whether posteroanterior (PA) or anteroposterior (AP) (B), erect or supine. (Portable films are taken AP and can magnify the mediastinum making comment on the heart size inaccurate. Supine films can make the recognition of pleural fluid and air more difficult.) An AP film should be marked as such
- Try and determine whether male or female (breast shadows (E)) and young or old (bone quality (D))
- Check for:
  - inspiration – adequate inspiration should be diaphragm at the level of the 6th rib anteriorly (or count 9–10 posterior ribs); determine if hyperexpansion or inadequate inspiration
  - rotation – spinous processes of the thoracic vertebrae should be midway between the medial ends of the clavicles (F)
  - penetration (lower thoracic vertebral bodies should be visible through the mediastinum (G))
  - inclusion of the appropriate anatomy (e.g. the apices have not been missed (H))
- If the above points are all alright, then state that the film is *technically adequate*
- There are three densities on plain film:
  - bone = white
  - air = black
  - soft tissue = grey

Diagnosis

- If there is an obvious abnormality then mention it now, describing the zones of the lungs and the lobe involved if possible
- The right lung has three lobes (upper, middle and lower (RUL, RML and RUL, respectively))
- The left lung has two lobes (upper (LUL) and lower (LLL)), plus the lingula which corresponds anatomically to the right middle lobe
- Remember there may be more than one abnormality so review the other areas following this
- If the abnormality is not obvious then use a systematic approach to cover all anatomy (see below)
- White on radiograph = increased opacity
- Black on radiograph = increased lucency
- Opacification can be air space (alveolar) or interstitial

Systematic approach to the chest radiograph

- Technicalities (as above)
- Heart
- Mediastinum
- Trachea
- Apices
- Hilar
- Lung fields
- Diaphragm
- Soft tissues
- Bone
- Tubes and lines

- *Please present this chest radiograph*
- *Please describe the abnormality on this chest radiograph*
- *In light of the respiratory examination you have just done, please interpret the patient's chest radiograph*
- *Please describe the abnormality on this chest radiograph and discuss how you would manage this patient*

Common chest radiograph abnormalities

- Consolidation of any lobe
- Pulmonary oedema
- Pneumothorax
- Interstitial lung disease
- Pleural effusion
- Atelectasis (collapse) of any lobe
- Lobectomy/pneumonectomy
- Neoplastic lesion (primary or secondary)
- TB
- Hilar enlargement
- Nasogastric tube in situ
- Central line in situ
- Endotrachial tube in situ

Example answers

- This is a PA chest radiograph of patient X, taken on (date). The film is technically adequate. The most striking abnormality is a large area of opacity in the left lower zone. There is a meniscus present and this would be consistent with a left-sided pleural effusion. There are no other obvious abnormalities that I can see
- This is an AP portable chest radiograph of patient X, taken on (date). It is technically adequate. The heart size appears normal, as does the mediastinum. The trachea and mediastinum are central. The apices and lung bases are clear and the costophrenic and cardiophrenic angles are visible. The heart borders are also clear. On closer inspection there are fractures of the 5th and 6th ribs on the right side but no evidence of a pneumothorax
- This is a PA chest radiograph of Mr Gowering taken yesterday. Technically the film is inadequate as the apices are missing and the film is underexposed. The most striking abnormality is a well-demarcated area of opacity in the right lower zone with loss of the diaphragm markings on this side. The right heart border is visible. There appears to be an air bronchogram visible within this opacity and so my conclusion is that the findings would be consistent with a right lower lobe consolidation
- This is a PA chest radiograph of patient X, taken on (date). There is increased opacity in the left mid zone with loss of the left heart border. This would be consistent with consolidation of the lingula lobe. On viewing the rest of the radiograph I could not see any further abnormalities

Causes of breathlessness without major radiograph changes

- Asthma
- COPD
- *Pneumocystis* pneumonia
- Pulmonary embolism
- Left lower lobe collapse
- Foreign body
- Toxic gas/fume inhalation
- Metabolic acidosis

Station 59: Chest radiograph interpretation

Station 60: Chest radiograph interpretation

Station 61: Chest radiograph interpretation

Station 62: Chest radiograph interpretation

Station 63: Chest radiograph interpretation

Station 64: Chest radiograph interpretation

Station 59: Chest radiograph interpretation – pleural effusion

- PA chest radiograph of a female patient
- No demographic information
- Slightly rotated and underpenetrated
- Most striking abnormality is an area of opacity in the right middle and lower zones
- There is a meniscus
- There is no obvious loss of volume of the hemithorax and no mediastinal shift
- This would be consistent with a large right-sided pleural effusion
- On closer inspection there is also some blunting of the left costophrenic angle
- I would like to review this patient clinically to determine the cause and commence management

Discussion points

- What are the causes of a pleural effusion?
- What further investigations would you like to perform?
- What further management would you consider?

Station 60: Chest radiograph interpretation – pneumothorax

- AP chest radiograph
- No demographic information
- Technically adequate
- The heart size is within normal limits and there is no mediastinal shift
- There are no obvious bone or soft tissue abnormalities
- On closer inspection there appears to be loss of lung markings in the periphery of the left lung field
- This finding would be consistent with a left-sided pneumothorax
- There is no evidence of tensioning but I would want to review this patient clinically, initially assessing ABCDE and then taking a history and performing a full examination

Discussion points

- What are the causes of a pneumothorax?
- What is the management of a pneumothorax?
- Are you aware of the British Thoracic Society guidelines?
- What information needs to be given to the patient?

Station 61: Chest radiograph interpretation – atelectasis

- PA chest radiograph
- Minimal rotation but adequate penetration
- The most striking abnormality is an area of opacity in the right upper zone
- There is an associated loss of volume of the right lung field with tenting of the diaphragm and some mediastinal shift towards the right
- This would be consistent with right upper lobe collapse, possibly caused by an obstructing lesion such as a lung neoplasm
- I would like to review this patient clinically including full history and examination

Discussion points

- What are the causes of atelectasis?
- What further investigations should be performed?
- What symptoms might this patient have presented with?
- What complications can occur as a result of local spread of a lung neoplasm?

Station 62: Chest radiograph interpretation – lung metastases

- Supine chest radiograph, underpenetrated
- The most striking abnormality is the presence of several areas of circular, well-demarcated opacification in both lung fields
- The two largest areas measure 2×2 cm and are in the right middle and lower zones
- The most likely diagnosis is multiple lung metastases
- A full history and examination is necessary to determine the primary

Discussion points

- What are the causes of a coin lesion on a chest radiograph?
- Which primary cancers metastasise commonly to the lung?
- What other investigations would need to be considered?
- What treatment options are available for metastatic cancer?

Station 63: Chest radiograph interpretation – critical care patient

- AP portable supine chest radiograph
- The patient is acutely unwell and the film is likely to have been taken on the intensive care unit as there is an endotracheal tube in situ
- Technical aspects are adequate for such a film
- Patient is attached to an ECG monitor
- As well as the endotracheal tube, there are right and left internal jugular central lines and a nasogastric tube
- There is widespread air space shadowing and the most likely explanation in such an unwell patient would be acute respiratory distress syndrome (ARDS; pulmonary oedema is unlikely as there are no pleural effusions or other signs of heart failure)

Discussion points

- Is this patient critically unwell? What features are consistent with this?
- What can cause cavitation on a chest radiograph?
- What other investigations would need to be considered?
- What might be the next stage in management to improve this patient's oxygenation?

Station 64: Chest radiograph interpretation – pulmonary oedema

- AP erect chest radiograph of an elderly female patient on oxygen
- Slight rotation
- There appears to be cardiomegaly, even taking into account this is an AP film
- There is widespread alveolar shadowing throughout both lung fields with upper lobe diversion
- There also appears to be opacification at the left lower zone with loss of the costodiaphragmatic angle
- These findings would be consistent with a diagnosis of pulmonary oedema and a possible left pleural effusion
- This patient needs to be reviewed clinically

Discussion points

- What are the radiographic findings of left ventricular failure?
- What causes upper lobe diversion?
- What is the difference between cardiogenic and non-cardiogenic pulmonary oedema?

Gastrointestinal symptoms

Anorexia	Haematemesis	Diarrhoea
Weight loss	Melaena	Constipation
Abdominal pain	Dysphagia	Abdominal distension
Change in bowel habit	Dyspepsia/indigestion	Jaundice
Nausea and vomiting	PR bleeding	

Specific gastrointestinal history points

Travel history	Previous GI operations
Sexual history	Family history
Detailed alcohol history	
Dietary history	
Current and previous drugs (e.g. NSAIDs, antibiotics, IV drug use)	

Station 65: Weight loss

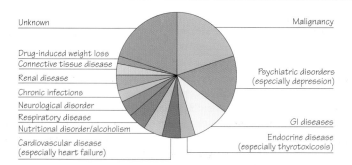

Unknown
Drug-induced weight loss
Connective tissue disease
Renal disease
Chronic infections
Neurological disorder
Respiratory disease
Nutritional disorder/alcoholism
Cardiovascular disease (especially heart failure)

Malignancy
Psychiatric disorders (especially depression)
GI diseases
Endocrine disease (especially thyrotoxicosis)

Chronic diarrhoea

Underlying pathology suggested by:
• Weight loss
• Nocturnal diarrhoea
• Abnormal FBC, B_{12}, folate, Fe, albumin

Pathological site

Pancreas
Chronic pancreatitis
Steatorrhoea
Pale, bulky, offensive fat-soluble vitamin deficiency
↓A, D, E, K

Small intestine
May have weight loss ++ and/or steatorrhoea e.g. coeliac, giardiasis, hypolactasia

Colon
Watery stool
Blood and mucus
Rectal urge
• Colitis
• Colonic neoplasm e.g. villous adenoma

Station 66: Diarrhoea

Causes of diarrhoea
Acute
Infective: bacterial, viral, amoebic
Drugs, e.g. antibiotics

Chronic
Inflammatory bowel disease (IBD)
Parasite infections, e.g. giardiasis
Malabsorption, e.g. coeliac disease
Drugs, e.g. proton pump inhibitors
Neoplasia
Faecal impaction (with overflow diarrhoea)
Endocrine, e.g. hyperthyroidism, carcinoid
Ischaemic bowel
Irritable bowel syndrome (IBS)

Bloody
Infective, e.g. Campylobacter, Salmonella
IBD
Neoplasia
Colitis, e.g. ischaemic

Station 67: Dysphagia

Causes of dysphagia
Oral/pharyngeal
• Poor dentition
• Ill-fitting dentures
• Pharyngeal pouch

Oesophageal
• Oesophagitis
• Benign stricture, e.g. peptic stricture
• Malignant stricture

Neuromuscular
• Cerebrovascular disease
• Bulbar palsy
• Myasthenia gravis
• Oesophageal motility problem
• Achalasia

Extrinsic pressure
• Goitre
• Mediastinal lymphadenopathy

Causes of dysphagia

Carcinoma
• Progressive history
• Solids (before liquids)
• Weight loss ++
• 'Apple core' lesion
• Usually lower 1/3
• Oesophageal or gastric origin

Peptic stricture
• Associated symptoms of reflux
• Commonest cause of benign strictures
• Other causes: after corrosives after radiotherapy after variceal injection

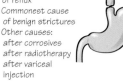

Systemic disease
• Scleroderma: often associated severe reflux → peptic stricture
• Dermatomyositis
• Connective tissue disorders, especially if Raynaud's present

Extrinsic compression
• Aortic arch aneurysm
• Lymph nodes: lymphoma lung cancer
• Enlarged L-atrium e.g. mitral stenosis

Neuromuscular dysphagia
• Cause usually obvious, CVA, motor neuron disease, progressive suprabulbar palsy
• If cause unclear, consider myasthenia gravis
• Usually liquids and solids

Achalasia — Progressive dilatation above sphincter — May cause aspiration pneumonia

Local nerve → **Hypertonic sphincter** → Prevent any symptoms of reflux

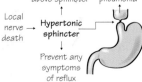

• Rare, 1 in 100,000
• Idiopathic, or Chagas' disease (Trypanosoma cruzi)
• Long history of intermittent dysphagia
• Occasionally attacks of severe chest pain due to oesophageal spasm ('vigorous achalasia')

Station 65: Weight loss

Student info: *Mrs GI is 39 and has been referred with weight loss. She was diagnosed as having an anxiety disorder recently and has now noticed an increase in frequency of bowel movements. Please take a full history and discuss a differential diagnosis and management plan*

Patient info: *You are Mrs GI, who is 39 years old. Your usual weight of 60 kg has fallen to 52 kg over 6 months. You are eating normally with a good diet with an increased frequency of bowel movements up to 4 times/day over the last 2 months. Your GP diagnosed anxiety 3 months ago but otherwise there is no PMH of note. Your father died of stomach cancer aged 72. There has been no abdominal pain or PR bleeding. You smoke 15/day and drink 4 bottles of wine per week, and live with your husband and two children who are all well. You feel your anxiety is due to the fact that you think you have cancer*

Hints and tips

- Determine patient's reason for visiting GP and ascertain current knowledge of the situation
- Determine symptomatology, full gastrointestinal history
- Associated history questions looking at other causes of weight loss
- Determine if weight loss is intentional
- Drug history looking for possible causes, e.g. laxative abuse
- Determine the patient's mood and assess the anxiety diagnosis
- Establish FH of stomach cancer, smoking and alcohol history
- Assess impact of the symptoms on the patient's life
- Address any fears and concerns the patient has

Discussion points

- Discuss the causes of weight loss in this patient
- What investigations would you request?

ΔΔ	Endocrine	Thyrotoxicosis
	GI	Coeliac disease; Crohn's disease
		Primary neoplasm
	Other	Depression/anxiety
Ix	Bloods	FBC, U&E, TFT, LFT, Glc, CRP
		Coeliac serology
	Micro	Stool culture
	Other	Gastroscopy + duodenal biopsy; colonoscopy

Station 66: Diarrhoea

Student info: *Mr LG is 28 and has been referred to hospital by his GP with a history of diarrhoea. You are the FY1 doctor who is seeing him on the assessment unit.*

Patient info: *You are a 28-year-old male with no PMH. You started having diarrhoea 5 months ago with loose stool on average 3 times/day. There is no blood PR. You went to India 4 months ago, and returned last week. You are now passing watery stool up to 5 times/day. There is some associated weight loss and you had a couple of episodes of probable gastroenteritis while away. You smoke 10/day but no alcohol. You are heterosexual with no HIV risk factors, no associated systemic symptoms and no FH of note*

Hints and tips

- Ascertain the patient's understanding of the reason the GP has referred him to hospital
- Ascertain the patient's meaning of diarrhoea (i.e. loose motions, increased frequency or both)
- Take an accurate history of the symptoms (frequency, colour, blood, mucus, flushability, volume, consistency)
- Establish the start of the diarrhoea was actually prior to the trip
- Ask about the weight loss; any other associated systemic symptoms?
- Ask about dietary intake and activities while in India
- Ask about close contacts (points to infection)
- Ask about nocturnal diarrhoea (presence usually indicates significant disease)
- Determine the impact of symptoms on quality of life
- Elicit any concerns the patient may have
- Offer a diagnosis and agree a management plan

Discussion points

- What investigations would you request?
- What are the causes of diarrhoea?

ΔΔ		Malabsorption, IBD, infective neoplasia, IBS
Ix	Bloods	FBC, U&E, LFT, haematinics, coeliac serology
	Micro	Stool culture
	Imaging	Consider an AXR if colitis is suspected
	Other	Small bowel enema, colonoscopy

Station 67: Dysphagia

Student info: *Mrs UG is 70 and has been referred to the gastro clinic on a 2-week wait with difficulty swallowing. Please assess and advise the patient on your management plan*

Patient info: *You are Mrs UG and are 70 years old. Your PMH is one of angina, which has been controlled for many years on medication alone. Over the last 12 months you have noticed problems with swallowing, which was initially intermittent but is now getting worse. There is no associated pain; the problem is worse with solids but has occasionally happened with liquids too. You get intermittent indigestion. Your appetite is good and there has been no weight loss or change in bowel habit. You are a non-smoker and do not drink alcohol. You live alone since your husband died 3 years ago, and were adopted. When pushed, you admit to worrying that it could be cancer. Your DH is: aspirin, clopidogrel, nitrate, omeprazole, bisoprolol, ramipril, ibuprofen prn*

Hints and tips

- Determine the patient's reason for coming to hospital and ascertain prior knowledge of the situation
- Determine symptomatology
- Elicit whether there is associated pain (odynophagia) and whether the problem is with solids or liquids
- Determine associated symptoms, e.g. weight loss?
- Elicit relevant PMH and the impact of the angina on her life
- Elicit the drug history, in particular those that could be contributing
- Elicit the patient's concerns and agree a management plan

Discussion points

- What investigations would you request?
- What are the causes of dysphagia?

Ix	Bloods	FBC, U&E, LFT, iron studies
	Imaging	CXR, consider barium swallow
	Other	Gastroscopy (first-line investigation for dysphagia unless suspecting pharyngeal pouch); video fluoroscopy swallow; 24-hour oesophageal manometry

Station 68: Abdominal examination

FACE
- Eyes — Sclera, Cornea
- Mouth — Breath, Lips, Gums, Tongue, Dentition

NECK
- Lymph nodes (especially left supraclavicular nodes)

CHEST
- Gynaecomastia
- Spider naevi
- Loss of chest and axillary hair

ABDOMEN
- Inspect — Scars, Distension, Dilated veins, Striae/bruising, Masses, Visible peristalsis
- Palpate (9 areas) — Superficial, Deep, Organs in turn (liver, spleen, kidneys, aorta)
- Percuss — Liver, Spleen, Ascites
- Auscultate — Bowel sounds

LEGS/FEET
- Oedema
- Scars
- Temperature/colour

TO COMPLETE
- Digital rectal examination (DRE)
- Urinalysis
- Genitalia
- Inguinal lymph nodes
- Hernial orifices

ARMS
- Radial pulse
- Spider naevi
- Muscle wasting
- Scratch marks
- Bruising

HANDS
- Clubbing
- Nail changes
- Arthropathy
- Liver flap
- Palmar erythema
- Dupuytren's contracture

GENERAL INSPECTION
(take a physical step back)
- Well/unwell
- General appearance
- Hydration/nutritional state
- Muscle bulk
- Mental state
- Signs of certain diseases
- Dyspnoea
- Sweaty
- Cyanosis/jaundice/pallor
- Cachexia
- Signs of chronic liver disease
- Body hair distribution
- Xanthelasma
- Bruising/tattoos

ESSENTIALS CHECKLIST
(WINCER)

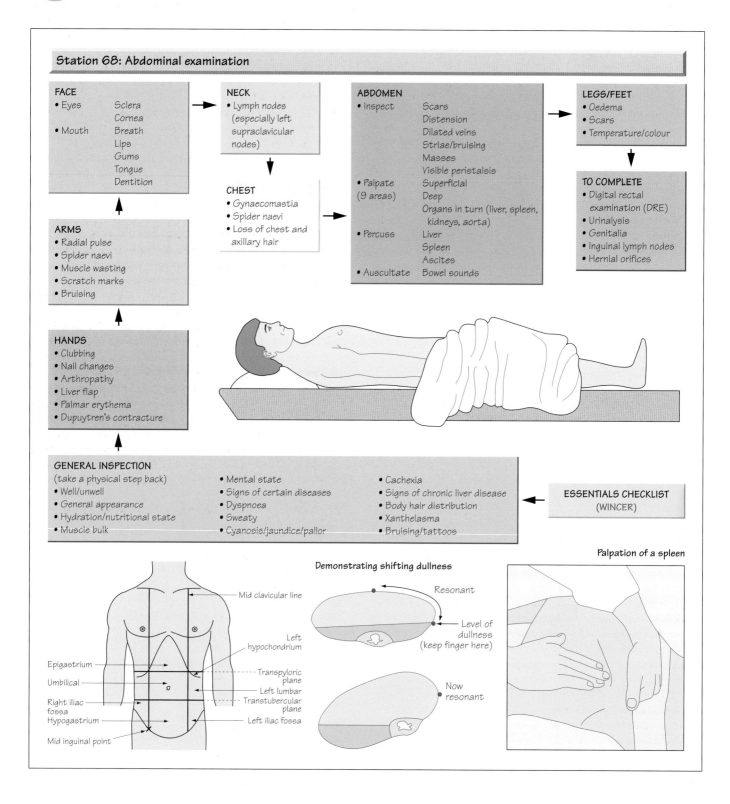

Mid clavicular line
Epigastrium
Umbilical
Right iliac fossa
Hypogastrium
Mid inguinal point
Left hypochondrium
Transpyloric plane
Left lumbar
Transtubercular plane
Left iliac fossa

Demonstrating shifting dullness
Resonant
Level of dullness (keep finger here)
Now resonant

Palpation of a spleen

Station 68: Abdominal examination

- *Please examine this man's abdominal system*
- *This middle-aged woman is complaining of itchy skin. Please examine her abdominal system*
- *This 44-year-old male is a known IV drug user and alcoholic. Please examine his abdomen*
- *Please palpate this patient's abdomen*

Examination routine

- Introduction/consent/ask about pain
- *Exposure*: officially the patient should be exposed from 'nipples to knees' but in practice underwear should be kept in place. It is also important to view the ankles and feet. Remember to respect dignity
- *Position*: lying flat with the head resting on a single pillow
- *General inspection*:
  - take a physical step back and observe the patient and surroundings
  - assess whether the patient is well/unwell, and comfortable lying at rest or dyspnoeic
  - observe the general appearance for evidence of specific diseases or syndromes, e.g. connective tissue disorders or congestive cardiac failure
  - assess the mental state for any evidence of encephalopathy
- *Screening test*: ask the patient to lift their head off the bed or give a cough. This may give useful information as to whether the patient is in any pain or if there is any evidence of a hernia
- *System-specific inspection*:
  - assess the nutritional status and determine if there is evidence of cachexia or muscle wasting
  - look at the skin for evidence of jaundice, scratch marks, tattoos, injection sites, rashes or changes in pigmentation
- *Hands*:
  - look for any signs of chronic liver disease (see Ch. 27)
  - palpate the radial artery briefly
  - check for evidence of a hepatic flap (asterixis)
- *Head and neck*:
  - look at the sclera for signs of jaundice, the conjunctivae for pallor and check for any iritis
  - check the periorbital region for xanthelasma
  - examine the teeth, tongue and mucous membranes, taking care to check for bad breath, gum hypertrophy, state of dentition, pigmentation, mouth ulcers and infections
  - sit the patient forward and palpate for lymphadenopathy (Virchow's node) and feel for salivary gland enlargement
- *Chest*: lie the patient supine once again and check the chest for evidence of gynaecomastia, spider naevi or loss of chest or axillary hair
- *Abdomen inspection*: note any scars (see Ch. 45), deformities, distension, swellings, visible pulsations, prominent veins, striae or skin discoloration
- *Abdomen palpation*: before beginning, check if the patient has any pain. If so examine this area last. Kneel down beside the patient to palpate. In your mind divide the abdomen into nine areas (see opposite). Lightly palpate in each of the nine areas with your palm keeping the fingers together and flexing slightly at the metacarpophalangeal (MCP) joints. Note any areas of tenderness or possible masses bearing in mind

the structures that are to be found in each of the areas. Next apply deeper palpation to help define the abnormalities. While palpating observe the patient's face for any sign of discomfort. Note any guarding or rebound tenderness although it would be unusual to have a patient with these signs in an exam. The abdominal organs should now be examined in turn

- *Liver*: start in the right iliac fossa with the hand parallel to the costal margin. Ask the patient to breathe in and out while using the border of the index finger to feel for the liver edge. Now percuss for the upper border of the liver starting in the right midclavicular line on the anterior chest wall above the level of the 5th intercostal space, and then the lower border by percussing up from the right iliac fossa (RIF)
- *Spleen*: commence palpation for the spleen in the RIF with the hand parallel to the left subcostal margin (otherwise a large spleen could be missed). Progress towards the costal margin at 2 cm intervals with the patient breathing in and out. If a spleen is not felt then roll the patient onto their right side and while palpating with the right hand, use your left hand to support the patient and pull the skin forward over the costal margin (see opposite). Percuss for the spleen starting from the RIF and moving proximally, concentrating over the lower costal margin and remembering to percuss in both inspiration and expiration
- *Kidneys*: use the bimanual method to palpate for the kidneys in turn
- *Aorta*: check for an expansile, pulsatile mass
- *Abdomen percussion*: examine for ascites by percussing for shifting dullness. Start with the patient lying supine. Percuss from the midline towards the flanks – away from you. If resonant in the midline and dull in the flanks then, keeping your hand in place, have the patient roll towards you. If now resonant then shifting dullness is present.
- *Abdomen auscultation*: listen for bowel sounds or any bruits. Check the legs and ankles for evidence of oedema, bruising or muscle wasting
- *Completion*: state to the examiners that you would like to complete your examination by checking the hernial orifices, external genitalia and by performing a digital rectal examination (see Ch. 45). Also check the observation chart and carry out a urinalysis

Summary of common gastrointestinal investigations

Bloods	FBC (anaemia)
	U&E
	LFT including albumin
	Clotting
	Amylase
	Iron studies
	Coeliac serology
Imaging	Abdominal radiograph
	Barium studies
	Ultrasound (US) of the abdomen
	CT of the abdomen
	Endoscopic ultrasound
Micro	Stool culture
	Ascitic fluid MC&S
	Urine MC&S
Other	Endoscopy (gastroscòpy, colonoscopy, sigmoidoscopy)
	Liver biopsy
	Capsule endoscopy

Station 69: Chronic liver disease

History hints

Alcohol intake
Drug history (prescribed and recreational)
Previous episodes of jaundice
Previous blood transfusions
Occupational (e.g. health care worker)/travel/sexual history
FH (e.g. Wilson's, haemochromatosis, α1AT deficiency)
Relevant PMH, e.g. diabetes (NAFLD, haemochromatosis), autoimmune disease (autoimmune hepatitis, primary biliary cirrhosis

Examination hints

General
Muscle wasting
Poor nutrition
Paucity of body hair
Scratch marks
Pallor/jaundice*
Tattoos/needle marks

Chest/abdomen
Spider naevi
Gynaecomastia
Hepatomegaly*
Splenomegaly*
Ascites*
Caput medusa

Hands
Clubbing
Palmar erythema
Leuconychia
Metabolic flap*
Dupuytren's

Other
Peripheral oedema*
Testicular atrophy

*also seen in acute liver disease

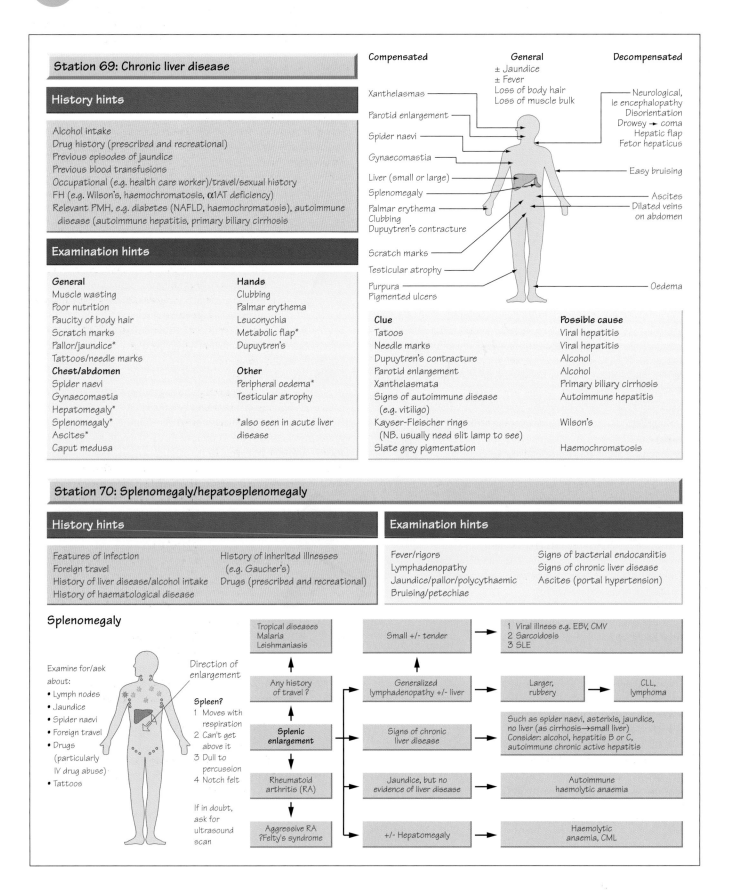

Compensated
Xanthelasmas
Parotid enlargement
Spider naevi
Gynaecomastia
Liver (small or large)
Splenomegaly
Palmar erythema
Clubbing
Dupuytren's contracture
Scratch marks
Testicular atrophy
Purpura
Pigmented ulcers

General
± Jaundice
± Fever
Loss of body hair
Loss of muscle bulk

Decompensated
Neurological,
ie encephalopathy
Disorientation
Drowsy → coma
Hepatic flap
Fetor hepaticus
Easy bruising
Ascites
Dilated veins on abdomen
Oedema

Clue	Possible cause
Tatoos	Viral hepatitis
Needle marks	Viral hepatitis
Dupuytren's contracture	Alcohol
Parotid enlargement	Alcohol
Xanthelasmata	Primary biliary cirrhosis
Signs of autoimmune disease (e.g. vitiligo)	Autoimmune hepatitis
Kayser-Fleischer rings (NB. usually need slit lamp to see)	Wilson's
Slate grey pigmentation	Haemochromatosis

Station 70: Splenomegaly/hepatosplenomegaly

History hints

Features of infection
Foreign travel
History of liver disease/alcohol intake
History of haematological disease
History of inherited illnesses (e.g. Gaucher's)
Drugs (prescribed and recreational)

Examination hints

Fever/rigors
Lymphadenopathy
Jaundice/pallor/polycythaemic
Bruising/petechiae
Signs of bacterial endocarditis
Signs of chronic liver disease
Ascites (portal hypertension)

Splenomegaly

Examine for/ask about:
• Lymph nodes
• Jaundice
• Spider naevi
• Foreign travel
• Drugs (particularly IV drug abuse)
• Tattoos

Direction of enlargement

Spleen?
1 Moves with respiration
2 Can't get above it
3 Dull to percussion
4 Notch felt

If in doubt, ask for ultrasound scan

Tropical diseases
Malaria
Leishmaniasis

Any history of travel?

Splenic enlargement

Rheumatoid arthritis (RA)

Aggressive RA
?Felty's syndrome

Small +/- tender → 1 Viral illness e.g. EBV, CMV
2 Sarcoidosis
3 SLE

Generalized lymphadenopathy +/- liver → Larger, rubbery → CLL, lymphoma

Signs of chronic liver disease → Such as spider naevi, asterixis, jaundice, no liver (as cirrhosis→small liver) Consider: alcohol, hepatitis B or C, autoimmune chronic active hepatitis

Jaundice, but no evidence of liver disease → Autoimmune haemolytic anaemia

+/- Hepatomegaly → Haemolytic anaemia, CML

Station 69: Chronic liver disease

- *Please examine this man's gastrointestinal system*
- *Please examine this 45-year-old female's abdomen. She is a non-drinker*

Hints and tips

- Examination as described in Chapter 26

Discussion points

- What are the causes of chronic liver disease?
- What are the causes of acute liver disease and how does the presentation differ from that of chronic liver disease?
- Name some complications of liver disease and discuss their management

Ix	*Bloods* (to assess severity)	LFTs (bilirubin, albumin) and clotting
		FBC (thrombocytopenia indicating hypersplenism from portal hypertension)
		U&Es (?hepatorenal syndrome, ?hyponatraemia)
	Bloods (to assess cause)	Viral serology (hepatitis B and C for chronic liver disease)
		Autoimmune profile (e.g. antimitochondrial antibodies)
		Iron and copper studies
		α_1-antitrypsin (AT) levels
		Lipids/glucose
	Imaging	US liver
	Micro	Diagnostic aspirate if ascites
	Other	Consider liver biopsy
Complications		Portal hypertension
		Variceal bleeding
		Ascites ± spontaneous bacterial peritonitis
		Coagulopathy
		Encephalopathy
		Hepatorenal syndrome
		Hepatocellular carcinoma

Causes of chronic liver disease

- Alcohol
- Toxins/drugs, e.g. methotrexate
- Viral hepatitis (B and C)
- Autoimmune chronic hepatitis
- Primary biliary cirrhosis
- Haemochromatosis
- Storage diseases
- Non-alcohol fatty liver disease (NAFLD)
- Wilsons disease
- α_1-antitrypsin deficiency

Causes of decompensation in liver disease

- Infection
- Gastrointestinal bleed
- Metabolic
- Drugs (including alcohol)

Station 70: Splenomegaly/hepatosplenomegaly

- *Please examine this patient's abdomen, skipping the peripheries*
- *This patient has been referred to the haematology clinic, please examine her neck and then proceed to abdominal palpation*

Hints and tips

- *Completion*:
  - examine the axillae and inguinal regions for lymphadenopathy (?lymphoproliferative disorder) *or*
  - perform a full cardiovascular examination (?endocarditis)

Discussion points

- What are the causes of splenomegaly?
- What is the commonest cause worldwide?
- How would you investigate a patient with an enlarged spleen?

Ix	*Bloods*	FBC + blood film:
		↑ haemoglobin (Hb) in polycythaemia rubra vera
		↓ Hb + ↑ retics + ↑ bilirubin = haemolytic anaemia
		Macrocytosis – liver disease
		↑ WCC – chronic myeloid leukaemia (CML), chronic lymphocytic leukaemia (CLL)
		↑ platelets in essential thrombocythaemia (ET)
		↓ platelets in portal hypertension
	Imaging	US abdomen
		CT abdomen
	Other	Lymph node biopsy
		Consider liver biopsy
		Consider bone marrow

Causes of splenomegaly

Infectious	Infectious mononucleosis (EBV/CMV)
	Subacute bacterial endocarditis
	Malaria
Lymphoproliferative disorders	CLL
	Lymphoma
Myeloproliferative disorders	Polycythaemia rubra vera
	CML
	ET
	Myelofibrosis
Cirrhosis + portal hypertension	
Benign infiltrative disorders	Gaucher's disease
	Amyloidosis
Autoimmune disease	SLE
Other	Haemolytic anaemia, e.g. thalassaemia, sickle cell

A further classification of splenomegaly

Massive	CML, myelofibrosis, malaria
Moderate	Portal hypertension, lymphoma, leukaemia
Mild	As per moderate and massive + infectious (endocarditis, EBV)

Station 71: Hepatomegaly

History hints

Alcohol/drug history
History of liver disease
Symptoms of heart failure/COPD (SOB/orthopnoea)
History of malignancy
Features of infection
Weight loss/poor appetite
Travel/sexual contacts/blood transfusions/drug abuse

Examination hints

Signs of chronic liver disease
Signs of heart failure
Cachexia, poor nutrition
Signs of an underlying malignancy, e.g. lymphadenopathy
Hepatomegaly – right upper quadrant mass that you cannot get above, that moves downwards on inspiration and is dull to percussion
Evidence of shifting dullness
Tattoos, needle marks

Station 73: Jaundice

History hints

Onset – acute/chronic	Systemic symptoms (weight loss, fever, etc.)
Painful or painless	Drug history (prescribed, over the counter, illicit)
History of liver disease	Alcohol history
History of gallstones	Family history
Travel	Features of obstruction (cholestasis) - dark urine, pale stools, itching

Examination hints

Yellow sclera	Hepatomegaly
Signs of anaemia (think haemolysis)	Splenomegaly
Signs of chronic liver disease (see Ch. 27)	Abdominal pain/masses
Scratch marks/bruising/petechiae	Ascites Liver flap

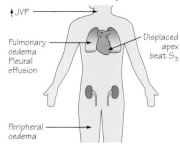

```
INVESTIGATIONS
```

Initial

Bloods	FBC (?haemolysis) LFT (↑ alk phos = cholestasis, ↑ transaminases = hepatocellular) Clotting
Imaging	Ultrasound of liver and gallbladder
Other	Urinary urobilinogen

Haemolysis	Hepatocellular	Obstructive
Bloods	Viral serology (hepatitis, EBV, CMV)	Imaging Ultrasound CT abdomen
Blood film ↑ Reticulocytes ↓ Haptoglobins ↑ Lactate dehydrogenase	Autoimmune profile Copper, iron, α_1-AT Imaging Ultrasound Other Liver biopsy	Other ERCP MRCP

Station 72: Ascites

History hints

Gradual increased swelling of abdomen
SOB/orthopnoea/peripheral oedema
Otherwise as per hepatomegaly/chronic liver disease

Examination hints

Transudates: SAAG > 11 g/L

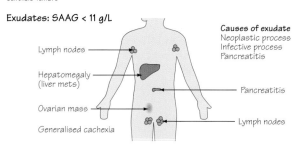

Causes of transudate
Cirrhosis   Alcoholic hepatitis
Cardiac failure

Cirrhosis with portal HT is the most common cause of ascites

Exudates: SAAG < 11 g/L

Causes of exudate
Neoplastic process
Infective process
Pancreatitis

Pathophysiology of jaundice

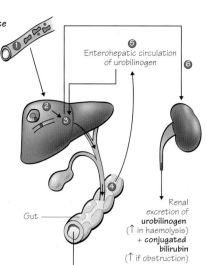

① Bilirubin from destruction of red cells circulates bound to **albumin**

② Hepatic conjugation into water soluble **bilirubin glucuronide** formed by **glucuronyl transferases**

③ Excretion into **bile**

④ Gut bacteria action Glucuronides → stercobilinogen → stool pigment (excreted)

⑤ Conjugated bilirubin from gut into blood → Urobilinogen

⑥ Urobilinogen excreted in urine

Renal excretion of **urobilinogen** (↑ in haemolysis) + **conjugated bilirubin** (↑ if obstruction)

Stool pigment-stercobilinogen

Station 71: Hepatomegaly

Hints and tips (examination as described in Chapter 26)
- Describe the size of the liver in finger breadths and then determine whether the edge is smooth, nodular, tender or pulsatile
- Middle-aged female + scratch marks – think primary biliary cirrhosis
- Hyperpigmentaion – think haemochromatosis
- Note that emphysema can cause an apparent hepatomegaly, so remember to percuss the upper border
- Riedel's lobe is a normal anatomical variant which is a projection of the liver from the right lobe
- Think – could you be feeling the gallbladder (especially if the patient has painless obstructive jaundice)?

Top three causes
- Cirrhosis (in early stages); CCF; carcinoma: primary or metastatic

Other causes
Infective	Acute viral hepatitis (A, B and E)
	EBV, CMV
	Liver abscess (pyogenic, amoebic)
	Hydatid cyst (tapeworm)
Infiltrative	Amyloid, sarcoidosis
Metabolic	Haemochromatosis, NAFLD
Autoimmune	Autoimmune hepatitis

Discussion points
- What are the causes of hepatomegaly?
- What investigations would you request to confirm your diagnosis?

Ix (depends on the underlying cause)
Bloods	See chronic liver disease (Ch. 27)
Imaging	CXR, US abdomen

Station 72: Ascites
- *Please examine this man's abdomen, there is no need to start with the peripheries*
- *This patient has increased swelling of his abdomen, please examine*

Hints and tips
- *Completion*: examine other relevant systems depending on the proposed cause, e.g. cardiovascular if suspecting heart failure

Discussion points
- What are the causes of ascites?
- How would you investigate a patient with ascites?
- What are the management principles for a patient with ascites?

Ix		
	Bloods	As for chronic liver disease + consider tumour markers
	Imaging	CXR, US abdomen, consider echo/CT abdomen
	ECG	
	Micro	Diagnostic aspirate sent for cell count/protein/albumin/LDH/cytology/Gram stain/MC&S/amylase

Commonest causes
- Cirrhosis with portal hypertension; intra-abdominal malignancy; CCF

Another classification
Measure the serum albumin–ascitic albumin gradient (SAAG) (g/L).

- Exudate = SAAG < 11 g/L
  Neoplasia (e.g. gynaecological malignancy); infection (e.g. TB peritonitis); pancreatic ascites
- Transudate = SAAG > 11 g/L
  Cirrhosis; alcoholic hepatitis; cardiac failure

Mx
Rx	Treat underlying cause
	Antibiotics for infection
	Fluid and salt restriction
	Diuretics, e.g. spironolactone
Procedures	Therapeutic paracentesis ± ascitic drain
Monitoring	Careful fluid management and strict fluid balance, weight
Specialists	Depending on cause (e.g. hepatologist)
Education	Reduce alcohol if necessary

Note on spontaneous bacterial peritonitis (SBP)
- Infection of ascites, mainly cirrhotics
- Clinical signs are often minimal but are often the cause of a cirrhotic patient deteriorating
- Always perform a diagnostic ascitic tap
- If raised neutrophils, commence IV antibiotics

Station 73: Jaundice
- *Look at this person's skin, eyes and then examine the abdomen*

Hints and tips
- Inspect carefully for signs of chronic liver disease, scratch marks, bruising, petechiae and cachexia
- Determine presence or absence of hepatomegaly, splenomegaly, ascites and abdominal mass
- *Completion*: perform urinalysis testing for bilirubin

Causes
1 *Prehepatic*:
- ↑ unconjugated bilirubin due to premature breakdown of red blood cells, i.e. haemolysis

2 *Hepatic (hepatocellular)*:
- Problem with uptake, metabolism or excretion of bilirubin
- Unconjugated and conjugated bilirubin:
  - Gilbert's syndrome (failure of conjugation, therefore unconjugated hyperbilirubinaemia)
  - acute hepatitis (alcohol, viral, drugs, toxins, infection, autoimmune)
- Chronic liver disease
  - infiltrative (malignancy, sarcoid, amyloid)

3 *Posthepatic (obstructive, cholestatic)*:
- Obstruction to bilirubin excretion
- Divided into intrahepatic (IHC) and extrahepatic (EHC):
  - primary biliary cirrhosis (IHC)
  - sclerosing cholangitis (IHC and/or EHC)
  - gallstones (EHC)
  - pancreatic carcinoma (EHC)

A classification of extrahepatic obstructive jaundice
- *In the lumen*	Gallstones
- *In the wall of the lumen*	Cholangiocarcinoma
	Stricture with sclerosing cholangitis
- *Outside the lumen*	Pancreatic neoplasm
	Lymph nodes

Station 74: Inflammatory bowel disease

History hints

Abdominal pain/diarrhoea/blood PR
Weight loss/fever

Local complications and extra colonic manifestations
Family history of irritable bowel disease/colon cancer

Smoking history

Examination hints

Features of ulcerative colitis		Extra intestinal manifestations common to UC and Crohn's	Features of Crohn's	
Extracolonic	*Local*		*Local*	*Extracolonic*
Uveitis Episcleritis Pallor Clubbing Hepatomegaly Pyoderma gangrenosum Erythema nodosum Ankylosing spondylitis	Colectomy scar Stoma	Uveitis Hepatitis Gallstones Primary sclerosing cholangitis Pyoderma gangrenosum (UC > Crohn's) Ankylosing spondylitis Sacro-iliitis Monoarthritis Erythema nodosum (Crohn's > UC)	Surgical scars Fistulae Evidence of current or previous stoma Perianal disease	Uveitis Episcleritis Pallor Swollen lips (due to granulomatous infiltration) Aphthous ulcers Clubbing Hepatomegaly Pyoderma gangrenosum Erythema nodosum Peripheral arthritis Ankylosing spondylitis

Station 75: Polycystic kidney disease

History hints

Family history
Hypertension
Dialysis

Previous history of subarachnoid haemorrhage
Drug history - antihypertensives

Examination hints

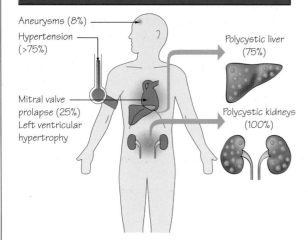

Aneurysms (8%)
Hypertension (>75%)
Mitral valve prolapse (25%)
Left ventricular hypertrophy

Polycystic liver (75%)
Polycystic kidneys (100%)

Station 76: Chronic kidney disease

History hints for renal disease

As for Station 75
PMH: hypertension, childhood renal infections, connective tissue disease, diabetes
DH: analgesics, antihypertensives
Full GUS systems review

FH: renal disease
Current management including dialysis

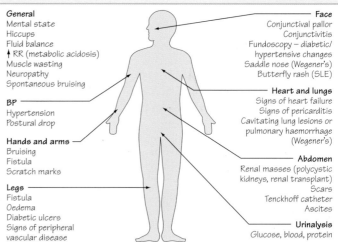

General
Mental state
Hiccups
Fluid balance
↑ RR (metabolic acidosis)
Muscle wasting
Neuropathy
Spontaneous bruising

BP
Hypertension
Postural drop

Hands and arms
Bruising
Fistula
Scratch marks

Legs
Fistula
Oedema
Diabetic ulcers
Signs of peripheral vascular disease

Face
Conjunctival pallor
Conjunctivitis
Fundoscopy – diabetic/hypertensive changes
Saddle nose (Wegener's)
Butterfly rash (SLE)

Heart and lungs
Signs of heart failure
Signs of pericarditis
Cavitating lung lesions or pulmonary haemorrhage (Wegener's)

Abdomen
Renal masses (polycystic kidneys, renal transplant)
Scars
Tenckhoff catheter
Ascites

Urinalysis
Glucose, blood, protein

Station 74: Inflammatory bowel disease

- *Please examine this patient's gastrointestinal system*
- *This 26-year-old patient has been suffering with bloody diarrhoea and abdominal pain, please examine his abdomen*

Hints and tips (examination as described in Chapter 26.)
- In a young patient with signs of multiple abdominal procedures, the diagnosis is most likely due to inflammatory bowel disease (IBD)
- Look carefully for evidence of both local and extraintestinal manifestations (see opposite)
- Inspection: signs of anaemia, clubbing, red eyes, swollen lips, mouth ulcers, Cushingoid appearance due to steroid treatment, slim build, skin lesions, surgical scars, stomas and fistulae
- *Completion*: perform a digital rectal exam

Discussion points
- What are the complications of IBD?
- What are the differences between Crohn's and ulcerative colitis?
- What treatment options are you aware of for IBD?
- What are the general management principles for a patient with IBD?
- How would you investigate a patient with a flare-up of their IBD?

Complications of ulcerative colitis
Toxic megacolon; perforation; colon cancer; primary sclerosing cholangitis (may lead to cirrhosis); anaemia (due to haemorrhage, chronic disease, iron deficiency); thromboembolism.

Complications of Crohn's disease
Perianal disease (fissures, fistulae, abscess); toxic megacolon (more usual in acute ulcerative colitis); perforation; fistulae; strictures (may lead to bowel obstruction); gallstones; renal disease (renal stones, pyelonephritis); malabsorption (small bowel involved).

Ix	Bloods	FBC, U&E, LFT, CRP, ESR
	Imaging	Abdominal X-ray (toxic megacolon)
		Consider CT abdomen, barium studies
	Micro	Stool culture, blood cultures
	Other	Flexible sigmoidoscopy, colonoscopy ± biopsy
Mx		
Rx	Medical	Drugs: topical (e.g suppositories/enemas) or systemic depending on location and extent of disease
		Steroids (IV for severe attacks)
		Acetylsalicylic acid (5-ASA) compounds, e.g. mesalazine
		Consider other immunosuppressant drugs, e.g. azathioprine
		Anti-tumour necrosis factor (anti-TNF) therapy in Crohn's disease, e.g. infliximab
	Surgery	
	Monitoring	Careful fluid balance, nutritional status
	MDT	Dietician, IBD nurse, stoma nurse
	Specialists	Gastroenterologist, GI surgeon
	Education	

Station 75: Polycystic kidney disease

- *Mr JK had a recent episode of haematuria, please examine his abdomen*
- *Mrs S has an inherited kidney problem, please examine her abdomen*

Hints and tips
- Examine the abdomen as described in Chapter 26, starting at the area instructed by the examiner
- Examine carefully for a liver as there is an association with liver cysts
- Observe carefully for any evidence of fistulae, transplant or Tenchkoff catheter insertion scars
- There may be bilateral masses in the flanks (NB you may only be able to feel one side)
- If kidney, the mass will be ballotable, resonant to percussion and it should be possible to get above it
- *Completion*: check blood pressure (75% have hypertension), and perform a urinalysis looking for haematuria and proteinuria

Discussion points
- What is the inheritance for adult polycystic kidney disease (APCKD)?
- Do you know of any associations?
- What are the management principles?

Ix	Bloods	FBC, U&E
	Imaging	US abdomen
	Othe	Urinalysis and protein estimation
Associations of APCKD		Cerebral aneurysms; hypertension; liver cysts (+ pancreas/spleen); mitral valve prolapse
Mx		
Rx		Control of hypertension
		Consider renal replacement therapy (dialysis) if renal function deteriorating
		Renal transplant if necessary
Monitoring		BP, renal function
MDT		Dialysis nurses
Specialists		Renal physicians
Education		Genetic counselling

Station 76: Chronic kidney disease

- *Mr JF has diabetes and some complications associated with this. Please perform a general examination and then discuss further aspects that you may want to examine*

Hints and tips
- Start with general observations as suggested opposite
- Look carefully for scars from previous fistulae, a Tenchkoff catheter or even a renal transplant
- *Completion*: it is important to know the causes of chronic kidney disease, so completion can include examination of all the necessary systems, e.g. in a diabetic patient think about CVS, fundoscopy, sensation

Discussion points
- What are the causes of chronic renal failure?
- Discuss some principles in the management of chronic renal failure
- What are the causes of acute renal failure?
- What is the management of hyperkalaemia?

Neurological symptoms

Headache
Change in taste/smell
Unsteady gait
Involuntary movements
Bowel and bladder problems

Dizzyness/vertigo
Altered hearing
Limb weakness
Memory impairment

Fit
Change in speech
Sensory disturbance
Confusion

Visual disturbance
Difficulty swallowing
Tremor
Change in personality

NB. To elicit some of these symptoms it may be necessary to gain a collateral history

Station 77: Transient ischaemic attack

TIA management

Commence secondary prevention (aspirin, statin)
Optimise vascular risk factors
Patient education
Smoking cessation
Refer to neurovascular/TIA clinic (within 1 week)
Ix
Bloods   FBC, U&E, ESR, lipids, glucose
         Consider clotting screen ± thrombophilia
         screen

ECG
Imaging   CT head (consider MRI head)
         Carotid Doppler
         Consider echocardiogram

Bamford classification for stroke

POCS (posterior circulation syndrome)
Cranial nerve palsy + contralateral motor/sensory deficit, or bilateral
     stroke, or disorders of conjugate eye movement, or isolated cerebellar
     stroke, or isolated homonymous hemianopia
LACS (Lacunar syndrome)
Pure motor or pure sensory deficit affecting two of three out of face,
     arm, and leg or acute-onset movement disorder
TACS (total anterior circulation syndrome) – need all three of:
1. Higher cortical dysfunction
     (dysphasia/dyscalculia/dyspraxia/neglect) +
2. Homonymous visual field defect +
3. Motor and/or sensory deficit contralateral to the lesion of at least
     two areas out of face, arm and leg
PACS (partial anterior circulation syndrome)
Two of three of TACS symptoms or isolated higher cortical dysfunction

Stroke classification

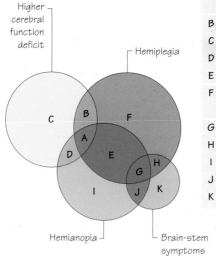

A	TACS, total anterior circulation syndrome
B	PACS, partial
C	anterior
D	circulation
E	syndromes
F	Lacunar syndromes, pure motor stroke
G	
H	POCS, posterior
I	circulation
J	syndromes
K	

Station 78: Acute confusion

Abbreviated mental test score (AMTS)

- Age
- Time
- Address to remember (42 West Street)
- Year
- Name of hospital
- Recognition of two people
- Date of birth
- Date of 1st WW
- Present monarch
- Count 20–1

Causes of acute confusional state (I WATCH DEATH)

	Examples
Infection	UTI, sepsis, meningitis
Withdrawal	Alcohol, barbiturates
Acute metabolic	Acidosis, electrolyte imbalance
Trauma	Head injury
CNS pathology	Space-occupying lesion, seizure
Hypoxia/hypotension	
Deficiencies	B_{12}, niacin
Endocrine	Hypo/hyperglycaemia, hypothyroidism
Acute vascular	Stroke, SAH, shock
Toxins/medications	Medications, illicit drugs
Heavy metals	Lead, mercury

Station 77: Transient ischaemic attack

Student info: *Mr TB is 74 and has a history of hypertension. He had an episode of right arm weakness this morning and his GP has sent him to hospital. The weakness has now resolved. Please take a full history, and formulate a differential diagnosis and management plan. There is no need to perform an examination*

Patient info: *You are Mr TB, aged 74 years. You have had hypertension controlled on tablets for 5 years. You smoke 2 cigarettes a day although your previous use was much heavier. You had an episode of transient loss of vision in the left eye 4 weeks ago, that lasted only 30 minutes. While having a cup of coffee this morning, you noticed that your right hand became clumsy and then your whole arm became weak.*

You made an appointment to see your GP who sent you into hospital. The weakness has now resolved. You do not suffer with diabetes, heart disease or raised cholesterol. You take a water tablet and another tablet for blood pressure control. You live with your wife who is not well and suffers with early dementia and arthritis. You are her main carer and up to now you have been completely independent. You still drive. Your major concern is who would look after your wife if anything happened to you. You do not have any children

Hints and tips
• Ascertain the patient's reason for coming to hospital and what the GP has already explained
• Determine symptomatology
• Determine timing of symptoms
• Determine the resulting disability
• Elicit a full neurological history
• Determine cerebrovascular disease risk factors
• Establish associated symptoms, in particular realise the possible connection with the transient loss of vision
• Establish smoking history
• Ascertain the patient's social history and in particular note that he is the main carer for his wife who suffers with dementia
• Assess impact of the symptoms on the patient's life
• Address any concerns the patient has, in particular his thoughts regarding the diagnosis and the impact that loss of independence would have on both him and his wife
• Discuss the suspected diagnosis and a management plan

Discussion points
• Discuss a differential diagnosis
• Following your history, it is necessary for you to perform an examination – what would you examine for?
• What investigations would you request?
• Discuss some management principles for this patient
• Can you discuss a clinical classification for stroke?

Station 78: Acute confusion

Student info: *You are an FY1 doctor in surgery. A 78-year-old female patient was admitted over the weekend with abdominal pain. A diagnosis of constipation was made and the pain has now settled. Your SpR has stated that she can now be discharged home and you have completed the paperwork. However, the nursing staff are concerned about this lady's cognitive state. They feel she is intermittently confused and at times has been acting inappropriately. You have not really noticed this but appreciate you have not spent any great time with the patient. Her son is visiting and the nurses have asked if you can reassess the situation. You perform a 10 point abbreviated mental test score and Mrs MG scores 6. Please take a collateral history from Mrs MG's son to determine the extent of confusion.*

Patient info: *You are Mrs MG, aged 78 years, and were admitted with abdominal pain that has been diagnosed as constipation. Your son is visiting and the junior doctor has come to reassess your suitability to return home. Your son will take the lead in this scenario as you are unclear of any specific details but are quite happy about the doctor talking with your son. You have a history of hypertension, osteoarthritis and have had a cholecystectomy. Your DH is: aspirin 75 mg OD, amlodipine 10 mg OD, paracetamol 1 g qds and codeine phosphate*

30 mg qds. You have lived alone since your husband died of bowel cancer 2 years ago.

Relative info: *You are Mrs MG's son and have noticed a fairly dramatic decline in your mother's health since your father died 2 years ago. The main problem has been a deterioration in her memory and you have noticed that she forgets dates and is never clear of what day it is. You pop in every day and take your mother shopping once a week. Your mother is able to manage activities of daily living, including cooking, although you are worried about her having both a gas fire and cooker. Over the last 6 months she has taken to staying indoors. Since admission to hospital your mother has seemed even more confused to you; she has had no falls or neurological symptoms.*

Alternative instructions
• *Please perform a mini mental state examination (MMSE) on this patient using the form provided*
• *Please perform an abbreviated mental test score (AMTS) on this patient*

Hints and tips
• Gain the patient's permission to talk with her son
• Ascertain the son's prior knowledge of the situation
• Confirm the history of confusion
• Determine timing of deterioration in memory
• Elicit PMH
• Elicit the social history and in particular the fact that this lady does not leave her house but currently manages with ADLs
• Address any concerns the son has and in particular the fact that he is worried about the progressive decline in his mother's memory and the fact she has a gas cooker and fire
• Discuss a differential diagnosis with the examiner and a management plan

Discussion points
• What are the causes of an acute confusional state?
• What would your differential include?
• How would you investigate a patient with suspected dementia?
• Do you know of any causes of dementia?

Ix	Bloods	FBC, U&E, Ca, LFT, albumin, Glc
		Consider ABG to assess oxygenation and metabolic state
	ECG	
	Imaging	CXR
	Micro	Urine MC&S
		Blood cultures
	Other	Further investigations may be necessary to determine the underlying cause
Mx		Diagnose the underlying cause
		Treat the underlying cause
		Maintain adequate hydration and nutrition
		Optimise nursing care (quiet, well lit environment)
		Enlist supportive help from family members
		Full medication review
		Close monitoring of mental state
		Be aware of drug withdrawal as a cause, e.g. alcohol
		Consider low-dose antipsychotics

Station 79: Upper limb motor examination

Inspection
Signs of specific diseases
Posture
Muscle bulk
Abnormal movements
Fasciculations
Screening test
Arms outstretched with eyes closed
Look for drift of the arms
Tone
Power (see table)
Reflexes
Coordination (see Ch. 37)
Completion

Movement	Muscle	Nerve	Root
Shoulder abduction	Deltoid	Axillary	C5
Elbow flexion	Biceps	Musculocutaneous	C5, C6
Elbow extension	Triceps	Radial	C7, C8
Finger extension	Extensor digitorum	(Radial)	C7, C8
Finger flexion	Flexor digitorum superficialis	Median and ulnar	C8
Finger abduction	1st dorsal interosseous	Ulnar	T1
Finger adduction	2nd palmar interosseous	Ulnar	T1
Thumb abduction	Abductor pollicis brevis	Median	T1

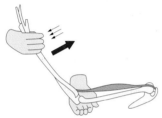

Elbow flexion

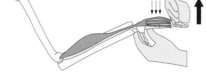

Finger extension

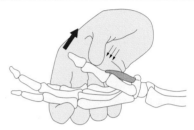

Thumb abduction

Station 80: Lower limb motor examination

Inspection
Signs of specific diseases
Posture
Muscle bulk
Abnormal movements
Fasciculations
High arch foot/pes cavus
Catheter
Walking aids
Screening test
Gait/ask patient to bend their legs
Tone
Power (see table)
Reflexes
Coordination (see Ch. 37)
Completion

Movement	Muscle	Nerve	Root
Hip flexion	Iliopsoas	Lumbar sacral plexus	L1, L2
Hip extension	Gluteus maximus	Inferior gluteal	L5, S1
Knee flexion	Hamstrings	Sciatic	L5, S1
Knee extension	Quadriceps femoris	Femoral	L3, L4
Foot dorsiflexion	Tibialis anterior	Deep peroneal	L4, L5
Foot plantarflexion	Gastrocnemius	Posterior tibial	S1
Great toe extension	Extensor hallucis longus	Deep peroneal	L5

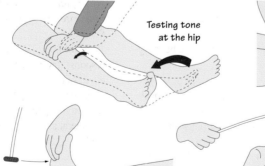

Testing tone at the hip

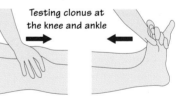

Testing clonus at the knee and ankle

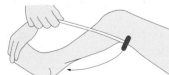

Testing the ankle reflex

Station 79: Upper limb motor examination

- *Please examine this patient's upper limb neurology*
- *This patient has noticed some weakness in their right arm, please examine and report your findings*

Examination routine

- Introduction/consent/ask about pain:
  - shake the patient's hand as part of your introduction and note if there is difficulty relaxing the grip (i.e. myotonia)
  - note if there is any abnormality with the patient's speech during the introductions (e.g. dysarthria or dysphasia; see Ch. 34)
- *Exposure*: the arms and shoulders need to be completely exposed but it is also useful to be able to examine the neck and cervical spine
- *Position*: sitting on the edge of the bed or lying on the examination couch at 45°
- *General inspection*:
  - take a physical step back and observe the patient and surroundings
  - note any features around the bedside, e.g. walking aids, glasses
  - note any facial features that could be consistent with a neurological diagnosis, e.g. Parkinsonian facies, facial palsy
- *Screening test*: ask the patient to raise their arms out in front of them with palms facing up and then close their eyes. Any weakness should be obvious. Also look carefully for any evidence of a drift and if this is more pronounced with the eyes shut
- *System-specific inspection*:
  - look for evidence of an abnormal posture, muscle wasting, involuntary movements or fasciculations, assess symmetry
  - include a glance at the neck both anteriorly and posteriorly, looking for any scars
- *Causes of arm drift*:
  - pronator drift – arm may drift downwards and pronate if evidence of subtle pyramidal weakness
  - sensory drift – loss of joint position sense can lead to a searching movement of the fingers (pseudoathetosis)
- *Tone*: test at wrists and elbows. Take the patient's hand as if shaking it and support the patient's elbow with your other hand. Pronate and supinate the forearm and then roll the hand round at the wrist. Next move the wrist and elbow through the full range of flexion and extension
- *Power*: grade power using the MRC scale. It is important to isolate the muscles when testing so the patient cannot 'cheat' by using other muscle groups. Compare right and left for each muscle. A screening routine involves testing the muscles shown opposite:
  - *shoulder abduction* – 'put your arms out to the side like a bird's wing, stop me pushing them down' (shoulder abducted to 90° with elbows flexed)
  - *elbow flexion* – 'bend your elbow, pull me towards you'
  - *elbow extension* – 'now push me away'
  - *finger extension* – 'hold your fingers out straight, stop me bending them'
  - *finger flexion* – 'squeeze my fingers'
  - *finger abduction* – 'spread your fingers apart and don't let me push them together' (test the index finger first and then the little finger)
  - *finger adduction* – 'try to prevent me pulling this piece of paper from between your fingers'
  - *thumb abduction* – 'place your palm facing upwards and point your thumb up towards the ceiling, try to stop me pushing it down'
- *Reflexes*:
  - have the patient relaxed with elbows flexed and hands in their lap (or place on a pillow). Test the biceps, triceps and brachioradialis (supinator) reflexes. If there is no response then try using a reinforcement manoeuvre (ask patient to clench teeth)
  - test for Hoffman's sign – tap the nail on the third or fourth finger. A positive Hoffman's is the involuntary flexing of the end of the thumb and index finger; normally, there should be no reflex response (upper motor neurone sign)
- *Coordination* (see Ch. 37)
- *Completion*: state to the examiners that you would like to complete your examination by completing any of the neurological routine you have not already done. Also offer other examinations depending on the diagnosis (e.g. cardiovascular assessment if a hemiparesis is noted)

Station 80: Lower limb motor examination

- *Please examine this patient's lower limb neurology*
- *This patient has noticed some weakness in their legs, please examine and report your findings*

Examination routine

- Introduction/consent/ask about pain: note if there is any abnormality with the patient's speech, e.g. dysarthria or dysphasia
- *Exposure and position*: the legs should be fully exposed with the patient lying on the examination couch
- General inspection: as per upper limbs
- *Screening test*:
  - assess the patient's gait if allowed and if they are able to walk (be sensitive if walking aids are present) (see Ch. 32)
  - otherwise ask the patient to bend each leg in turn
- *System-specific inspection*:
  - as per upper limb
  - note the presence of a catheter (may indicate spinal cord pathology)
- *Tone*: test at the hip (with the patient lying with straight legs, roll the knees from side to side), knee (put your hand under the knee and lift quickly, watching the heel) and ankle (dorsiflex and plantarflex the ankle). If the patient does not relax, distract them by asking them to count down from 20
- *Power*: hints as per upper limb:
  - *hip flexion* – 'keep your leg straight and lift it up, don't let me push it down' (push down with your hand on the thigh)
  - *hip extension* – 'push your leg down into the bed; don't let me push it up'
  - *knee flexion* – 'bend your knee and bring your heel towards your bottom, don't let me straighten it'
  - *knee extension* – 'now try to straighten it'
  - *foot dorsiflexion* – 'bend your foot up and don't let me push it down'
  - *foot plantarflexion* – 'now push it down'
  - *toe extension* – 'pull your big toe up and stop me pushing it down'
- *Reflexes*:
  - test the knee, ankle and plantar reflexes (see opposite). If there is no response, try using a reinforcement manoeuvre (e.g. ask the patient to clasp their hands)
  - before checking the plantar response, explain the procedure carefully to the patient, as it can be uncomfortable. Stroke the foot up the lateral aspect and curve in towards the great toe using an orange stick
  - *Clonus*: test for clonus at the ankle (± knee) by dorsiflexing the joint briskly and inspecting for prolonged rhythmic contraction (more than 3 beats is abnormal)
- *Coordination*: see Chapter 37
- *Completion*: as per upper limb

Station 81: Sensory examination

Routine
Inspection
Pin prick ⎫ Spinothalamic
Temperature ⎬ tract
Vibration sense ⎫ Posterior
Proprioception ⎬ columns
Light touch — Not a single column
Completion

Patterns of sensory deficit
Mononeuropathy – single nerve
Radiculopathy – root problem
Peripheral nerve – glove and stocking
Spinal cord – complete transverse lesion
 – hemisection
 – central cord
 – posterior column loss
 – anterior spinal lesion

Brainstem
Thalamic

Spinal cord section
Lateral corticospinal tract
Posterior column
Anterior corticospinal tract
Spinothalamic tract

Key to figures below
PP Pin prick
T Temp
V Vibration
PR Proprioception
(labels in red indicate loss of modality)

Dermatomes

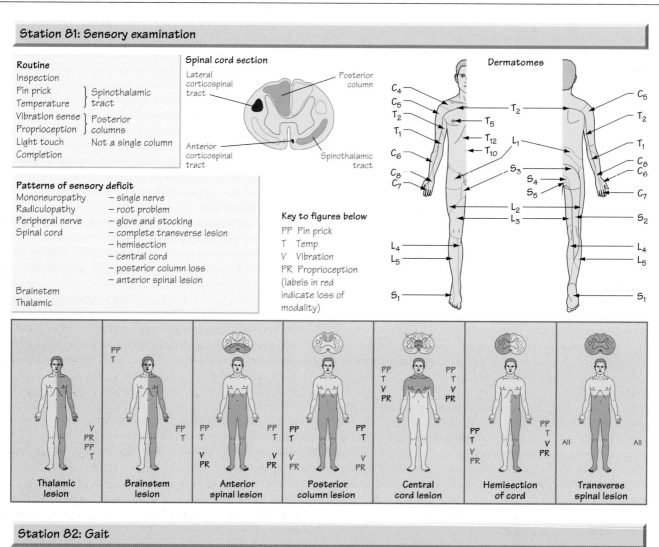

| Thalamic lesion | Brainstem lesion | Anterior spinal lesion | Posterior column lesion | Central cord lesion | Hemisection of cord | Transverse spinal lesion |

Station 82: Gait

Routine
General inspection
If appropriate ask the patient if they can stand/walk without assistance
Let them use their walking aid if present
Ask them to stand first
Ask the patient to walk for a few metres, turn around and walk back
Walk heel to toe/walk on heels/walk on toes
Completion

Gait disorders
Apraxic = frontal lobe problem = feet glued to floor
Cerebellar ataxia
Hemiplegic
Marche à petits pas (widespread cerebrovascular disease)
Myopathic = waddling = proximal muscle weakness
Neuropathic = foot drop = high stepping
Parkinsonian
Sensory ataxia = posterior column loss = stamping of feet
Spastic paraparesis = scissoring

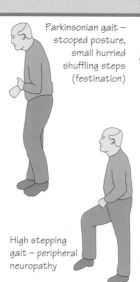

Parkinsonian gait – stooped posture, small hurried shuffling steps (festination)

A wide–based staggering gait – cerebellar or labyrinthine disease

High stepping gait – peripheral neuropathy

Waddling gait
• Wide based gait
• Body sway
• Lumbar lordosis and protuberant abdomen

Station 81: Sensory examination

- *Please examine the sensation of this man's arms*
- *This patient has a problem affecting their posterior columns, please examine their legs*

Examination routine

If you have already examined the motor system, then you may have a clue to the diagnosis or be able to predict your sensory findings.
- Introduction/consent/ask about pain
- *Exposure*: adequate exposure of the part to be tested (you *cannot* test sensation through socks!)
- Position: either have the patient at 45° or sitting on the edge of the bed, whichever is more comfortable. It is often easier when assessing sensation of the upper limbs to have the patient in the anatomical position
- *Inspection*: clues to the diagnosis may be apparent from the end of the bed (stroke, multiple sclerosis, diabetes, walking aids needed for ataxia). Look for evidence of abnormal posture, muscle wasting, involuntary movements or fasciculations. Glance at the spine looking for any scars

Spinothalamic pathway: pain and temperature

Use a disposable neurological pin (one end is sharp, the other is blunt) – *do not use a needle*! Demonstrate the sharpness on the patient's chest. Ask the patient to close their eyes and then ask them to tell you if they feel a sharp or dull sensation. Try to produce a stimulus of the same intensity each time. Start on the limb proximally, stimulating points within each dermatome and main nerve. This way it is possible to create a pattern of sensory loss that may fit into a dermatomal loss (representing a nerve root lesion), a peripheral nerve loss (e.g. the median), peripheral neuropathy (e.g. glove and stocking) or a hemisensory loss (cord or brain problem). Tap the pin several times in each area. Remember this is a test of pinprick sensation so the blunt end is used intermittently to check the patient recognises the difference. Start proximally and as always with examination, compare side to side. If a deficit is found, concentrate more accurately on this area, to determine the actual boundaries of sensory loss or sensory level.

Assessing temperature is not usually asked routinely in an OSCE. The formal way of testing is to have two test tubes, one filled with cold water and the other with hot water. Make sure the outside of the tubes are dry. Test first in an unaffected area and randomly apply either the hot or cold tube to areas on the upper and lower limbs.

Posterior columns: vibration and proprioception

Use a 128 Hz tuning fork to assess vibration sense. First demonstrate by placing the vibrating tuning fork onto the patient's sternum and check they understand the feeling of vibration. Ask them to close their eyes and tell you when the vibration stops (stop the vibration with your finger tips). Repeat this process on a distal bony prominence (thumb for upper limb, great toe for lower). If sensation is intact distally then there is no need to test proximally; if not, work up the limb proximally placing the tuning fork on each bony prominence.

To test proprioception (joint position sense), initially demonstrate to the patient the technique with their eyes open. Hold the distal phalanx at the sides between your thumb and index finger. Move their finger up and down. Next get them to close their eyes and repeat the movement asking if they can sense which direction the movement is in. Again start distally and move proximally.

Romberg's test is also a test of proprioception – see below.

Light touch

These fibres are not unique to an individual pathway and so this test is not discriminating. Either use a piece of cotton wool or your finger tip, applied lightly. Examine each of the areas as per pinprick. Use a tapping motion rather than a stroking one.

Important peripheral nerves

- Upper limb: axillary, median, radial and ulnar nerves
- Lower limb: lateral cutaneous nerve of the thigh, common peroneal, femoral and sciatic nerves

Station 82: Gait

- *Please examine this patient's lower limbs*
- *This patient has noticed some unsteadiness when walking, please examine and report your findings*

Examination routine

- Introduction/consent/ask about pain
- *Exposure*: adequate exposure of the lower limbs
- *Position*: standing
- *Inspection*: initially inspect the patient on the couch or chair for any obvious signs of disease. Look around the bed for any walking aids. Note if there is a catheter (may indicate spinal cord disease)
- *Gait*: ask the patient if they are ok to stand and walk unaided. Be sensitive if there are walking aids around the bed. Make sure you walk with the patient if they are unsteady. Ask the patient to walk a few metres, turn round and come back. Look for: ability to initiate movement; symmetry (shoulders, hips, knees and feet); posture; stride length; distance between feet; arm swing; evidence of pain on movement.
- If a diagnosis is not clear, it may be necessary to try some of the following: ask the patient to sit from standing; ask the patient to walk heel to toe; ask the patient to walk on their heels and then their toes.

Gait disorders

- Cerebellar ataxia: broad-based gait, unsteady, veer towards side of lesion, difficult to perform heel to toe (see Ch. 37)
- Hemiplegic: unilateral upper motor neurone lesion
- Marche à petits pas: short stride, normal arm swing, no stooping
- Myopathic: waddling gait, rotation of pelvis and shoulder, protuberant abdomen
- Neuropathic: knees lifted higher, foot drop
- Parkinsonism: loss of arm swing, short shuffling gait, difficulty initiating movement, festinant gait (hurrying) (see Ch. 37)
- Sensory ataxia: wide based, stamping, patient concentrates on their feet and the floor
- Spastic paraparesis: scissoring or crossing over of legs, diplegic gait

Romberg's test

- Ask the patient to stand with their feet together
- If they are unsteady like this, then you cannot proceed with the test. This test cannot be performed if the patient cannot stand unaided
- Now ask the patient to close their eyes stating prior to this that you will not let them fall. Romberg's test is positive if the patient becomes unsteady with their eyes closed (i.e. a proprioceptive problem NOT a cerebellar problem)
- Causes of unsteadiness:
  - posterior column loss
  - peripheral neuropathy

NB. Romberg's test is *not* positive in cerebellar disease as these patients are unsteady when standing with their eyes open.

Station 83: Cranial nerve examination

GENERAL INSPECTION
- Well/unwell
- Mental state
- Evidence of hemiplegia
- General appearance
- Speech abnormality
- Evidence of ataxia
- Asymmetry
- Muscle wasting/drooping/ptosis
- Squint/Horner's/head tilt

I
'Have you noticed any change in your sense of smell?' Formal testing is not usually required (see opposite).

Visual field testing

Patient

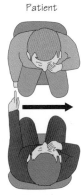

Examiner

Looking left

Normal

Left lateral rectus palsy (VI nerve)

Looking ahead

Normal

Left III nerve palsy

THE EYES (II, III, IV, VI)
Visual Acuity (II)
Ask the patient to wear glasses if used
Ask them to cover one of their eyes. Test each eye in turn.
Visual Fields
Screening test
Formal test
Pupils
Direct and consensual light reflexes
Size
Shape
Accommodation reflex
Fundoscopy
Eye Movements
Full range
Smooth
In unison
Nystagmus

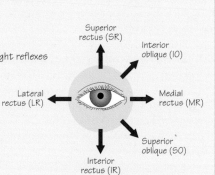

Superior rectus (SR)
Interior oblique (IO)
Lateral rectus (LR)
Medial rectus (MR)
Superior oblique (SO)
Interior rectus (IR)

V MOTOR
'Clench your teeth'
'Open your mouth against resistance'

V Sensory
Light touch and pin prick over the three areas
Corneal reflex

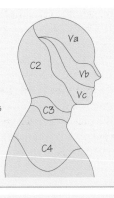

Va
Vb
Vc
C2
C3
C4

VII
'Raise your eyebrows'
'Screw up your eyes'
'Show me your teeth'
'Blow out your cheeks'
'Smile'
'Whistle'

VIII
Whisper a number in each ear while occluding the opposite one

IX & X
'Open your mouth and say ah'
'Please can you give me a cough'
'Please can you swallow this water'
Gag reflex

Visual field testing – screening test

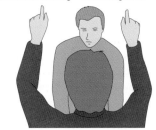

Move each finger in turn, then both together, in each quadrant of the patient's (binocular) visual field

Left XII palsy

XII
'Stick out your tongue and wiggle it from side to side'
'Push your tongue into your cheek and try and resist me pushing on it'

XI
'Shrug your shoulders, don't let me push them down'
'Turn your head to the left and try and resist me pushing it back' (repeat for the right)

Station 83: Cranial nerve examination

- *This 78-year-old man has recently had a stroke, please examine his cranial nerves*
- *Please examine this patient's eyes*

Examination routine
- Introduction/consent
- *Exposure*: expose the face and neck
- *Position*: ask the patient to sit on the edge of the bed or have them sitting in a chair. Sit opposite the patient at a similar height.
- *General inspection*: look in particular for any evidence of hemiparesis, ataxia, muscle wasting, drooping of the face, ptosis, acromegaly, Parkinsonism or walking aids

- *System-specific inspection*:
  - note any asymmetry of the face
  - some abnormalities may be more obvious from a little distance away, e.g. facial droop, Horner's, ptosis and forehead wrinkling

I
- 'Have you noticed any change in your sense of smell'
If the examiners would like you to formally asses smell, then a selection of substances should be available in bottles. Most cases of anosmia are not due to a cranial nerve lesion.

The eyes (II, III, IV, VI)
1 *Visual acuity*: test with glasses in place. Ask patient to cover one of their eyes and test each eye in turn:

- Use a Snellen chart if available (see Ch. 98) *or*
- Use a newspaper or equivalent printed material

If vision appears poor then:
- Ask the patient to count fingers
- See if the patient can perceive movement of your hand
- See if the patient can perceive light

2 *Visual fields*:
- *Screening test*: test for inattention (see opposite). Ask the patient to look at your nose. Place your extended index fingers towards the limit of your upper temporal fields. Ask the patient to indicate which finger you move (move them individually and then both together). If there is visual inattention, one finger will be ignored when both are moved together, although it will be seen when moved alone. This is a higher cortical function rather than an actual cranial nerve test although it will demonstrate a gross visual field defect
- *Formal test*: Ask the patient to stare at your nose. Ask them to cover one of their eyes. Test their left temporal field against your right temporal field by moving your index finger (flexing) from the periphery towards the centre (see opposite). Test the upper and lower quadrants (move your finger slowly so as not to miss subtle deficits). Now swap hands and test the nasal field. Complete by testing the other eye. Ask the patient to specifically state when they can see your finger moving. A red pin is needed to test for a central scotoma or the blind spot. Ask the patient to stare at your nose as above, and with the pin equidistant between you, move it on the horizontal plane until the pin disappears

3 *The pupils*:
- Check for equal size and shape
- Test direct and consensual light reflexes (afferent II, efferent III)
- Check the accommodation reflex (afferent arises frontal lobes, efferent III) and consider swinging light test

4 *Fundoscopy*: see Chapter 98

5 *Eye movements*: on inspection, check more carefully for ptosis and the position of the eyes in primary gaze (divergence or convergence). Hold your index finger about 50 cm away from the patient in the centre of gaze and ask him to follow it without moving his head. Ask if there is double vision (diplopia) at any point and if so describe the false image. Also look for evidence of nystagmus. Check that both eyes move through the full range and that the movements are smooth and in unison

V

1 *Motor*:
- Look for wasting of the temporalis muscle
- Ask the patient to clench their teeth while feeling the masseter and temporalis muscles; ask the patient to open their mouth, and try and close it against resistance

2 *Sensory* (V1, ophthalmic branch; V2, maxillary; V3, mandibular):
- Test light touch using your finger tip in each of the divisions of the trigeminal nerve bilaterally (see opposite)

3 *Reflexes*:
- State you would test the corneal reflex (afferent V1; efferent VII)
- Jaw jerk: place your thumb on the patient's chin and tap with the tendon hammer

VII

Look for asymmetry especially when patient blinks. There may be loss of forehead wrinkles or nasolabial folds. Ask the patient to raise their eyebrows (demonstrate if necessary), screw up their eyes (try and open them), blow out their cheeks, smile, show you their teeth and whistle.

Functions of the VII nerve: muscles of facial expression; stapedius; taste: anterior two-thirds of tongue; parasympathetic supply to lacrimal glands; efferent limb of the corneal reflex

VIII

Remember there are two components to this nerve – cochlear (hearing) and vestibular. For the purposes of the screening cranial nerve examination it is routine to just perform a gross test of hearing.
- Test each ear in turn. Block one ear by pressing on the tragus while whispering a number in the other ear. Increase in volume until the patient can hear
- If there is an abnormality in hearing, state to the examiners that you would perform Rinne's and Weber's tests (see Ch. 103)

IX and X

Functions of the glossopharyngeal (IX):
- Sensory: posterior one-third of the tongue and pharynx
- Motor: stylopharyngeus (not able to test clinically)
- Autonomic: salivary glands

Functions of the vagus (X):
- Sensory: tympanic membrane and external auditory canal
- Motor: palatal muscles, pharynx and larynx
- Autonomic: parasympathetic supply to chest and abdomen

These two nerves are tested together.
- Ask the patient to open their mouth and say 'ahh'. Look for symmetry of the uvula and palate
- Listen to the patient's speech for volume, ask them to cough and then ask them to swallow some water
- State to the examiners that you would also perform a gag reflex by touching the back of the pharynx on either side with an orange stick (afferent is IX and efferent is X)

XI

The accessory nerve innervates the sternomastoid and the trapezius.
- Check for muscle wasting
- Ask the patient to shrug their shoulders while you press down. Then ask the patient to turn their head to one side and try and move it back against resistance while looking at the sternomastoid on the opposite side

XII

The hypoglossal innervates the muscles of the tongue.
- Observe for fasciculation or wasting while the tongue is in the mouth
- Ask the patient to poke out their tongue and waggle it from side to side. Check for deviation. Next ask the patient to push his tongue into his cheek and push against it to check power. Repeat on both sides

NB. Where is the pathology? Tongue towards, jaw towards and palate away (i.e. the tongue and jaw deviate towards the side of the lesion and the palate deviates away from the site of the lesion)?

Completion

State you would complete your examination by performing any areas that you skipped, e.g. fundoscopy. Otherwise completion of this examination routine will depend on the findings. In general you would want to examine the rest of the neurological system including speech, higher cortical function and the peripheries. This may confirm upper or lower motor neurone lesions or cerebellar findings.

Station 84: Speech

Inspection	Look for spot diagnoses
General questions	'What is your name and address?'
	'What have you eaten today?'
	'How did you get to the hospital?'
Understanding	'Is this a pen?' (show an object that is not a pen)
	'Close your eyes'
	'Cover your right eye with your left hand'
Fluency	'Do you have difficulty finding the right words to say?'
Naming objects	'What is this called?' (point to your watch and then the strap and then the hands)
	'Name as many animals as you can'
Repetition	'Please repeat the following: the weather is warm; no ifs, ands or buts'
Articulation	'Please repeat the following phrases: royal artillery; British constitution; bbb, ppp; sss, ttt; ka, ka, ka'

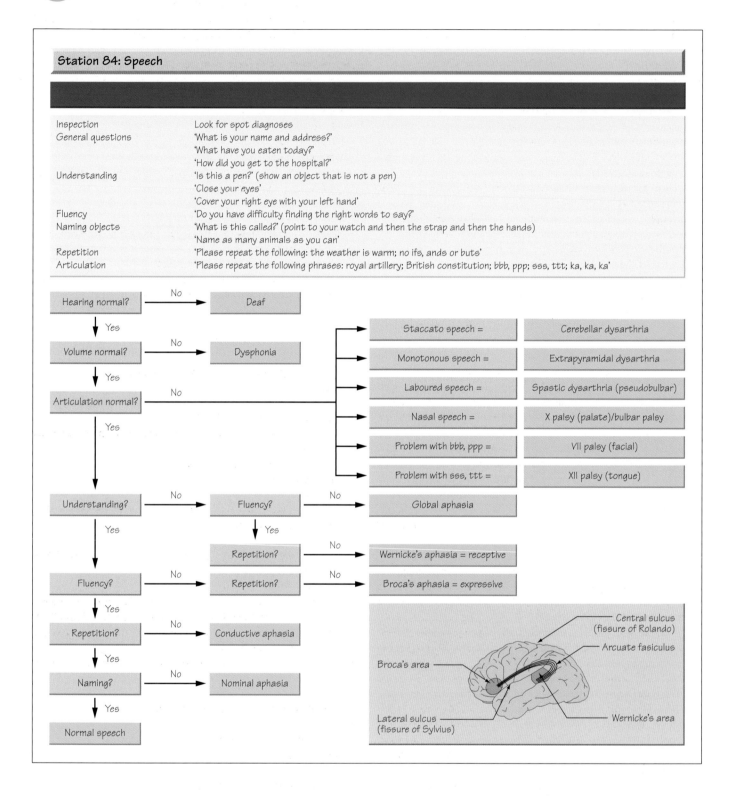

- *This lady has recently suffered a stroke, please assess her speech*
- *Ask this patient a few questions and discuss your findings*
- *Please examine this patient's speech*
- *Mr Smith has noticed his wife is talking nonsense, please assess*

Hints and tips

This is one of the stations that students fear and for this reason it is often a discriminator. Use all the clues possible in front of you. The most important aspect is to keep to a sensible, logical order and be able to attempt a sensible diagnosis using the flow chart opposite.

- *Remember the essentials checklist* (see Ch. 1)
- Introduction/consent
- *Position*: make sure the patient is comfortable
- *General inspection*: look for signs of other neurological problems that might point you to a diagnosis:
  - hemiplegia might suggest a dysphasia if higher cortical function has been affected *or* a dysarthria if the facial nerve is affected
  - Parkinsonian facies might suggest dysarthria
  - the patient may not follow your instructions if a receptive dysphasia is present
  - a wide-based gait may suggest a cerebellar dysarthria
- *General questions*:
  - ask some general questions. It is essential to get the patient to say a few sentences in order to fully assess their speech. Yes/no answers are not helpful
  - during this time quickly assess hearing and volume of speech
  - next determine articulation, understanding, spontaneity and fluency
- *Articulation*: if it is an articulation problem then check there are no mechanical reasons, e.g. poor fitting dentures or *Candida*. Proceed assessing for a dysarthria asking the patient to repeat:
  - the phrases 'British constitution' and 'royal artillery' (staccato speech of cerebellar dysarthria may be noticed)
  - the sounds BBB, PPP (facial nerve lesion)
  - the sounds TTT, SSS (hypoglossal nerve lesion)
  - the sounds Ka, Ka, Ka (palatal nerve palsy)
- If articulation is normal then it is necessary to assess in more detail for a dysphasia
- *Understanding*: you may have discovered the patient has a receptive dysphasia by this stage if they have not understood some of your requests. To test understanding start with simple instructions and proceed to more complicated ones (see opposite). If understanding is affected, it suggests a receptive dysphasia
- *Expression*: while the patient is speaking try and assess if their speech is spontaneous and fluent; the lack of these features suggests an expressive dysphasia. Patients are often frustrated by this so it is useful to ask 'are you having difficulty finding the right words?'
- *Naming*: test the ability of the patient to name objects (as opposite). An inability to name objects may suggest a nominal dysphasia which is a specific type of expressive dysphasia. Start with easy objects and progressively get more difficult (e.g. ask the patient if they recognise a watch and then break it down into several bits, i.e. strap, second hand, numerals etc.)
- *Repetition*: test the ability of the patient to repeat phrases (as opposite)
- *Completion*: explain you would like to complete a full neurological examination including mental state, higher cognitive function, reading and writing

Discussion points

- Discuss the abnormalities and what they might mean
- What are the possible causes of the abnormalities?
- How would you investigate and manage a patient with a speech problem?
- What other aspects of higher cognitive function can be tested?

Possible cases 1: dysphasia/aphasia

- *Wernicke's aphasia* (superior posterior temporal lobe): receptive or sensory aphasia
  - poor comprehension
  - fluent
  - often meaningless
  - absent repetition
- *Broca's aphasia* (posterior frontal lobe): expressive or motor aphasia
  - preserved comprehension
  - non-fluent speech
  - absent repetition
- *Global aphasia:* lesion in dominant hemisphere affecting both Wernicke's and Broca's areas
- *Nominal aphasia* (rare to have this alone)
- *Conductive aphasia*: understanding and expression normal but lack of ability to repeat (lesion in the arcuate fasciculus)

Causes of aphasia

- Cerebrovascular accident (CVA)
- Trauma
- Space-occupying lesions (e.g. tumour, abscess)
- Degenerative brain conditions

Possible cases 2: dysarthria

- *Cerebellar dysarthria*: slurred, scanning speech (emphasis equal on each syllable)
  - causes: alcohol, multiple sclerosis
- *Spastic dysarthria*
  - slurred
  - poor mouth opening (↑ tone with upper motor neurone (UMN) lesion, so tight muscles)
  - laboured
  - causes: any cause of a pseudobulbar palsy (i.e. bilateral UMN lesion of IX, X and XII)
- *Lower motor neurone dysarthria*
  - findings and causes depend on the cranial nerve involved (see opposite)
  - bulbar palsy is a bilateral lower motor neurone (LMN) lesion of IX, X and XII which causes nasal speech due to reduced tone of the musculature
  - isolated XII nerve palsy is rare
- *Extrapyramidal dysarthria*: look for other features of Parkinsonism (see Ch. 37)

Causes of pseudobulbar palsy (UMN signs)

- Multiple sclerosis
- Bilateral cerebrovascular disease
- Motor neurone disease

Causes of bulbar palsy (LMN signs)

- Motor neurone disease
- Brainstem lesion
- Poliomyelitis
- Guillain–Barre
- Myasthenia gravis

Station 85: Upper motor neurone lesion

Examination hints

Increased tone/spasticity	Weakness
Increased reflexes	Clonus
Up-going plantar response	Hoffman's sign

Wasting is minimal but there can be some atrophy secondary to disuse
Upper limb weakness is more marked in abductors and extensors
Lower limb weakness in more marked in flexors and abductors

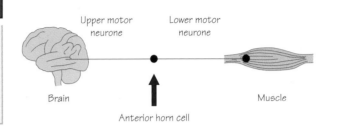

Station 86: Lower motor neurone lesion

Examination hints

Fasciculations	Reduced tone
Marked muscle wasting	Reduced or absent reflexes
Plantar response normal or absent	

Weakness often more obvious distally
Flexor and extensor muscles affected equally

Anatomical stations
A. Anterior horn cell
B. Peripheral nerve
C. Neuromuscular junction
D. Muscle

Dorsal root ganglion

Ventral root

A. Anterior horn cell disease
Examination as above
Example = poliomyelitis

C. Neuromuscular junction disease
Fatiguable weakness, no wasting
Symmetrical pattern of weakness
Ocular and bulbar muscles commonly affected
Normal or decreased tone
Normal reflexes
Example = myasthenia gravis

D. Muscle disease
Wasting
Symmetrical pattern of weakness, usually proximal
Decreased tone
Reduced or absent reflexes
Example = myopathy or dystrophy

B. Peripheral nerve disease
Weakness can be focal or diffuse depending on the extent of nerve involvement and the cause
These conditions can be pure motor, pure sensory or combined sensorimotor

Two patterns – FOCAL and DIFFUSE
Focal

Spinal nerve root disease	= radiculopathy
Plexus disease	= plexopathy
Specific peripheral nerve disease	= mononeuropathy
Several discrete nerves affected	= mononeuritis multiplex

Example mononeuropathy	= carpal tunnel syndrome

Diffuse
Peripheral neuropathy (polyneuropathy)
Example = diabetic neuropathy

Station 85: Upper motor neurone lesion

Hints and tips
• Upper motor neurone disease is a clinical term
• Denotes interruption of the corticospinal tract somewhere along its course
• If the lesion is above the pyramidal decussation, the clinical signs will be contralateral and if the lesion is below the decussation, the signs will be ipsilateral
• Many causes of an UMN lesion can be made with the initial inspection, e.g. stroke, multiple sclerosis
• Monoparesis is weakness of one limb
• Hemiparesis involves the arm and leg on one side (CVA)
• Tetraparesis invoves all four limbs (high cervical cord lesion, bilateral brainstem lesion)
• Paraparesis involves both legs (spinal cord disease below arm level)

Causes
• *Hemiparesis* (i.e. unilateral):
  • cerebrovascular accident
  • space-occupying lesion, e.g. subdural haematoma, abscess
  • multiple sclerosis
  • trauma
• *Spastic paraparesis* (i.e. bilateral):

- multiple sclerosis
- spinal cord compression, e.g. tumour, disc, abscess
- motor neurone disease
- subacute combined degeneration of the cord
- cerebral palsy

Station 86: Lower motor neurone lesion

Hints and tips
- Lower motor neurone disease is a further clinical term that refers to an abnormality distal to the anterior horn cell
- The anatomical stations that can be affected are summarised opposite
- Examine the part of the body requested, looking out for the general findings of a LMN lesion
- Inspection may give clues to the diagnosis, e.g. signs of myotonic dystrophy (see Ch. 38) or ulcers on the lower limbs related to diabetic neuropathy

Anterior horn cell disease
Causes are: poliomyelitis; motor neurone disease (see Ch. 38)

Peripheral nerve disease
Hints and tips
- Know the classification, the speed of onset and the disease associations
- Peripheral neuropathies may be predominantly sensory, predominantly motor, mixed or autonomic
- If sensory then all modalities of sensation are affected (ascending problem)
- Legs are more often affected than arms
- Bulbar involvement is rare
- A neuropathy should be confirmed by nerve conduction studies and electromyography (demyelinating vs axonal neuropathies)

Classification
- Polyneuropathy: sensory, motor, mixed, autonomic
- Radiculopathy
- Plexopathy
- Mononeuropathy

Timing
- Acute: vascular, inflammatory, toxic
- Subacute: toxic, nutritional, systemic
- Chronic: hereditary, metabolic

Causes of polyneuropathy
- *Hereditary*: Charcot–Marie–Tooth disease (hereditary motor and sensory neuropathy)
- *Metabolic*: diabetes mellitus, vitamin deficiencies (e.g. B_{12}), chronic renal failure
- *Toxic*: alcohol, other drugs (e.g. amiodarone)
- *Inflammatory/immune*: Guillain–Barré syndrome, acute inflammatory demyelinating polyneuropathy (AIDP), chronic inflammatory demyelinating polyneuropathy (CIDP), critical care polyneuropathy, diphtheria, vasculitis, paraneoplastic

Investigations of peripheral nerve disease
Bloods   FBC, ESR, B_{12}, folate, U&E, LFT, TFT, Glc, immunoglobulins and protein electrophoresis, ANA, ANCA, autoimmune screen
Other   Nerve conduction studies

Demyelinating neuropathy
- Usually motor
- Slowing of conduction but normal action potential
- Causes:
  - Hereditary motor and sensory neuropathy type 1
  - Guillain–Barre syndrome
  - CIDP
  - drugs (amiodarone)

Axonal neuropathy
- Sensory or mixed
- Normal conduction
- Reduced compound muscle action potential
- Causes:
  - diabetes mellitus
  - alcohol
  - metabolic disturbances (renal failure, B_{12} deficiency)
  - paraneoplastic
  - vasculitis
  - drugs, except amiodarone (e.g. chemotherapy, statins)

Common mononeuropathies
Median nerve; ulnar nerve; common peroneal nerve; radial nerve

Conditions associated with mononeuropathies
- Diabetes mellitus/acromegaly/RA/hypothyroidism

Causes of mononeuritis multiplex
- *Endocrine*: diabetes mellitus
- *Vasculitis*: polyarteritis nodosa
- *Connective tissue disease*: rheumatoid arthritis, sarcoidosis
- *Infective*: HIV
- *Neoplastic*: araneoplastic

Causes of a radiculopathy
- Cervical or lumbar disc protrusion
- Space-occupying lesions

Management of peripheral neuropathy
- Treatment and optimisation of any underlying medical problem, e.g. diabetes, thyroid disease
- Removal of causative agent
- Pain relief (anticonvulsants for neuropathic pain)
- Specific management depending on the cause, e.g. podiatry, physiotherapy, surgery, immunosuppressive drugs

Neuromuscular junction disease
Causes
- Myasthenia gravis (see Ch. 38)
- Eaton–Lambert syndrome

Muscle disease
Causes of myopathy
- *Inherited*: muscular dystrophies (Duchenne's, Becker's, myotonic)
- *Inflammatory*: polymyositis
- *Endocrine*: steroid induced, hyper-/hypothyroid
- *Metabolic*: storage diseases
- *Toxic*: alcohol

Station 87: Cerebrovascular disease

History hints

Sudden-onset neurological deficit
Associated symptoms – headache, fits
Motor/sensory deficit

Higher function deficit
Vascular risk factors
DH: anticoagulants

Examination hints

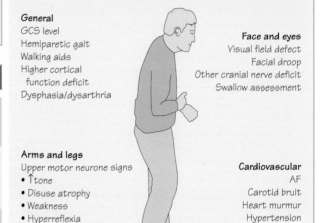

General
GCS level
Hemiparetic gait
Walking aids
Higher cortical
  function deficit
Dysphasia/dysarthria

Face and eyes
Visual field defect
Facial droop
Other cranial nerve deficit
Swallow assessment

Arms and legs
Upper motor neurone signs
• ↑tone
• Disuse atrophy
• Weakness
• Hyperreflexia
• Babinski reflex

± Sensory deficit

Cardiovascular
AF
Carotid bruit
Heart murmur
Hypertension

Station 88: Glasgow Coma Scale assessment

Eye opening	Spontaneous	4
	To verbal command	3
	To painful stimulus	2
	Not at all	1
Best verbal response	Orientated	5
	Disorientated	4
	Incoherent words	3
	Incomprehensible vocalisations	2
	No response	1
Best motor response	Obey commands	6
	Localising to pain	5
	Withdraws	4
	Flexes to pain	3
	Extends to pain	2
	No response	1

Station 89: Multiple sclerosis

History hints

History of neurological deficits at different times
  and at varying sites
Blurred vision   Eye discomfort
Weakness   Numbness
Unsteadiness   Bladder problems
Functional limitation   Memory problems
Mood disturbance

Uthoff's phenomenon – symptoms worsen with hot
  temperature or exercise
Lhermitte's sign – neck flexion causes lightening
  pains down the spine (due to cervical cord plaques)

**Left internuclear ophthalmoplegia
(dysconjugate eye gaze)**

On looking to the right, the right eye abducts
normally but the left eye is unable to adduct.
The right eye has nystagmus

Both eyes look to the left normally

Examination hints

Intellectual loss ('dementia')
in long-standing MS
• Mood changes e.g. depression

Optic neuritis
Acute phase
• Central visual field defect
• 'Scotoma' —'like cotton wool'
• Discomfort—worse on eye movement
• Often normal fundoscopy
• Usually recovers in 10–20 days
Chronic phase
• Fundoscopy shows optic atrophy
  i.e. very pale disc,
• Visual loss often minor
  i.e. ↓ colour vision

Motor weakness
Due to pyramidal tract damage
  (in spinal cord or higher):
• Weakness
• Arm extension
• Leg flexion
• Spasticity i.e. ↑tone ('clasp knife') pattern
• Increased reflexes +/- clonus +/- upgoing plantar

Sensory loss
Difficult to describe—anaesthesia or
  paraesthesia (i.e. altered sensation)
If isolated symptom, differential
  diagnosis is hyperventilation, or
  peripheral neuropathy
Can occur anywhere in the body

Cerebellar signs often prominent

Brain-stem involvement
• Dysconjugate eye gaze due to
  internuclear ophthalmoplegia
• Trigeminal neuralgia-like syndrome
• Recurrent facial nerve palsy

Spinal cord damage
• Gradual onset spastic
  para- or tetraparesis
• Acute 'transverse myelitis'
  – leads to flaccid
  paralysis in acute phase,
  spasticity in chronic phase
• Dorsal column damage
  → Abnormal gait
  ('sensory ataxia') due to
  loss of position sense

• Lhermitte phenomena
  bending neck forward
  → 'Electric shock'
  passing along spine

• Brown–Sequard-like syndrome

Station 87: Cerebrovascular disease

- *Please examine this patient's upper limbs/gait/speech*

Hints and tips

The examination routine will depend on the instruction but will involve one of the core neurology routines described on the preceding pages.
- *Completion*: examine the rest of the neurological system including gait, speech and cognition. Examine the cardiovascular system

Discussion points

- What are the risk factors for stroke disease?
- Name some causes of stroke in younger patients
- Do you know of any classification systems for stroke?
- How would you investigate this patient?
- Discuss some management principles of stroke

Ix *Bloods* FBC, ESR, U&E, Glc, lipids, clotting
ECG
Imaging CT head (consider MRI)
Consider carotid doppler
Consider echocardiogram

Causes of 'young stroke' Vasculitis; carotid/vertebral artery dissection; antiphospholipid syndrome; inherited thrombophilias; drug induced

RF for stroke Hypertension; smoking; diabetes; family history; heart disease (valvular, ischaemic, AF); excess alcohol; raised cholesterol; polycythaemia; clotting abnormalities

Mx: acute
ABCDE (see Ch. 11)
Rx Aspirin (need to rule out haemorrhage)
Consider thrombolysis if proven ischaemic stroke within 3 hours of onset of symptoms
Deep vein thrombosis (DVT) prophylaxis
Optimise nutrition, oxygenation, fluid balance, vascular risk factors and glycaemic control
Procedures May need nasogastric tube
MDT Physiotherapy, occupational therapy, social worker, speech and language (swallow assessment), dietician
Location Stroke unit
Monitoring Regular observation, pressure areas, fluid balance, nutrition
Specialists Stroke physician and nurse specialist
Mx: chronic
Rx Optimise vascular risk factors
Antiplatelet therapy
Consider anticoagulation for cardiac thromboembolism or AF
Consider carotid endarterectomy if carotid stenosis on Doppler
Continued MDT approach
Prevention of pressure sores and contractures
Optimise nutrition
Complications Infections; venous thromboembolism; pressure sores; joint contractures; depression and anxiety; falls and fractures; dependent oedema; shoulder pain/subluxation

Station 88: Glasgow Coma Scale assessment

- *A 75-year-old man has been brought to A&E and is drowsy. Please demonstrate to the examiner how you would assess his GCS, using the mannequin (see opposite)*

Station 89: Multiple sclerosis

- *Please examine this patient's cerebellar system*
- *This patient has had several episodes of blurred vision in the past and has noticed some weakness of her arms, please examine the upper limbs and discuss your findings*

Hints and tips

The examination routine will depend on the instruction. If you are asked to examine the arms, legs or gait then initially follow the appropriate routine described previously.
- *Completion*: examine remaining neurology (gait, speech and eyes)
- Common examination findings will be UMN or cerebellar signs
- The eye signs found are summarised opposite

Internuclear ophthalmoplegia

Indicates a problem with conjugate eye movements (i.e. the eyes do not move together when looking either to the right or left). To allow the eyes to move together, there is a connection between the VI nerve of one eye and the III nerve of the opposite eye – this connection is called the medial longitudinal fasciculus. Demyelination of this connection can occur in multiple sclerosis.

Gait

Examination of the gait may reveal a spastic paraparesis (UMN) or cerebellar ataxia. Take care when asking the patient to walk and ask if they are able to do so first. Look around the bed for any walking aids.

Discussion points

- What would you include in a differential diagnosis?
- How would you investigate a patient with suspected multiple sclerosis?
- What patterns of disease are you aware of?
- Do you know of any treatments?

Ix *Imaging* MRI scan – white matter hyperintensities (plaques)
Micro Lumbar puncture – oligoclonal bands in the CSF
Other Visual evoked potentials – test the conduction of the optic nerve
ΔΔ Multiple strokes
Cerebral vasculitis
Sarcoidosis
Metastases
Patterns of disease Relapsing and remitting
Secondary progressive
Relapsing progressive
Primary progressive
Mx
Rx Steroids during the acute phase may reduce the severity of the attack
Disease-modifying agents – interferon
Baclofen for spasticity
Anticonvulsants for neuropathic pain
Antidepressants
Monitoring Bowel and bladder care – laxatives and intermittent catheterisation if necessary
MDT
Specialists Neurologist
Education

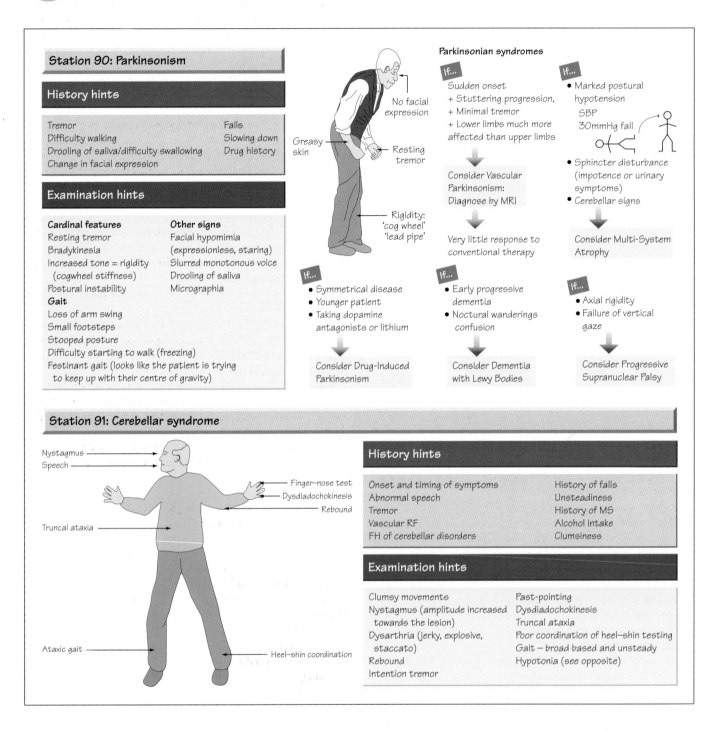

Station 90: Parkinsonism

History hints

Tremor	Falls
Difficulty walking	Slowing down
Drooling of saliva/difficulty swallowing	Drug history
Change in facial expression	

Examination hints

Cardinal features
Resting tremor
Bradykinesia
Increased tone = rigidity
  (cogwheel stiffness)
Postural instability

Gait
Loss of arm swing
Small footsteps
Stooped posture
Difficulty starting to walk (freezing)
Festinant gait (looks like the patient is trying
  to keep up with their centre of gravity)

Other signs
Facial hypomimia
(expressionless, staring)
Slurred monotonous voice
Drooling of saliva
Micrographia

No facial expression
Greasy skin
Resting tremor
Rigidity: 'cog wheel' 'lead pipe'

Parkinsonian syndromes

If... Sudden onset + Stuttering progression, + Minimal tremor + Lower limbs much more affected than upper limbs → Consider Vascular Parkinsonism: Diagnose by MRI → Very little response to conventional therapy

If... • Marked postural hypotension SBP 30mmHg fall • Sphincter disturbance (impotence or urinary symptoms) • Cerebellar signs → Consider Multi-System Atrophy

If... • Symmetrical disease • Younger patient • Taking dopamine antagonists or lithium → Consider Drug-Induced Parkinsonism

If... • Early progressive dementia • Noctural wanderings confusion → Consider Dementia with Lewy Bodies

If... • Axial rigidity • Failure of vertical gaze → Consider Progressive Supranuclear Palsy

Station 91: Cerebellar syndrome

Nystagmus
Speech
Finger–nose test
Dysdiadochokinesis
Rebound
Truncal ataxia
Ataxic gait
Heel–shin coordination

History hints

Onset and timing of symptoms	History of falls
Abnormal speech	Unsteadiness
Tremor	History of MS
Vascular RF	Alcohol intake
FH of cerebellar disorders	Clumsiness

Examination hints

Clumsy movements
Nystagmus (amplitude increased
  towards the lesion)
Dysarthria (jerky, explosive,
  staccato)
Rebound
Intention tremor

Past-pointing
Dysdiadochokinesis
Truncal ataxia
Poor coordination of heel–shin testing
Gait – broad based and unsteady
Hypotonia (see opposite)

Station 90: Parkinsonism

- *Please examine this patient's upper limbs*
- *Please examine this patient's gait*
- *This patient has noticed a tremor of his right hand, please assess*

Hints and tips

The examination routine will depend on the instruction but will involve one of the core neurology routines described previously.

- Once you feel confident of your diagnosis, state to the examiner that you would like to perform some specific tests to help confirm your thoughts:
  - demonstrate bradykinesia: ask the patient to open and close their hands rapidly (like the birdie song)
  - observe for tremor: ask the patient to rest one hand in their lap while tapping the other hand up and down on the chair arm (this distraction technique causes the tremor to become more intense)

- tone: if rigidity is not obvious ask the patient to move the contra-lateral arm up and down as a distraction (synkinesis)
- glabellar tap: although documented in several textbooks, do not perform this test as it is not pleasant for the patient
- gait: examine the patient's gait if not already done. Offer to demonstrate loss of postural reflexes (i.e. stand behind the patient and pull their shoulders back, reassuring them that you will not let them fall)
- writing: to demonstrate micrographia
- *Completion*:
  - postural blood pressure: side effect of L-dopa or multiple system atrophy (MSA)
  - cranial nerves: vertical gaze palsy in progressive supranuclear palsy or nystagmus in MSA
  - MMSE: dementia with Lewy bodies

Discussion points
- What are the causes of Parkinsonism?
- What features are more likely to suggest a diagnosis of idiopathic Parkinson's disease?
- Discuss some management principles

Ix	*Imaging*	CT and MRI may help with a diagnosis of vascular Parkinsonism Positron emission tomography (PET)/single photon emission CT (SPECT) scan may help differentiate between the tremor of Parkinsonism vs essential tremor
Mx		
Rx		Levodopa replacement (given in combination with a peripheral dopa decarboxylase inhibitor) Dopamine agonists
Monitoring		Impact of illness on patient
MDT		
Education		

Causes
- *Idiopathic Parkinson's disease*: symmetry, slow progression, upper body initially, fluctuation in severity, good response to L-dopa
- *Drug-induced Parkinsonism*: phenothiazines, antiemetics
- *Vascular Parkinsonism*: pyramidal signs, brisk reflexes, predominant gait disturbance
- *Postencephalitic* (now rare)
- *Brain damage from anoxia* (e.g. post cardiac arrest)
- *Multiple system atrophy* (degeneration of the nigrostriatal pathway)
- *Progressive supranuclear palsy*
- *Wilson's disease* (younger patient)
- *Corticobasal degeneration*

Station 91: Cerebellar syndrome
- *Mr GH has noticed some unsteadiness while walking, please examine his cerebellar system*
- *Please examine this patient's arms/legs*
- *Please examine this patient's speech*
- *Mrs JK has noticed some clumsiness, please examine her coordination*

Hints and tips
The examination routine will depend on the instruction. If you are asked to examine the arms, legs or gait then initially follow the appropriate routine as described earlier. Once you feel confident of the diagnosis then ask the examiners if you can continue by examining the rest of the cerebellar system. If the instruction is to examine coordination then proceed as follows:
- *Inspection*: general inspection with the patient lying down
- *Speech*: assess for any sign of dysarthria (see Ch. 34)
- *Nystagmus*
- *Truncal ataxia*: ask the patient to cross their arms and sit up
- *Rebound*: ask the patient to stretch out their arms and close their eyes. Push down on the arms and then let go – the arms should return to the starting point. If there is a cerebellar problem they will oscillate before returning to rest (this is basically caused by uncoordination of antagonist and agonist actions of the muscles)
- *Finger–nose test*: look for an intention tremor (tremor increases further away from the patient's body) and past pointing (patient overshoots the finger)
- *Heel–shin testing*: ask the patient to slide their heel up and down their opposite leg from knee to shin)
- *Gait*: look for a broad-based gait with a stagger (towards the side of the lesion, if unilateral)
- *Tone*: there is mixed opinion in the literature as to whether hypotonia is a reliable sign in cerebellar disease but a student would be required to know how to examine tone in a neurology OSCE
- Try and assess gait first if the examiners will let you
- There are a couple of mnemonics to help remember the cerebellar signs (DANISH, DASHING). When students use these they look less slick as the order is not logical so we would recommend the routine above
- *Completion*: examine the remaining neurology and also consider a cardiovascular examination if the diagnosis is a likely stroke

Discussion points
- What are the causes of cerebellar syndrome?
- How would you investigate this patient further?

Ix: this depends on the proposed cause but consider:

Bloods	TFT (hypothyroidism)
Imaging	CT brain, MRI brain
Micro	Lumbar puncture for oligoclonal bands

Causes
- *Unilateral*:
  - space-occupying lesion
  - cerebrovascular disease
  - multiple sclerosis
  - trauma
- *Bilateral*:
  - alcohol
  - drugs, e.g. phenytoin, carbamazepine
  - multiple sclerosis
  - space-occupying lesion/paraneoplastic
  - cerebrovascular disease
  - Friedreich's ataxia

Station 92: Myotonic dystrophy

History hints

Family history
Autosomal dominant
Genetic anticipation – successive generations more severely affected
Muscle weakness causing functional problems

Examination hints

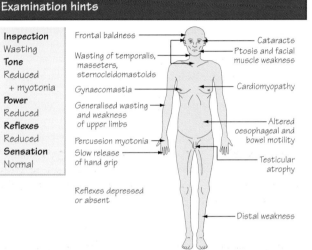

Inspection
Wasting
Tone
Reduced
  + myotonia
Power
Reduced
Reflexes
Reduced
Sensation
Normal

Frontal baldness
Wasting of temporalis, masseters, sternocleidomastoids
Gynaecomastia
Generalised wasting and weakness of upper limbs
Percussion myotonia
Slow release of hand grip

Cataracts
Ptosis and facial muscle weakness
Cardiomyopathy
Altered oesophageal and bowel motility
Testicular atrophy

Reflexes depressed or absent

Distal weakness

Station 93: Motor neurone disease

History hints

Gradually increasing weakness
Swallowing problems
Functional status
Speech problems

Examination hints

N.B. Signs will depend on whether upper or lower motor neurones are predominantly affected

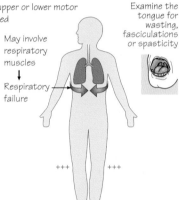

Inspection
Wasting
Fasciculations
Tone
Increased (usually)
Power
Reduced
Reflexes
Absent or brisk
Sensation
Normal
Bulbar muscles often affected
Mix of UMN and LMN
NO SENSORY SIGNS
NO BLADDER DISTURBANCE

May involve respiratory muscles
↓
Respiratory failure

Examine the tongue for wasting, fasciculations or spasticity

+++   +++

↑+++   +++↑

Station 94: Myasthenia gravis

History hints

Weakness that worsens during the day or after activity
Double vision
Speech, swallow problems   History of autoimmune conditions

Examination hints

Bilateral ptosis
Extraocular muscle palsies
Symmetrical proximal muscle weakness that fatigues on exertion
Dysarthria if bulbar involvement
Look for evidence of previous tracheostomy
Look for sternotomy scar (thymectomy)

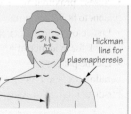

Hickman line for plasmapheresis

Station 95: Cervical myelopathy

History hints

Neck pain   Weakness
Parasthesia of upper limbs   Gait abnormalities

Examination hints

Middle age/elderly
UMN signs in the lower limb
  (i.e. below the lesion)
Radiculopathy at the level
  (commonest level C5/C6)
May be sensory impairment
  (posterior columns)
Spastic paraparetic gait
Often asymmetrical

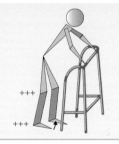

+++

+++

Station 92: Myotonic dystrophy

• *Please examine this man's upper limbs*
• *Please assess this patient's strength and discuss your findings*

Hints and tips

• The key as always is with your inspection
• The diagnosis may be clear as soon as you have shaken the patient's hand – look for evidence of myotonia (delayed relaxation)
• To confirm this myotonia consider asking the patient to make a fist or close his eyes tightly
• Consider testing for percussion myotonia (tap the thenar eminence and a dimple should appear which is slow to resolve)
• The patient often has a typical face – frontal balding, ptosis and 'droopy expression' due to muscle wasting
• On examination of the muscles there is widespread weakness and wasting
• Reflexes are reduced
• *Completion*: examine other relevant systems, e.g. eyes (cataracts), CVS (cardiomyopathy), urinalysis (glucose)

Discussion points

• What are the management principles for a patient with myotonic dystrophy?
• Do you know of any medication that can be used to help?
• Name some associations with this condition

Associations

Cataracts; cardiomyopathy; gynaecomastia; testicular atrophy; diabetes; dysarthria; mild cognitive impairment; sleep apnoea

Mx

Rx	No treatment for the weakness
	Treatment of associations, e.g. diabetes
	Phenytoin for myotonia (rarely needs treatment)
Monitoring	For the above associations
	Monitor respiratory and cardiac function
MDT	Ankle splints, physio, swallowing assessment
Specialists	Neurologist
	Ophthalmology input for ptosis and cataracts
	Other specialists as needed for associations
Education	Caution with general anaesthetic
	Genetic counselling

Station 93: Motor neurone disease

• *This man has noticed a gradual weakness of his arms and problems swallowing. Please examine his upper limbs*

Hints and tips

• The key as always is with your inspection
• The diagnosis may be clear if there is marked global muscle wasting
• Look carefully for fasciculations, including the tongue
• There may be a combination of upper and lower motor signs
• This could be manifest as brisk knee reflexes and normal plantar reflex or absent ankle jerks and upgoing plantars
• There is no sensory involvement
• There will not be evidence of cerebellar, extrapyramidal or ocular signs
• Sphincter disturbance is rare
• Cognitive function is rarely affected
• *Completion*: complete the neurological assessment including speech and also request a swallow assessment. The speech abnormality could be bulbar (LMN) or pseudobulbar (UMN) palsy

Discussion points

• What are the management principles for a patient with motor neurone disease (MND)?
• Do you know any classifications for MND?
• What are the complications of MND?

Ix

	Diagnosis is clinical
Imaging	Consider MRI spine ± brain to rule out other causes
Other	Electromyography
	Nerve conduction studies

Mx

Rx	Supportive
	Riluzole – prolongs time to ventilation
	Non-invasive ventilation
Monitoring	Respiratory function, swallow
MDT	Nutritional review
Specialists	Neurologist

Classification of motor neurone disease

• Amyotrophic lateral sclerosis (≈ 50%): UMN and LMN signs
• Progressive muscular atrophy: predominantly LMN
• Primary lateral sclerosis: predominantly UMN
• Progressive bulbar palsy

Causes of absent ankle reflex and upgoing plantar

MND; Friedreich's ataxia; subacute combined degeneration of the cord; cauda equina lesion, and mixed pathology, e.g. cervical myelopathy + diabetic neuropathy

Station 94: Myasthenia gravis

• *This patient has been complaining of double vision, please examine her eyes*

Hints and tips

• The majority of patients (two-thirds) have ptosis ± extraocular muscle involvement
• The ptosis may be obvious (think about the differential for bilateral ptosis), but will become worse by asking the patient to look upwards for a prolonged time
• Examine for strabismus and abnormal eye movements
• Following the eye examination ask the patient to count to 30 to help assess for a dysarthria
• Assess proximal muscle weakness and fatigability by getting the patient to hold their arms above their head
• Look closely at the neck to see if their has been a previous tracheostomy
• Look for evidence of a sternotomy scar (thymectomy)
• Lie the patient flat and ask them to breathe, looking for an abdominal paradox (i.e. the abdomen is sucked in on inspiration indicating possible diaphragmatic weakness)
• Note that it is unusual for there to be significant limb weakness without ocular involvement
• Reflexes are normal

Discussion points

• What is the cause of myasthenia gravis?
• Do you know any associations?
• How do you investigate a patient with suspected myasthenia gravis?
• How do you treat myasthenia gravis?

Ix *Bloods* Acetylcholine receptor antibodies (present in 90%)
    Imaging Mediastinal imaging (CT or MRI)
    Other Edrophonium (Tensilon) test – short-acting anticholinesterase, increases concentration of acetylcholine at the motor end plate and therefore produces a rapid (but transient) improvement in signs (i.e. the ptosis)
        NB. The patient should be on a cardiac monitor as edrophonium may cause heart block
        Electromyography – decreased amplitudes with repetitive stimulation
Association   Graves' disease
        Diabetes mellitus
        Rheumatoid arthritis
        SLE
        Thymoma
        Thymic hyperplasia

Mx

Rx Long-acting cholinesterase inhibitors (e.g. pyridostigmine)
    Immunosuppresive therapy (e.g. steroids, azathioprine)
    Consider thymectomy
Specialist referral

NB. These patients can develop myasthenic crises, which can lead to respiratory failure requiring intubation and ventilation. In this acute phase, treatment with IV immunoglobulin or plasmapharesis should be considered.

Causes of bilateral ptosis

- Congenital
- Myasthenia gravis
- Myotonic dystrophy
- Bilateral Horner's syndrome

Station 95: Cervical myelopathy

- *This elderly female has been complaining of neck pain. Please examine her lower limbs*

Hints and tips

- Usually middle-aged to elderly patients
- Degenerative changes in the cervical vertebrae lead to a slowly progressive compression of the cord
- The nerve roots can be involved causing a radiculopathy at that spinal level
- The main features are of an UMN lesion below the spinal level

Ix *Imaging* MRI spine

Station 96: Facial nerve palsy

History hints

Onset   Associated symptoms, e.g. weakness elsewhere
Hearing problems   Previous parotid surgery

Examination hints

Upper motor neuron facial weakness - left side

Upper face unaffected
Slight droop of mouth and flattening of nasolabial fold

Lower motor neuron facial weakness - left side

Affects upper and lower face
Weakness of forehead, eye closure and mouth

Bell's phenomenon = eyeball rolls upwards on attempting to close the eye

Lower vs upper motor neurone facial weakness

Lower   = facial nerve palsy
           Paralysis of the upper and lower parts of the face
Upper   = lesion above the VII nerve nucleus
           The upper face is spared due to bilateral innervation

Station 97: Horner's syndrome

History hints

History of neck surgery   History of lung cancer
History of stroke or MS

Examination hints

Horner's syndrome

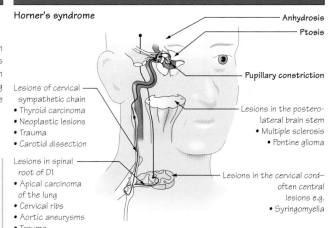

- Anhydrosis
- Ptosis
- Pupillary constriction

Lesions of cervical sympathetic chain
• Thyroid carcinoma
• Neoplastic lesions
• Trauma
• Carotid dissection

Lesions in spinal root of D1
• Apical carcinoma of the lung
• Cervical ribs
• Aortic aneurysms
• Trauma

Lesions in the postero-lateral brain stem
• Multiple sclerosis
• Pontine glioma

Lesions in the cervical cord– often central lesions e.g.
• Syringomyelia

Station 98: Ocular palsy

History hints

Double vision
Blurred vision
History of DM / CVA or demyelinating disease
History of posterior communicating artery aneurysm

Examination hints

Right third nerve palsy–neutral gaze

Ptosis (usually complete)

Dilated (mydriatic pupil)

Downward and outward deviation of eye

Right sixth nerve palsy–gaze to right

Third nerve palsy divided into complete (dilated pupil) or partial. The pupil becomes dilated if there is parasympathetic damage. This is caused by compressive lesions as the parasympathetic fibres are on the outside of the nerve. Complete = surgical. Partial = medical.

Station 99: Visual field defect

Examination hints

Visual field defects

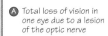
Ⓐ Total loss of vision in one eye due to a lesion of the optic nerve

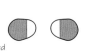
Ⓑ Bitemporal hemianopia due to compression of the optic chiasma. The upper quadrants are usually first affected

Ⓒ Right homonymous hemianopia from a lesion of the optic tracts

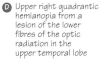
Ⓓ Upper right quadrantic hemianopia from a lesion of the lower fibres of the optic radiation in the upper temporal lobe

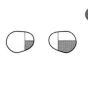
Ⓔ Less commonly a lower quadrantic hemianopia occurs from a lesion of the upper fibres of the optic radiation in the anterior part of the parietal lobe

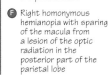
Ⓕ Right homonymous hemianopia with sparing of the macula from a lesion of the optic radiation in the posterior part of the parietal lobe

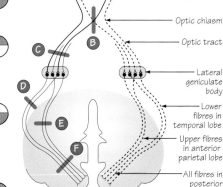

Visual fields

- Retina
- Optic nerve
- Optic chiasm
- Optic tract
- Lateral geniculate body
- Lower fibres in temporal lobe
- Upper fibres in anterior parietal lobe
- All fibres in posterior parietal lobe
- Occipital cortex

Station 96: Facial nerve palsy

Hints and tips

- *Completion*: complete the neurological examination, in particular speech
- The patient may have an isolated VII nerve palsy or one associated with other cranial nerve deficits, for example:
  - VI and VII: pons lesion
  - V, VII and VIII: cerebellopontine lesion
- A VII nerve palsy can cause a dysarthria (see Ch. 34)
- There may be UMN signs of the limbs if associated with a stroke or multiple sclerosis

NB. Ptosis is *not* due to weakness of muscles supplied by the VII nerve.

Discussion points

- How do you distinguish between a lower and upper motor neurone facial weakness?
- What are the causes of a VII nerve palsy?
- What is the treatment for a Bell's palsy?
- Can you tell me about Bell's phenomenon?

Causes

- *Unilateral LMN*:
  - Bell's palsy
  - cerebellopontine angle lesion
  - herpes zoster – Ramsey–Hunt syndrome
  - parotid tumours
- *Bilateral LMN*:
  - sarcoidosis
  - Guillain–Barre syndrome
  - myasthenia gravis – fatiguable weakness
  - myopathies
- *Unilateral UMN*:
  - cerebrovascular accident
  - demyelination
  - space-occupying lesions
- *Bilateral UMN*:
  - pseudobulbar palsy
  - motor neurone disease

Rx Bell's palsy: steroids
Herpes zoster: aciclovir
Eye protection
Specific treatment of the underlying cause, e.g. surgery if acoustic neuroma

Station 97: Horner's syndrome

- *Please examine this patient's eyes*

Hints and tips

The instruction could be to examine the cranial nerves, but is more likely to ask you to concentrate on the eyes.

- Look carefully for ptosis and miosis, which are not always obvious at first glance
- If you are confident with the diagnosis then state to the examiners that you would like to test for anhydrosis (absence of sweating) on the forehead and look carefully for evidence of scars around the neck and, if allowed, palpate for any masses around the neck
- *Completion*: you may want to finish a neurological routine (looking for other evidence of stroke or demyelinating diasease) or perform a brief respiratory examination looking for evidence of lung cancer and its complications

Discussion points

- What are the causes of Horner's syndrome?

Causes

Horner's syndrome is caused by the interruption of some part of the sympathetic chain.

1 First neurone (travels from hypothalamus to spinal cord C8/T1 and through the brainstem). Causes include:

- Brainstem strokes
- Demyelinating lesion
- Space-occupying lesion
- Trauma

2 Second neurone (preganglionic neurone, travels from C8/T1 to the superior cervical ganglion (SCG)). Causes include:

- Pancoast's tumour
- Cervical rib
- Following neck surgery
- Mediastinal mass
- Thyroid enlargement
- Cervical lymphadenopathy

3 Third neurone (postganglionic, travels from the SCG via different fibres to innervate the pupil and eyelid muscles). Causes include:

- Carotid artery aneurysms or dissection
- Trauma
- Surgery

Station 98: Ocular palsy

- *Please examine this woman's eye movements*

Hints and tips

The most likely abnormalities that could be included in an OSCE are isolated III or VI nerve palsies. Isolated IV nerve palsies are rare.

- *Completion*: this will depend on your differential diagnosis, e.g. if you feel the lesion is due to diabetes (mononeuritis multiplex), then state to the examiner that you would check for diabetic retinopathy, peripheral neuropathy and perform urinalysis to look for glucose

Oculomotor palsy (III)

- Ptosis
- Divergent strabismus – eye is fixed 'down and out'
- Dilated pupil (if complete nerve palsy, i.e. parasympathetic damage)
- Eye points down and out due to the unopposed action of lateral rectus (VI) and superior oblique (IV)

Causes of a complete III nerve palsy (surgical)

- Posterior communicating artery aneurysm
- Space-occupying lesion
- Trauma
- Cavernous sinus disease (infection, tumour)

Causes of a partial III nerve palsy (medical)

- Mononeuritis multiplex, e.g. diabetes
- Cerebrovascular disease
- Demyelination
- Vasculitis

Abducens palsy (VI)

- Convergent strabismus
- Failure of adduction
- Diplopia (outermost image is from the affected eye)

Causes

- Mononeuritis multiplex
- Demyelination
- Cerebrovascular disease
- Space-occupying lesion
- Raised intracranial pressure
- Infection – subacute meningitis (TB, fungal, bacteria)

Trochlear palsy (IV)

- Rare
- Adducted eye cannot look inferiorly
- Diplopia – the added image is in the vertical plane

Station 99: Visual field defect

- *Please examine this man's eyes*
- *This patient has had a recent stroke, please examine the visual fields*
- *Please examine this patient's cranial nerves*

Hints and tips

The abnormalities possible are summarised opposite. In reality the most likely abnormality that you would encounter is a homonymous hemianopia.

Causes of a homonymous hemianopia

- Cerebrovascular disease
- Space-occupying lesion

Causes of a bitemporal hemianopia

- Pituitary tumour
- Meningioma
- Aneurysm

Endocrine symptoms

Symptom	Type 1 diabetes	Hyperthyroid	Hypothyroid	Acromegaly	Cushing's	Addison's	Hypercalcaemia
Weight gain			Yes	Yes	Yes		
Weight loss	Yes	Yes				Yes	Yes
Malaise	Yes		Yes			Yes	Yes
Polydipsia	Yes			Yes			Yes
Polyuria	Yes			Yes			Yes
Appearance change		Yes	Yes	Yes	Yes		
Diarrhoea	Yes	Yes				Yes	
Constipation			Yes	Yes			Yes
Infertility		Yes		Yes			
Irritability		Yes		Yes			
Depression			Yes	Yes		Yes	Yes
Cold intolerance			Yes			Yes	
Heat intolerance		Yes					
Abdominal pain	Yes			Yes		Yes	Yes
Menorrhagia			Yes				
Impotence				Yes	Yes		
Hirsutism				Yes	Yes		
Amenorrhoea		Yes			Yes		
Muscle weakness		Yes		Yes	Yes		Yes

Station 100: Diabetes

Presenting symptoms in type 1 diabetes
Polyuria
Polydipsia
Weight loss
Fatigue
Recurrent infection
Presentation with features of ketoacidosis (vomiting, abdominal pain, SOB, drowsiness)

Diagnostic criteria for diabetes
Diabetes
• Fasting plasma venous glucose > 7.0 mmol/L
• 2-hour OGTT plasma venous glucose > 11.1 mmol/L
Impaired glucose tolerance
• 2-hour OGTT plasma venous glucose ⩾ 7.8 mmol/L and < 11.1 mmol/L
Impaired fasting glucose
• Fasting plasma venous glucose measurement 6.1–6.9 mmol/L

History in a known diabetic patient
Date of diagnosis
Treatment to date
Monitoring (urine/blood)
HbA1C
Monitoring charts
Awareness of hypos
Current treatment
Smoking and alcohol history
Complications – macrovascular/microvascular
FH of diabetes and other autoimmune conditions
Hypertension
Diet/weight/exercise
Previous history of other autoimmune conditions
Impact of the illness on the patient's life

Station 101: Hypercalcaemia

Signs and symptoms of hypercalcaemia

Abdominal pain	Constipation	Nausea
Polyuria	Polydipsia	Anorexia
Weight loss	Lethargy	Confusion
Renal stones	Renal failure	Hypertension
Weakness	Depression	Peptic ulcer

Signs or symptoms from an underlying malignancy
'Bones, stones, groans and psychic moans'

Causes of hypercalcaemia
Primary hyperparathyroidism
Malignancy
Increased vitamin D (e.g. ingestion, sarcoidosis)
Increased bone turnover (e.g. hyperthyroidism, thiazide diuretics)
Renal failure
Drugs (e.g. lithium)

Station 100: Diabetes

Student info: *Miss DM is 19 and has attended her GP with a history of thirst and weight loss. Please take a full history and formulate a management plan. There is no need to perform an examination. A blood sugar level is 14*

Patient info: *You are Miss DM, 19 years old. You have no PMH, but there is a FH of your maternal grandmother having type 2 diabetes. You remember she took tablets and also started on some injections before she died. You have no other knowledge about diabetes. You are due to attend university next year, enjoy an active social life and consume 24 units of alcohol per week and smoke 15/day. You have been unwell for 3 months with increasing thirst and polyuria and have also noted some unintentional weight loss. You are not aware of the cause of diabetes or of any of the complications. You hate needles and do not wish to take any regular medications. You are concerned that this diagnosis will mean it is difficult for you to attend university*

Hints and tips

- Ascertain the patient's reason for visiting GP
- Determine symptomatology and timing of symptoms
- Establish FH of diabetes
- Ascertain the patient's prior knowledge of the illness
- Establish the smoking and alcohol history
- Assess impact of the symptoms on the patient's life and the impact of a diagnosis of diabetes
- Address any concerns the patient has (i.e. her fears)
- Discuss the suspected diagnosis and agree a management plan including support groups and information leaflets
- Arrange a follow-up appointment and for her to see the diabetes specialist nurse and to have training in insulin injecting

Discussion points

- What investigations would you consider?
- Describe the oral glucose tolerance test (OGTT)
- Discuss the treatment options and complications of diabetes

Ix	*Bloods*	FBC, U&E, TFT, LFT, Glc
Mx		
Rx		Optimise glycaemic control
Monitoring		Urine or blood glucose testing
MDT		Diabetes nurse
Specialists		Diabetologist
Education		Important – educate about the complications of diabetes and the importance of tight sugar control

Station 101: Hypercalcaemia

Student info: *Mrs VD (52 years) has been referred to hospital with a calcium of 3.5. You are the FY1 doctor on the medical admissions ward. Please take a full history and formulate a differential diagnosis*

Patient info: *You are Mrs VD, 52 years old. You have a PMH of mild depression diagnosed 2 years ago following your divorce and the death of your mother. A water tablet has also recently been started due to some ankle swelling which has now improved. You have been suffering with constipation for about 6 months although have always had rather stubborn bowels. Leg cramps started at a similar time but one of the main problems is lethargy. You have been complaining of thirst. Your DH is bendro-flumethiazide 2.5 mg OD; no FH of note; no allergies. You smoke 10/day and have a glass of sherry each night. There is no PMH of cancer or pancreatitis*

Hints and tips

- Ascertain the patient's prior knowledge of the situation
- Determine symptomatology and timing of symptoms
- Ascertain PMH of depression and ankle swelling
- Enquire about a history of renal stones or peptic ulcer disease
- Enquire if there is a FH of high calcium
- Complete a full systems enquiry looking for any clues for an underlying cause of the raised calcium (e.g. malignancy)
- Address any concerns the patient has (i.e. her fears)

Discussion points

- What are the causes and treatment of hypercalcaemia?

Ix	*Bloods*	Ca, Alb, U&E, FBC, PTH, LFT
		Protein electrophoresis
	Imaging	CXR, parathyroid imaging (sestamibi scan)
	Other	24-hour urinary calcium
		Consider investigation for underlying malignancy

Station 102: Hypothyroidism

Student info: *You are the FY1 doctor on the admissions ward. An 82-year-old female has been referred. She has had two falls in the last month. She has recently been complaining of tiredness. On examination her pulse is 40 and regular*

Patient info: *You are Mrs HG, 82 years old. Over the last 6 months you have been feeling lethargic, mentally slowed and suffering with constipation. You have been experiencing intermittent dizziness which has not necessarily been worse on standing. Twice you have fallen, although no loss of consciousness, which can be confirmed by your husband. Your PMH includes a right hemicolectomy 6 years previously for bowel cancer, but no other serious medical conditions and no history of cardiac or autoimmune disease. DH: nil. You live with your husband in a bungalow and are independent in ADL*

Hints and tips

- Ascertain the patient's prior knowledge of the situation
- Determine the exact nature of the falls
- Take a full cardiac and neurological history
- Determine the negative history of loss of consciousness but realise the importance of confirming with her husband
- Determine the timing of symptoms
- Appreciate that the association of lethargy, bradycardia and mental slowing could indicate hypothyroidism and complete an endocrine systems enquiry
- Establish PMH, home circumstances and SH
- Address any concerns the patient has (i.e. her fears)
- Discuss a differential diagnosis and a management plan

Discussion points

- What is your differential diagnosis from this history?
- What investigations would you request?

ΔΔ	*Endocrine causes*	Hypothyroidism
	Cardiac causes	Heart block, sick sinus syndrome, postural hypotension, aortic stenosis
	Neurological causes	Cerebrovascular disease, SOL
Ix	*Bloods*	FBC, U&E, Glu, LFT, Ca, TFTs
	ECG	
	Imaging	CXR
	Other	Consider 24-hour heart monitor

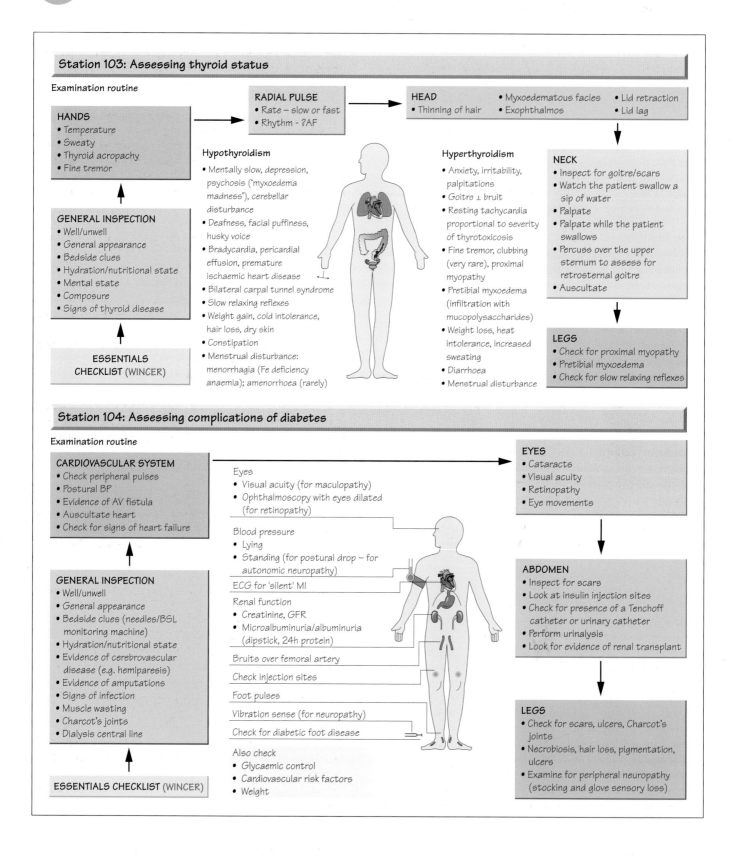

Station 103: Assessing thyroid status

Examination routine

HANDS
- Temperature
- Sweaty
- Thyroid acropachy
- Fine tremor

RADIAL PULSE
- Rate – slow or fast
- Rhythm - ?AF

HEAD
- Thinning of hair
- Myxoedematous facies
- Exophthalmos
- Lid retraction
- Lid lag

GENERAL INSPECTION
- Well/unwell
- General appearance
- Bedside clues
- Hydration/nutritional state
- Mental state
- Composure
- Signs of thyroid disease

ESSENTIALS CHECKLIST (WINCER)

Hypothyroidism
- Mentally slow, depression, psychosis ('myxoedema madness'), cerebellar disturbance
- Deafness, facial puffiness, husky voice
- Bradycardia, pericardial effusion, premature ischaemic heart disease
- Bilateral carpal tunnel syndrome
- Slow relaxing reflexes
- Weight gain, cold intolerance, hair loss, dry skin
- Constipation
- Menstrual disturbance: menorrhagia (Fe deficiency anaemia); amenorrhoea (rarely)

Hyperthyroidism
- Anxiety, irritability, palpitations
- Goitre ⊥ bruit
- Resting tachycardia proportional to severity of thyrotoxicosis
- Fine tremor, clubbing (very rare), proximal myopathy
- Pretibial myxoedema (infiltration with mucopolysaccharides)
- Weight loss, heat intolerance, increased sweating
- Diarrhoea
- Menstrual disturbance

NECK
- Inspect for goitre/scars
- Watch the patient swallow a sip of water
- Palpate
- Palpate while the patient swallows
- Percuss over the upper sternum to assess for retrosternal goitre
- Auscultate

LEGS
- Check for proximal myopathy
- Pretibial myxoedema
- Check for slow relaxing reflexes

Station 104: Assessing complications of diabetes

Examination routine

CARDIOVASCULAR SYSTEM
- Check peripheral pulses
- Postural BP
- Evidence of AV fistula
- Auscultate heart
- Check for signs of heart failure

GENERAL INSPECTION
- Well/unwell
- General appearance
- Bedside clues (needles/BSL monitoring machine)
- Hydration/nutritional state
- Evidence of cerebrovascular disease (e.g. hemiparesis)
- Evidence of amputations
- Signs of infection
- Muscle wasting
- Charcot's joints
- Dialysis central line

ESSENTIALS CHECKLIST (WINCER)

Eyes
- Visual acuity (for maculopathy)
- Ophthalmoscopy with eyes dilated (for retinopathy)

Blood pressure
- Lying
- Standing (for postural drop – for autonomic neuropathy)

ECG for 'silent' MI

Renal function
- Creatinine, GFR
- Microalbuminuria/albuminuria (dipstick, 24h protein)

Bruits over femoral artery

Check injection sites

Foot pulses

Vibration sense (for neuropathy)

Check for diabetic foot disease

Also check
- Glycaemic control
- Cardiovascular risk factors
- Weight

EYES
- Cataracts
- Visual acuity
- Retinopathy
- Eye movements

ABDOMEN
- Inspect for scars
- Look at insulin injection sites
- Check for presence of a Tenchoff catheter or urinary catheter
- Perform urinalysis
- Look for evidence of renal transplant

LEGS
- Check for scars, ulcers, Charcot's joints
- Necrobiosis, hair loss, pigmentation, ulcers
- Examine for peripheral neuropathy (stocking and glove sensory loss)

Station 103: Assessing thyroid status

• *Please examine this patient's thyroid status*
• *Please examine this patient's neck and then determine their thyroid status*

Examination routine

It is important to listen carefully to the instruction, but if asked to determine thyroid status, perform the following routine.

• Introduction/consent
• *Exposure*: adequate exposure of the head and neck is essential
• *Position*: the ideal position will depend on which aspect of the routine you are performing, but as a general guide have the patient initially sitting in a chair
• *General inspection*:
  • take a physical step back and observe the patient and surroundings
  • assess the composure of the patient (agitated vs immobile) and observe for any inappropriate clothing for the current weather
  • during introductions, assess for a hoarse voice
• *System-specific inspection*: now check for any particular signs of thyroid disease (e.g. goitre, eye signs)
• *Hands*:
  • assess temperature and presence of sweating
  • check for palmar erythema, clubbing (thyroid acropachy)
  • check for a tremor: place a piece of paper on outstretched hands
  • check the radial pulse for rate and rhythm
• *Head*:
  • look for evidence of hair thinning, particularly the lateral third of the eyebrows
  • myxoedematous facies (puffy cheeks, oedema, 'peaches and cream' complexion)
• *Eyes*:
  • exophthalmos – sclera visible above the lower lid
  • lid retraction – sclera visible above the cornea
  • proptosis – protrusion of the eyeball best seen from above
  • periorbital oedema (chemosis)
  • lid lag – keeping the patient's head still assess upwards vertical gaze and then drop the examining finger quickly and watch for a delay in the drop of the eyelid
• *Neck* (see Ch. 48):
  • inspect for a goitre
  • ask the patient to take a sip of water, hold it in their mouth and then swallow on command (look for evidence of movement on swallowing)
  • stand behind the patient and check permission to palpate their neck, explaining that there may be some discomfort
  • start by palpating the isthmus just below the thyroid cartilage with your right index and middle fingers. Next feel the lobes to either side and ask the patient to swallow a sip of water again
  • note size, texture: is the enlargement diffuse or nodular?
• *Legs*:
  • check for a proximal myopathy by asking the patient to stand up without the use of their hands
  • examine the shins for evidence of pretibial myxoedema
  • test the reflexes looking for slow relaxation
• Depending on findings to date, the routine could be completed by examining the cardiorespiratory systems for evidence of heart failure or pleural effusions

Discussion points

• What are the causes of hypothyroidism and hyperthyroidism?

• What symptoms might point towards a diagnosis of thyroid disease?
• What are the causes of a goitre?

Station 104: Assessing complications of diabetes

• *Mr ID is 63 and has had insulin-dependent diabetes since he was 19. Please examine him for any complications that may have occurred*

Examination routine

It is important to listen carefully to the instruction given and examine the appropriate part of the patient. In general a candidate will be asked to perform some aspect of a cardiovascular or neurological routine. However a station could test a candidate further by asking for them to examine a patient for evidence of complications of diabetes. It will involve picking the relevant parts out of other examination routines. A suggested routine is given.

• Introduction/consent
• *Exposure*: adequate exposure of the patient's peripheries is essential
• *Position*: examine the patient either on the bed at 45° or seated
• *General inspection*: take a physical step back and observe the patient and surroundings. Look for:
  • body habitus and nutritional status
  • evidence of previous cerebrovascular accident, amputations and operations
  • signs of infection, muscle wasting, dialysis lines, arteriovenous (AV) fistulae and Charcot's joints
  • walking aids, white stick or glasses
• *Cardiovascular system*:
  • check peripheral pulses, looking carefully for any scars from previous vascular procedures (e.g. old fistula, femoropopliteal bypass)
  • check BP for hypertension and also for a postural drop (autonomic neuropathy)
  • check AV fistula for palpable thrill and listen for bruit
• *Eyes*:
  • check visual acuity for evidence of maculopathy
  • check eye movements for any evidence of ophthalmoplegia (mononeuritis multiplex)
  • perform fundoscopy looking for evidence of cataracts (loss of red reflex) or retinopathy
• *Abdomen*:
  • check for evidence of a Tenchkoff catheter (peritoneal dialysis) or scars from previous ones
  • inspect for renal transplant scar and if found state you would perform a full abdominal palpation
  • check for evidence of a urinary catheter (atonic bladder)
  • state you would perform urinalysis to check for protein and glucose
• *Legs*: look for evidence of scars, ulcers, peripheral vascular disease, charcot joints
• *Neurology*:
  • look for evidence of muscle wasting (i.e. possible motor neuropathy) and if found state you would perform a motor examination of the affected limb
  • check for sensory peripheral neuropathy (glove and stocking sensory loss)

Discussion points

• Describe the complications of diabetes mellitus
• How would you manage these complications?

Station 105: Hypothyroidism

History hints

Weight gain	Constipation	Dry skin
Hair loss	Change in voice	Menorrhagia
Depression	Cold intolerance	Psychosis

PMH of thyroid disease
Previous treatment for hyperthyroidism
  (thyroidectomy, radioiodine)
Use of amiodarone or history of arrythmias
PMH of autoimmune disease
FH of thyroid or autoimmune problems

Station 106: Hyperthyroidism

History hints

Weight loss
Increased appetite
Diarrhoea
Tremor
Irritability
Sweating
Itch
Heat intolerance
Palpitations
Oligomenorrhoea

Thyroid eye disease

Swollen extra-ocular muscles
Compression of optic nerve → blindness

Eye projects beyond line (proptosis)
Eyelids retract
Cornea exposed
Eye moves forward
Corneal ulcers
Blindness

Eyelid retraction

↑T4   Normal

- 50% Graves' disease at presentation
- ↑ rate in smokers

Examination hints

Hypothyroidism

Heart and lungs
Bradycardia
Pericardial effusion
Pleural effusion

Hands and arms
Carpal tunnel syndrome

Legs
Peripheral oedema
Slow relaxing reflexes
Peripheral neuropathy

General
Increased body habitus
Mentally slow, psychosis
Hoarse voice, hair loss, dry skin
Warm clothes
Vitiligo (associated autoimmune problem)

Face and neck
Myxoedematous facies (puffy face, periorbital oedema)
Thin eyebrows (lateral 1/3rd)
Goitre
Deafness
Conjunctival pallor

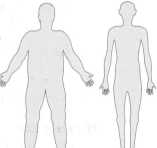

Hyperthyroidism

General
Thin
Anxious, irritable
T-shirt (heat tolerance)
Sweaty

Face and neck
Staring face
Goitre ± bruit
Thyroid scar

Heart and lungs
Tachycardia ± AF
Signs of cardiac failure

Eyes
Staring face
Exophthalmos, proptosis
Ophthalmoplegia
Lid retraction. Lid lag

Hands and arms
Carpal tunnel syndrome
Thyroid acropachy
Palmar erythema
Tremor

Legs
Pretibial myxoedema
Proximal myopathy
Brisk reflexes

Specific to Graves'
Exophthalmos
Pretibial myxoedema
Thyroid acropachy
Ophthalmoplegia

Station 107: Type 1 diabetes mellitus

History hints

Acute (diabetic ketoacidosis) or subacute presentation
Generally unwell   Polyuria   Polydipsia   Weight loss
FH of autoimmune disease
Complications: retinopathy, neuropathy, nephropathy

Examination hints

Young, thin patient
Lipoatrophy of skin following repeated injection sites
Unwell
Hyperventilation
Reduced conscious level
Abdominal pain
Ketotic breath
Ketones + glucose on urinalysis

Causes of DKA
First presentation   Infection
Non-compliance   MI
Intercurrent illness   Surgery

Diabetic ketoacidosis (DKA)

Normal → drowsy → coma

Ketotic 'fetor'

↓ Blood pressure
Postural hypotension

↑ Respiratory rate and depth (Kussmaul breathing)

↑ Heart rate

Gastroparesis (succussion splash)

Urine
- Ketones +++
- Glucose +++

Mortality rate < 5%

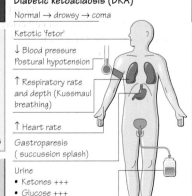

Station 108: Type 2 diabetes mellitus

History hints

Acute presentation (hyperosmolar hyperglycaemic state (HHS))
Insidious onset (polyuria/polydipsia)
20% present with a complication (e.g. MI or CVA)   Middle age/elderly
Incidental finding   Overweight

Examination hints

Increased BMI
Unwell
Drowsy
Tachycardic
Possible thrombotic complications due to hyperviscosity
Urinalysis: glucose, -ve ketones

Hyperosmolar hyperglycaemic state

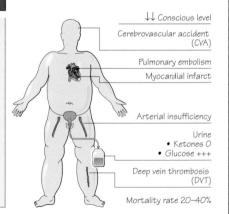

↓↓ Conscious level
Cerebrovascular accident (CVA)
Pulmonary embolism
Myocardial infarct
Arterial insufficiency
Urine
- Ketones 0
- Glucose +++
Deep vein thrombosis (DVT)

Mortality rate 20–40%

Station 105: Hypothyroidism

• *This patient has noticed some weight gain, please assess their thyroid status*

Hints and tips

• If suspecting hypothyroidism, look particularly for the features opposite

Discussion points

• What are the causes of hypothyroidism?
• What investigations would you consider for a patient with newly diagnosed hypothyroidism?
• Name some conditions associated with hypothyroidism
• What abnormalities could be found on testing the FBC in a patient with hypothyroidism?
• What are the management principles for a hypothyroid patient?

Causes

• Congenital
• Primary (disease of the thyroid):
  • autoimmune: Hashimoto's thyroiditis (goitre), atrophic thyroiditis (no goitre)
  • iodine deficiency
  • drugs: amiodarone, lithium
  • iatrogenic: post thyroidectomy, post radio-iodine
• Secondary (disease of the pituitary)
• Tertiary (disease of the hypothalamus)

Associations		Type 1 diabetes
		Vitiligo
		Pernicious anaemia
		Addison's disease
Ix	*Bloods*	FBC: macrocytic anaemia (MCV 95–115 fl)
		If MCV > 115 consider pernicious anaemia
		If MCV < 85 check iron levels (?menorrhagia)
		U&Es, lipids
		TFTs: ↓ thyroxine (T4)
		↑ thyroid-stimulating hormone (TSH) if primary, or low/normal TSH if secondary or tertiary
		Thyroid autoantibodies
	ECG	?Bradycardia
Rx		Thyroxine 50 μg/day (caution in elderly or those with heart disease)

Station 106: Hyperthyroidism

• *This woman has noticed a tremor, please examine her thyroid status*

Hints and tips

• If suspecting hyperthyroidism, look particularly for the features opposite
• Grave's disease is associatied with thyroid eye disease, but remember the patient may be biochemically hypo-, hyper- or euthyroid

Discussion points

• What are the causes of hyperthyroidism?
• What investigations would you organise?
• What possible treatments can you describe?

Causes

• *Primary*:
  • autoimmune: Graves' disease, Hashimoto's thyroiditis (may produce hyperthyroidism first)
  • toxic: multinodular goitre, single hot nodule
  • obstetric: postpartum thyroiditis, hyperemesis gravidarum, ovarian teratoma containing thyroid tissue
  • infective: viral thyroiditis (de Quervain's)
  • drugs: amiodarone
  • exogenous iodine
• *Secondary*:
  • pituitary disease: TSH-producing tumour

Associations with Graves'		Type 1 diabetes
		Pernicious anaemia
Ix	*Bloods*	FBC: normocytic anaemia (Graves')
		ESR, Ca (can be raised in Graves'), U&Es
		TFTs: ↓ TSH, free T3 and T4 ↑
		Thyroid autoantibodies (TSH receptor antibodies in Graves')
	ECG	Tachycardia, AF
	Imaging	Thyroid scan
Rx	*Medical*	Symptom control – β-blocker
		Thyroid suppression – carbimazole
		Radioiodine
	Surgery	Partial thyroidectomy

Station 107: Type 1 diabetes mellitus

• *Please examine this diabetic patient, looking for signs of complications*

Hints and tips

Listen to the instruction clearly. If looking for complications of diabetes follow the suggested routine in Chapter 41. Other common instructions would include fundoscopy and sensory testing.

Discussion points

• What is the treatment of diabetic ketoacidosis (DKA)?
• What may precipitate DKA in a known diabetic patient?

Mx of DKA

ABCDE (see Ch. 11)

Rx	Oxygen, fluid resuscitation, insulin sliding scale, K$^+$ replacement, thromboembolic prophylaxis
	Treat any precipitating cause, e.g. antibiotics for infection
Procedures	Consider urinary catheter, central line and arterial line
Monitoring	Strict fluid balance, regular U&E and bicarbarbonates, ABGs
	Consider CVP measurements
Location	Endocrine ward, consider HDU
Specialists	Diabetes nurse, diabetologist
Ix *Bloods*	FBC, Glc, CRP, U&E, LFT, bicarbonate
	ABG (metabolic acidosis)
ECG	
Imaging	CXR
Micro	Urine and blood for MC&S

Station 108: Type 2 diabetes mellitus

• *This patient has recently been diagnosed as having diabetes, please talk me through the relevant examination aspects*

Hints and tips

Again, listen to the instruction carefully. At this station the examiner may want a full cardiovascular or other focused routine.

Discussion points

• Please describe the management principles of a diabetic patient
• What are the treatment options for controlling diabetes?

Mx

Rx	Optimise glycaemic control to prevent macrovascular and microvascular complications (diet, oral hypoglycaemic agents or insulin)
	Optimise cardiovascular RF
Monitoring	Regular monitoring and follow-up
	Monitor urine or blood sugar
	Monitor for signs of complications

MDT	GP, podiatrist, dietician
Specialists	Diabetologist, nephrologist, ophthalmologist
Education	Information on monitoring sugar levels
	Information about diabetes and how to control, especially during intercurrent illness
	Smoking cessation

Summary of common endocrine investigations

Bloods	General: FBC, U&E, LFT
	Specific blood levels according to clinical suspicion, e.g. glucose, thyroid function, calcium, prolactin
	Specific stimulation or inhibition tests, e.g. glucose tolerance test, short synacthen test, dexamethasone suppression test
	Autoantibodies, e.g. thyroid
Imaging	Specific to proposed diagnosis, e.g. CXR (thyroid), AXR (calcified adrenals), US (thyroid), CT or MRI head (pituitary), radioisotope scans (e.g. sestamibi parathyroid scan)

Station 109: Acromegaly

History hints

Age 30-50 years	Blurred vision	Headache
Fatigue	Weight increase	Sweating
Impotence	Erectile dysfunction	Change in voice
Galactorrhoea	Menstrual irregularities	
Tingling in the hands	Symptoms of hyperglycaemia	
Hand and feet enlargement (rings do not fit)		
Gradual change in facial appearance (in photos)		

Examination hints

Face
Characteristic facies
Prominent supraorbital ridges
Large jaw with prognathism
  (lower jaw protrudes)
Teeth separation
Enlargement of nose, ears,
  and tongue
Coarse features and
  thickened skin
Hirsutism

Axillae and chest
Acanthosis nigricans
Skin tags
Gynaecomastia

Abdomen
Organomegaly
Hypogonadism

Urinalysis
Glucose

Eyes
Visual field defect
Diabetic, hypertensive changes

Neck
Goitre
Large collar size

Heart
Hypertension
Signs of cardiac failure

Hands
Large hands
Sweaty
Carpal tunnel syndrome
(look for thenar wasting) –
perform Phalens test

Legs and feet
Arthropathy
Proximal myopathy
Foot drop (entrapment
  neuropathy)

Station 110: Gynaecomastia

History hints

Enlargement of breast tissue	
Drug history	
PMH of chronic liver disease or pituitary disorder	Middle age/elderly
PMH of prostate or testicular cancer	Overweight

Examination hints

Unilateral or bilateral enlargement of breasts due to increased glandular
  tissue
Obesity
Evidence of other endocrine disorder
Atrial fibrillation (digoxin)
Heart failure (spironolactone)
Clubbing, cachexia (lung cancer)
Signs of chronic liver disease

Causes

Nutritional	Obesity
Hepatology	Chronic liver disease
Neoplastic	Lung, liver or testicular carcinoma
Endocrine	Pituitary disease
Drugs	Oestrogens, antiandrogens, digoxin, spironolactone, alcohol, Ca blockers, metoclopramide, benzodiazepines, opiates, marijuana, cimetidine, ranitidine, isoniazid, ketoconazole

Station 111: Cushing's syndrome

History hints

Steroid use	Weight increase	Hirsutism
Amenorrhea	Easy bruising	Depression
PMH of asthma/COPD/IBD/renal transplant		
Previous fractures or back pain		

Station 112: Hypoadrenalism/Addison's disease

History hints

Fatigue	Anorexia	Abdominal pain
Weight loss	Diarrhoea	Dizzyness
Weakness	Arthralgia	Myalgia
Long-term steroid use		

Examination hints

Cushing's syndrome

General
Easy bruising
Thin skin
Low mood/psychosis
Signs of steroid dependent
  disease, e.g. COPD

Face and neck
Acne, hirsutism, thin hair
Thickening of facial fat
  (moon face)
Supraclavicular fat pad
Visual field defect

Back
Intrascapular fat pad
  (buffalo hump)
Kyphoscoliosis (osteoporosis)

Heart
Hypertension
Signs of cardiac failure

Abdomen
Truncal obesity
Scars (adrenalectomy)
Adrenal mass
Purple striae

Urinalysis
Glucose

Legs
Peripheral oedema
Proximal myopathy
Peripheral neuropathy

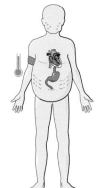
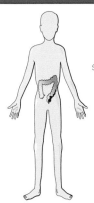

Addison's disease

General
Thin
Vitiligo
Pigmentation
Signs of other autoimmune disease (e.g. thyroid)

Face and neck
Buccal mucosa pigmentation

Heart
Postural hypotension

Hands and arms
Palmar crease pigmentation

Urinalysis
Glucose

Abdomen
Abdominal pain
Diarrhoea

Station 109: Acromegaly

• *This woman has recently had to alter the size of her wedding ring. Please perform a general examination of this patient and discuss your findings*

Hints and tips

• Some cases in the OSCE will basically involve spotting a diagnosis from the end of the bed
• There may not be a set routine but it is still important to have a logical order, so start as always with inspection (which may give the answer) and proceed to examine the peripheries and face
• The instruction (as in the example above) may well give you a hint!
• Avoid possibly insulting comments such as 'spade-like' hands and 'big forehead'

Discussion points

• What causes acromegaly?
• What investigations would you perform to aid your diagnosis?
• Name some complications associated with acromegaly
• What is the treatment of acromegaly?

Causes Benign pituitary macroadenoma (or micro-) causing hypersecretion of growth hormone; associated features may be present due to hypopituitarism or local pressure effects of the tumour
Pituitary carcinoma (rare)

Associations

Cardiovascular	Hypertension, cardiomyopathy, heart failure
Respiratory	Obstructive sleep apnoea
Endocrine	Impaired glucose tolerance
Neurological	Carpal tunnel syndrome, bitemporal hemianopia, cerebrovascular disease
Neoplastic	Colonic polyps and carcinoma

Ix	*Bloods*	Glucose, prolactin, testosterone, luteinising hormone (LH), TFTs
		$\uparrow$ insulin-like growth factor 1
		Oral glucose tolerance test – failure of suppression of growth hormone (GH)
		Consider other tests of pituitary function
	ECG	
	Imaging	MRI pituitary fossa
		Consider echocardiogram
	Other	Colonoscopy

Mx		
Rx	*Surgical*	Trans-sphenoidal resection
		Transcranial resection
	Medical	Somatostatin analogues, e.g. octreotide
		Dopamine agonists (cabergoline)
	Radiotherapy	
	Monitoring	Optimise BP
		Optimise glycaemic control

Station 110: Gynaecomastia

• *This patient has a history of heart failure, please examine their praecordium and discuss your findings*

Hints and tips

The importance of inspection is once again demonstrated in this station. With the above instruction it would be easy for a student to merely focus on the auscultatory findings. However, this patient has heart failure and atrial fibrillation and has developed gynaecomastia as a result of digoxin and spironolactone.

Discussion points

• What are the causes of gynaecomastia?

Station 111: Cushing's syndrome

• *Please examine this patient who has had steroid-dependent COPD for many years*

Hints and tips

For hints on the approach see Station 109.

Discussion points

• What are the causes of Cushing's syndrome?
• What investigations would you organise?
• What possible treatments can you describe?

Causes

ACTH independent	Corticosteroid treatment
	Adrenal adenoma
	Adrenal carcinoma
ACTH dependent	Cushing's disease (adrenocorticotrophic hormone (ACTH) secreting pituitary microadenoma)
	Ectopic ACTH (e.g. small cell lung cancer or carcinoid)

Associations

Cardiovascular	Hypertension, ischaemic heart disease
Endocrine	Impaired glucose tolerance
Neoplastic	Small cell lung cancer
Musculoskeletal	Osteoporosis
Infective	Recurrent infections
Psychiatric	Depression, psychosis
Gynaecological	Infertility

Ix	This involves initially confirming the diagnosis of Cushing's syndrome and then identifying the actual cause	
	Screening	Overnight dexamethasone suppression test (positive if the cortisol level is still high in the morning)
		24-hour urinary free cortisol
	Localisation	Check plasma ACTH (if undetectable = adrenal cause, if high either ectopic ACTH production or pituitary cause)
		High-dose dexamethasone suppression test (ectopic ACTH will not suppress)
	Imaging	MRI pituitary
		Abdominal CT

Mx		
Rx	*Medical*	Review need for steroids if possible
		Metyrapone decreases plasma cortisol
	Surgery	Transphenoidal hypophysectomy for Cushing's disease
		Adrenalectomy for adrenal adenoma/carcinoma
		Surgical removal of ectopic tumour
	Radiotheraopy	
	Monitoring	Optimise BP
		Optimise glycaemic control
		Optimise osteoporosis risk factors and prescribe prophylaxis

Station 112: Hypoadrenalism/Addison's disease

- *Please examine this patient who has noticed fatigue and weight loss*

Hints and tips

This is yet another station that will involve careful inspection and concentration on the instruction given. From the above instruction it would seem relevant, if given no other hints, to perform a full abdominal system examination; the clues may be found in the palmar creases and buccal mucosa. If considering this diagnosis, state you would complete your examination by performing a postural BP measurement.

Discussion points

- What are the causes of hypoadrenalism?
- What investigations would you request?
- Do you know any management options?

Causes of hypoadrenalism

Autoimmune	Addison's
Infective	Tuberculosis, HIV
Haematological	Lymphoma
Neoplastic	Metastases
Infiltration	Sarcoidosis
Congenital	Adrenal hyperplasia
Ix *Bloods*	U&E ($\downarrow$ Na, $\uparrow$ K$^+$), Glc ($\downarrow$)
	FBC ($\downarrow$ Hb), Ca ($\uparrow$), LFT
	Short synacthen test
	ABG (mild metabolic acidosis)

ECG	
Imaging	Abdominal X-ray/CXR (calcification)
	CT abdomen
Micro	Septic screen
Associations of Addison's	Thyroid disease
	Vitiligo
	Diabetes mellitus
	Pernicious anaemia
	Coeliac disease

Mx

Rx	*Medical*	Steroid replacement (hydrocortisone PO)
		Mineralocorticoid replacement (fludrocortisone PO)
	Education	Advise of need to increase steroids if vomiting/unwell
		Medic bracelet
		Alert dentists and health professionals to problem

Mx: acute

Acute adrenal failure is a medical emergency
ABCDE (see Ch. 11)

Rx	Aggressive fluid resuscitation
	IV steroid replacement
	Treat precipitant, e.g. antibiotics
Procedures	Consider urinary catheter
	Consider invasive monitoring
Location	Endocrine ward, consider HDU

Station 113: Acute abdominal pain

Remember non-surgical causes of abdominal pain

Gynaecological causes can include:
- Ectopic pregnancy
- Salpingitis
- Uterine fibroids
- Ovarian cyst

Medical causes can include:
- Pneumonia (referred pain)
- Gastroenteritis
- Urinary tract infection
- Irritable bowel syndrome
- Diabetic ketoacidosis

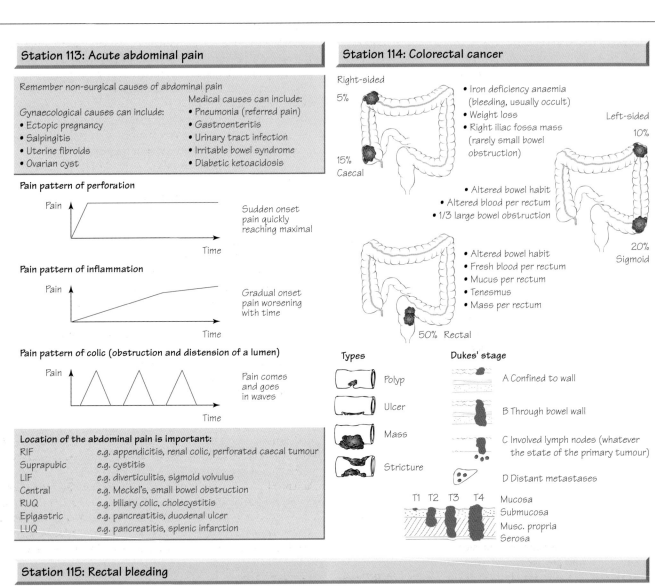

Pain pattern of perforation

Sudden onset pain quickly reaching maximal

Pain pattern of inflammation

Gradual onset pain worsening with time

Pain pattern of colic (obstruction and distension of a lumen)

Pain comes and goes in waves

Location of the abdominal pain is important:

RIF	e.g. appendicitis, renal colic, perforated caecal tumour
Suprapubic	e.g. cystitis
LIF	e.g. diverticulitis, sigmoid volvulus
Central	e.g. Meckel's, small bowel obstruction
RUQ	e.g. biliary colic, cholecystitis
Epigastric	e.g. pancreatitis, duodenal ulcer
LUQ	e.g. pancreatitis, splenic infarction

Station 114: Colorectal cancer

Right-sided 5%

15% Caecal

- Iron deficiency anaemia (bleeding, usually occult)
- Weight loss
- Right iliac fossa mass (rarely small bowel obstruction)

Left-sided 10%

- Altered bowel habit
- Altered blood per rectum
- 1/3 large bowel obstruction

20% Sigmoid

- Altered bowel habit
- Fresh blood per rectum
- Mucus per rectum
- Tenesmus
- Mass per rectum

50% Rectal

Types
- Polyp
- Ulcer
- Mass
- Stricture

Dukes' stage
- A Confined to wall
- B Through bowel wall
- C Involved lymph nodes (whatever the state of the primary tumour)
- D Distant metastases

T1 T2 T3 T4
Mucosa
Submucosa
Musc. propria
Serosa

Station 115: Rectal bleeding

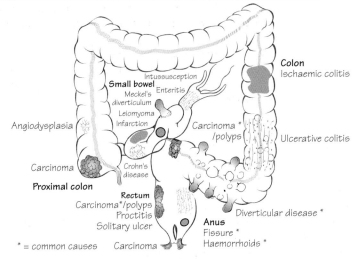

Colon
Ischaemic colitis

Small bowel
Intussusception
Meckel's diverticulum
Enteritis
Leiomyoma
Infarction

Angiodysplasia

Carcinoma*/polyps

Ulcerative colitis

Carcinoma

Crohn's disease

Proximal colon

Rectum
Carcinoma*/polyps
Proctitis
Solitary ulcer

Diverticular disease *

Anus
Fissure *
Haemorrhoids *

Carcinoma

* = common causes

Bright red: anorectal cause, or significant distal or proximal bleeding
Dark red: suggests distal colonic bleeding
Altered/occult: suggests proximal bleeding

In younger patients haemorrhoids and colitis are common causes
In older patients diverticular disease, cancer and angiodysplasia are common causes

Station 113: Acute abdominal pain

Student info: *Mr EF has been referred by his GP to the surgical assessment unit with abdominal pain. Please take a history and present your differential diagnosis and initial management plan*

Patient info: *You are Mr EF, a 29-year-old male with a 12-hour history of worsening abdominal pain and nausea. The pain started gradually and was general at first, though now is constant in your right iliac fossa (RIF). Movements make this worse. You have nausea and decreased appetite but no vomiting. Your health is otherwise normal and there are no other symptoms of gastrointestinal disease*

Hints and tips

- Take a full history of the pain
- Do not forget to ask about radiation and migration
- Remember the typical pain patterns (see opposite)
- Include a full gastrointestinal history
- Has the patient needed surgery for anything previously?
- Associated history questions such as fever and weight loss
- Remember gynaecological symptoms in females or if there is a chance of pregnancy (ectopic)
- Elicit medication history
- Remember smoking and alcohol history
- General questions regarding the patient's health
- Assess the impact of the symptoms on the patient's life
- Address any concerns the patient has (i.e. his fears)
- Discuss a differential and agree a management plan

Discussion points

- What are the possible causes of this pain?
- What else might you consider in a female patient?
- What investigations would you request?
- What are the causes of referred abdominal pain?

ΔΔ: male	Appendicitis
	Ileal Crohn's disease
	Meckel's diverticulitis
ΔΔ: female	As above plus:
	Ovarian cyst
	Salpingitis/pelvic inflammatory disease (PID)
	Ectopic pregnancy

NB. Remember for approximately one-third of patients with RIF pain no cause may be found!

Ix	*Bloods*	FBC, U&E, G&S
		β-human chorionic gonadotrophin (β-HCG) in females
	Micro	Stool/urine culture if symptoms
Mx		Analgesia, IV fluids, antiemetics for nausea
		Nil by mouth until review by senior surgical team
		Consider abdodominal/transvaginal US in females

Station 114: Colorectal cancer

Student info: *Mr PR is 67 and has been referred to hospital by his GP with a history of altered bowel habit. Please take a history and present your differential diagnosis and initial investigations*

Patient info: *You are a 67-year-old male with a 2-month history of irregular bowel habit. Your bowels were previously normal and regular. You have had some loose motions, suffer occasional abdominal discomfort and bloating, and have lost weight despite a normal appetite. You have had an unhealthy diet for many years, with a high fat content; despite the weight loss, you are still overweight. Your current problems do not seem to be related to diet. You are very anxious about the possible cause*

Hints and tips

- Ascertain the patient's understanding of the reason the GP has referred him to hospital
- Ascertain the patient's normal and current bowel habit
- Enquire about symptoms of rectal mucus, bleeding or tenesmus
- Take an accurate history of the associated symptoms (abdominal pain, bloating, weight loss)
- Enquire about other associated systemic symptoms
- Ask about dietary intake and activities
- Determine the impact of symptoms on quality of life
- Establish PMH, DH and SH
- Address any concerns the patient may have
- Discuss a differential and agree a management plan

Discussion points

- What is your differential diagnosis?
- What investigations would you request?
- What are the risk factors for colorectal cancer?
- What potentially curative operations are available?

ΔΔ	Colonic adenocarcinoma, diverticular disease, IBS
Ix	Rigid sigmoidoscopy and proctoscopy when examined
	Bloods FBC, U&E, LFT, haematinics
	Imaging Barium enema
	Other Colonoscopy + biopsy

Station 115: Rectal bleeding

Student info: *Miss FW has been referred to the out-patient clinic by her GP with rectal bleeding. Please assess and advise the patient on your management plan*

Patient info: *You are Miss FW and are 23 years old. Over the past few months you have noticed intermittent rectal bleeding associated with bowel movements. The blood is on the toilet paper. Your bowel habit is regular. You have no previous history of GI disease and no medication. Your PMH includes two normal child births and a tonsillectomy*

Hints and tips

- Ascertain the patient's knowledge of the reason for referral
- Quantify the blood loss; is it mixed in with the stool? What colour is it?
- What is the patient's normal bowel habit?
- Is there any pain on bowel opening?
- Determine the associated symptoms especially any further red flags, e.g. weight loss

Discussion points

- What is your differential diagnosis?
- What investigations would you request?
- What treatments are available?

ΔΔ	See opposite
Ix	Rigid sigmoidoscopy and proctoscopy when examined
	Bloods FBC
	Other Flexi-sigmoidoscopy/colonoscopy

Station 116: Surgical abdominal examination

Describing areas of the abdomen

Midclavicular line

Epigastric | Hypochondrial

Transpyloric plane

Umbilical | Lumbar

Intertubercular line

Suprapubic | Iliac fossa

The upper areas can also be described simply as right/left upper quadrant

Identification of stomas

Transverse loop colostomy

PEG (percutaneous endoscopic gastrostomy), e.g. for feeding

Ileal conduit: formed with spout Urine product, e.g. following cystectomy

End colostomy: Flush with skin Faeces product, e.g. following rectal resection or as emergency Hartmann's procedure

Ileostomy: formed with spout (corrosive product) Watery output, e.g. following resection of large bowel, or temporarily protecting distal bowel anastamosis

Mucous fistula: Rectal stump brought to skin following sigmoid colectomy

Identification of scars

Rooftop (double Kocher's)
Liver, splenic, radical pancreatic, radical gastric, and bilateral adrenal surgery

Right Kocher's
Open cholecystectomy
Nephrectomy

Left Kocher's
Splenectomy
Nephrectomy

Renal surgery
Nephrectomy
Open pelviureteric surgery
Open stone surgery

Midline laparotomy

Paramedian laparotomy

Transverse laparotomy
Open AAA repair

Mc Burney's/ gridiron
Appendicectomy

Inguinal incision
Hernia repair
Radical orchidectomy

Pfannenstiel
Caesarean section
Gynaecological procedures
Bladder surgery

Rutherford Morrison
Renal transplant (usually right side)

Station 117: Digital rectal examination

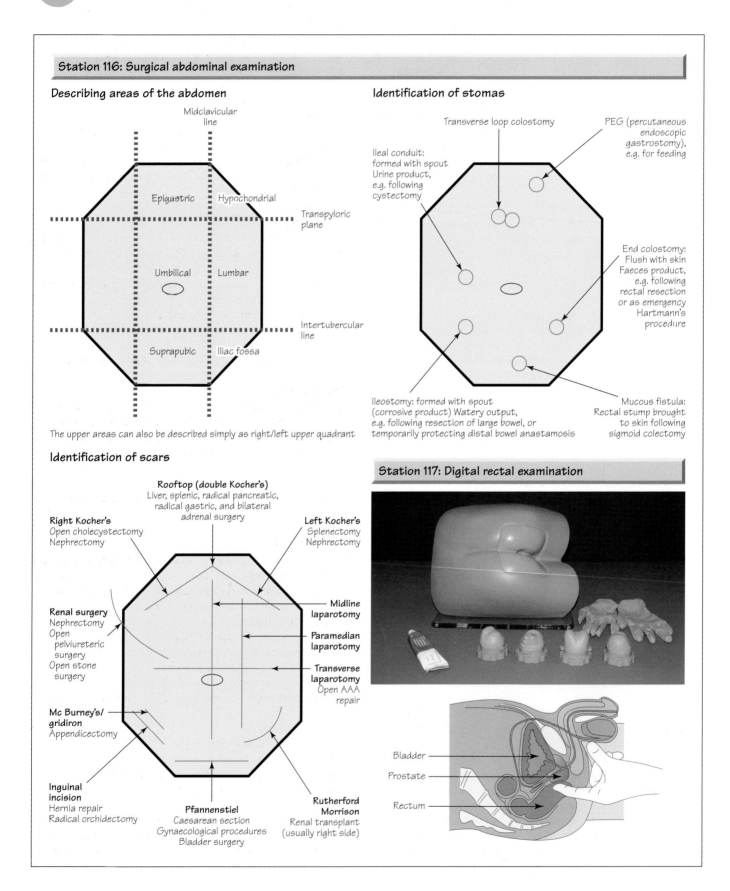

Bladder

Prostate

Rectum

Station 116: Surgical abdominal examination

- *This man had surgery last week. Please examine his abdomen*
- *Please inspect this woman's abdomen. Tell me what you see*
- *This man is coming for surgery next week, please examine his abdomen*

Examination routine

Listen carefully to the instruction: if asked to inspect then do not touch; if asked to examine the abdomen start peripherally. It is better to be moved on than to look as if you missed something out.

- Introduction/consent/ask about pain
- *Exposure*: traditionally the patient should be exposed 'from nipple to knees' but unless directed, adequate exposure is from xiphisternum to symphysis pubis
- *Position*: for surgical abdominal examination lie the patient flat – be prepared to lower the head of the bed yourself. Make sure the patient is comfortable with this position
- *General inspection*:
  - age of the patient
  - whether they are comfortable
  - their state of nutrition
  - jaundice
  - anaemia
  - venous lines for fluid/nutrition
  - appliances (e.g. stoma bags, urinary/suprapubic catheters)
- *Screening test*: ask the patient to lift their head off the bed (or to cough) to illicit any herniae
- *System-specific inspection*: specifically look at the abdomen for:
  - distension
  - asymmetry
  - pulsation
  - herniae
  - scars (operations, trauma, drain sites)
  - stomas
- Comment on your findings to the examiner as you see them if required. Note any dressings, and mention any tube drains you can see together with the colour/consistency of the draining fluid
- Proceed to examine the hands, looking for peripheral stigmata of abdominal disease (see Ch. 26). Continue to work more centrally as described in the medical examination of the abdomen. Do not worry if the examiner moves you on to focus on the abdomen to save time
- The majority of the information you need will be available on inspection alone in this part of the exam. Do not continue until you have really finished inspecting
- *Palpation*:
  - kneel down next to the bed so that you are at the same level as the patient
  - ask them clearly if they have any pain before starting. If they have ask them where, and make sure your examination initially starts as far away from this as possible
  - begin palpating superficially whilst looking at the patient's face and not your own hands. Gently palpate the nine areas of the abdomen in a methodical order. Repeat this again more deeply, examining carefully for tenderness and masses
  - if you encounter tenderness or cause the patient pain during your examination *stop!* Show that you have recognised this and apologise to the patient. If appropriate, ask them and/or the examiner whether you should continue with your examination. Failure to do this, blustering on,

or being unduly rough in your examination technique is a common cause of failing this OSCE station

  - make it clear that you are examining for both hepatomegaly and splenomegaly (both starting in right iliac fossa)
  - ballot the kidneys in turn
  - gently palpate in the epigastrium with your fingertips, feeling for the expansile mass of an abdominal aortic aneurysm
  - if appropriate, examine for the dome of a distended bladder
  - see Chapter 26 for more information
- *Percussion*:
  - you may be required to define the boundaries of a liver or spleen, assess ascites or define the boundaries of a large bladder
  - the principles of this are similar to those for any other percussion
  - ascites needs to be demonstrated by the presence of shifting dullness (see Ch. 26)
- *Auscultation*:
  - listen for bowel sounds and bruits
  - bowel sounds are variable and you should listen (or explain that you would normally listen) for 30 seconds. Note their presence, absence and pitch
- *Completion*: cover the patient and thank them. Inform the examiner that you would like to:
  - perform a digital rectal examination (DRE)
  - examine the external genitalia (if not already done)
  - review the observation charts
  - perform a urine dipstick test (?UTI ?renal colic ?renal function)

Hints and tips

- Let any scars present guide you – are they hiding an incisional hernia? Is there a transplanted kidney under a scar in the right iliac fossa?
- If you reach the end of your examination and you have not found any positive findings, do not panic – there may not necessarily be any!

Station 117: Digital rectal examination

- *Please explain the procedure of digital rectal examination to this patient and then demonstrate the technique using the mannequin provided*

Hints and tips

This is considered an essential part of the abdominal examination. Whilst it is very unlikely you would be asked to perform this, you should be able to describe the technique and be able to demonstrate on a model.

- Explain the procedure and why you need to do it
- Obtain verbal consent
- Request a chaperone and gather equipment
- Ask the patient to lower their clothing and roll onto their left side
- Ask them to bring knees up to their chest
- Inspect the perianal area, perineum and buttocks
- With a gloved lubricated index finger, gently enter the anal canal and rectum
- Note anal sphincter tone
- Check the contents of rectum – empty? hard faeces?
- Obvious mass (indentable? faeces?)
- Smoothly run your finger 360° over palpable mucosa
- Note prostate in men – sulcus palpable? size?
- Remove finger and examine glove – blood? melaena?

A DRE is not just looking for prostate or rectal cancer – it also useful for assessing constipation, per rectum (PR) bleeding, neurological injury, perianal fissure (this is so painful, DRE may not be possible) and pelvic appendicitis, amongst others.

Station 118: Abdominal stoma

Common conditions potentially requiring an operation and stoma

See Chapter 45 for typical stoma locations

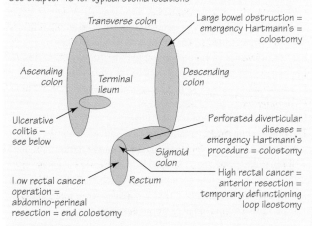

Transverse colon

Large bowel obstruction = emergency Hartmann's = colostomy

Ascending colon

Terminal ileum

Descending colon

Ulcerative colitis – see below

Perforated diverticular disease = emergency Hartmann's procedure = colostomy

Sigmoid colon

Low rectal cancer operation = abdomino-perineal resection = end colostomy

Rectum

High rectal cancer = anterior resection = temporary defunctioning loop ileostomy

Ulcerative colitis = ileostomy (temporary or permanent, depending on procedure). Operation may be either:
1. subtotal colectomy (rectum remains)
2. pan-proctocolectomy (all colon and rectum excised)
If stoma temporary → loop ileostomy (easier to reverse)
If permanent → end ileostomy

Hartmann's procedure is performed as a quick 'emergency stoma' in patients for whom a primary anastomosis of bowel is contraindicated. This may be due to local intra-abdominal contamination (e.g. pus, faeces) or systemic problems (e.g. generalised sepsis, cardiovascular instability). In these cases the anastamosis may not heal, hence a stoma is the preferred option. This may be reversible once the patient has recovered (if they wish and are fit for a further operation)

Identifying abdominal masses on examination

Liver
- Right upper quadrant – may extend to right iliac fossa
- Dull to percussion (as opposed to bowel which may be resonant)
- Moves towards right iliac fossa with inspiration
- Cannot palpate above it

Gallbladder
- Located in right upper quadrant below tip of ninth rib
- Moves with respiration (remember Murphy's sign when inflamed)

Spleen
- Left upper quadrant – may extend towards right iliac fossa
- Dull to percussion (as opposed to bowel which may be resonant)
- Moves inferiorly with respiration
- Cannot palpate above it
- May have a notch palpable on the medial border

Kidney
- Overlying bowel means this may be resonant to percussion
- Right kidney lies lower. Distal tip may be palpated in normal patient
- Can be bimanually palpated (balloted)

Bowel
- Generally mobile
- May be resonant to percussion if flatus present

Station 119: Abdominal mass

The six 'F's of abdominal swellings:

Fat
Centripetal obesity may give the impression of abdominal distension, and even when it is recognised it can make accurate palpation of the abdomen difficult

Fluid
Ascites: test for shifting dullness (see Chapter 26)

Flatus
This may be normal for the patient, or may result from abnormal retention of swallowed air as in the case of large or small bowel obstruction

Faeces
May be palpable in patients, particularly in the descending colon in the constipated. Faeces should be indentable

Fetus
In a woman of child-bearing age who may (or may not!) be aware she is pregnant. This mass will arise from the pelvis and you will not be able to get below it

'Flipping' big mass
An obviously abnormal mass may arise from within the abdomen, pelvis or abdominal wall

Fothergill's sign is used to distinguish between masses arising from within the pelvis or abdomen as opposed to those arising from within the abdominal wall (e.g. hernia or rectus sheath haematoma). Ask the supine patient to bend forward lifting their shoulders off the bed. Tensing the abdominal musculature to do this means a mass within the abdominal cavity becomes impalpable, whereas a mass arising from the abdominal wall may still be palpated

Possible causes of an abdominal mass

Right upper quadrant
Liver
Kidney
Colon
Gallbladder

Left upper quadrant
Spleen
Stomach
Pancreas
Kidney

Retroperitoneal masses
Lymphadenopathy
Sarcoma

Abdominal aortic aneurysm (AAA)
Palpable expansile swelling proximal to the aortic bifurcation (which is at the level of the umbilicus).

Omental swellings
Secondary cancer

Left iliac fossa
Descending colon/ sigmoid
Ovarian mass
Fallopian tube (eg ectopic)
Pelvic kidney

Right iliac fossa
Caecum and ascending colon
Appendix mass
Ovarian mass
Fallopian tube (e.g. ectopic)
Pelvic kidney (see station 3)

Umbilical and suprapubic
Bladder
Rectum
Fetus
Uterus

Station 118: Abdominal stoma

This is a common case in abdominal OSCE stations. Be familiar with different stomas, and be prepared to suggest the operation and possible indications for this given the type of stoma and age of the patient.

• *This patient had surgery 5 days ago. Please examine her abdomen and present your findings*

Examination routine

• Take plenty of time to inspect and describe your findings
• *Inspection*:
  • ensure the patient is recumbent
  • note any discomfort or peripheral stigmata of abdominal disease. Is there a recent midline laparotomy wound (note staples if used for abdominal closure)?
  • describe the stoma bag covering the stoma, e.g. 'stoma bag containing light brown liquid stool, stoma pink and healthy appears to be a . . .' (select appropriate): 'spouted end ileostomy in the right iliac fossa' *or* 'flush colostomy in the left iliac fossa'
• *Palpation*:
  • is the abdomen soft and non-tender?
  • are there any masses or organomegaly?
• Although you are unlikely to do this in an exam, at this stage you should offer to remove the stoma bag to inspect the stoma and surrounding skin ± perform a digital stoma examination depending on your findings and the patient's complaint
• *Percussion and auscultation*: are there any abnormalities?
• *Completion*:
  • offer to inspect the perineum and perform a PR as appropriate. Depending on the type of stoma the patient may not have an anus!
  • inspect the fluid balance chart/stoma output chart/blood results (new stomas may initially have a large fluid output affecting the patient's fluid balance)
  • offer to ask the patient some questions about how they are managing with their stoma, e.g. is it sited in the right position for them? Are they able to change the bag themselves? Do they have any leak from around it? NB. Be careful not to miss common complications, e.g. parastomal hernia.

Discussion points

• What type of stoma do you think this is? Why?
• What different types of stoma do you know about?
• What metabolic complications may follow an ileostomy?
• What operation might this patient have had?
• What stoma complications are you aware of?

Station 119: Abdominal mass

• *This man is awaiting surgery. Please examine his abdomen*

Examination routine

• *Inspection*:
  • ensure the patient is recumbent
  • note any discomfort or peripheral stigmata of abdominal disease. Are there signs of recent or previous surgery?
  • is the abdomen symmetrical?
  • describe clearly any obvious swelling and relation to abdominal scars

• ask the patient to cough to ensure this is not a hernial swelling (e.g. incisional hernia, which may obviously increase in size with such a rapid rise in intra-abdominal pressure)
• *Palpation*:
  • as for the previous examination
  • be methodical in your examination, as you would for any swelling (site, size, surface, shape, expansile, tenderness, etc.). Take time to try and identify the origin of the swelling (see opposite) and be prepared to justify why you think this is liver/stomach, etc. Ask the patient to lift their head and shoulders a little off the bed and see if the mass is still palpable (e.g. does the mass arise from the abdominal wall or from within the abdominal cavity – Fothergill's sign)
• *Percussion*: as normal, including over the swelling to test for resonance
• *Auscultation*: be sure to listen over the swelling for bowel sounds
• *Completion*: as for previous station

Discussion points

• What is the differential diagnosis for a right-sided abdominal mass?
• What is the classic triad of symptoms for patients presenting with a renal tumour?
• How can you differentiate a left renal mass from splenomegaly?
• How can you differentiate a liver mass from colonic?

Station 120: Renal transplant

• *Mr FT has an inherited kidney problem, please examine his abdomen*

Hints and tips

• Examine the abdomen as per Chapter 26
• Observe carefully for any evidence of fistulae, transplant scar or previous Tenckhoff catheter insertion sites
• Inspect for signs of anaemia
• Look for evidence of immunosuppressive treatment, e.g. Cushingoid appearance if on steroids or gum hypertrophy if on cyclosporin
• There may be bilateral masses in the flanks (NB you may only be able to feel one side) if the reason for transplant was acute polycystic kidney disease
• There may be a typical curved inguinal incision present overlying the transplanted kidney (Rutherford–Morrison incision)
• Palpate the scar for the underlying kidney as they are sometimes removed
• There may be a previous nephrectomy scar in the flank

Discussion points

• What are the most common reasons for renal transplantation?
• What are the complications of renal transplant?

Complications   Rejection – acute/chronic
Increased incidence of infections due to immunosuppression
Increased incidence of malignancy (skin, lymphoma)
Increased incidence of cardiovascular disease
Side effects of drugs
Recurrence of the original underlying disease

Station 121: Groin examination

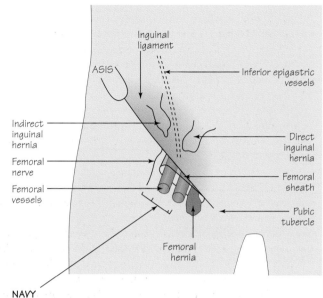

NAVY
Order of structures can be remembered with this mnemonic:
Nerve, **A**rtery, **V**ein, **Y**-fronts! (from lateral to medial)

Anatomy

• Examination relies heavily on anatomical knowledge. You will be expected to demonstrate your knowledge of this in order to differentiate an inguinal from a femoral hernia, and a direct from an indirect inguinal hernia

• Key surface landmarks are:
    – anterior superior iliac spine (ASIS)
    – pubic tubercle

• The inguinal ligament runs between the two
• This is formed from the fibres of the external oblique aponeurosis and reflects to form the inguinal canal
• The spermatic cord enters the inguinal canal half way along the ligament – the mid-point of the inguinal ligament
• This is the location of the deep inguinal ring
• Not to be confused with the mid-inguinal point which is half way between the symphysis pubis and the ASIS and which marks the surface landmark of the femoral artery

• The pubic tubercle is a small bony projection on the crest of the pubis. It can be difficult to find below overlying fat! Practise on yourself. A useful trick is to locate the easily palpable adductor longus tendon in the medial proximal thigh and follow this up into its insertion on the crest of the pubis just below the tubercle

Station 122: Groin swellings

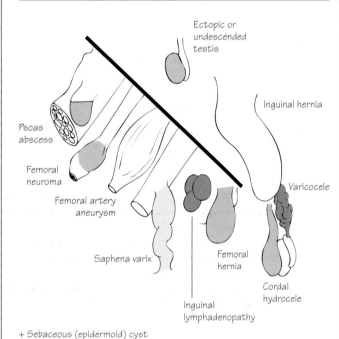

+ Sebaceous (epidermoid) cyst
+ Lipoma

Differentiating hernias

Femoral hernia
• Lie below and lateral to pubic tubercle
• May be small and can be difficult to palpate
• More common in women
• Strangulation is frequent

Boundaries of the femoral ring
Anterior: inguinal ligament
Posterior: pectineus muscle overlying crest of pubis
Medial: lacunar ligament
Lateral: femoral vein
NB. The femoral ring forms the opening of the femoral canal

Inguinal hernia
• Lie above and medial to the pubic tubercle
• May become very large
• Indirect hernias may pass along a patent processus vaginalis to descend into the scrotum

Deep ring = opening in transversalis fascia

Superficial ring = opening in external oblique

Walls of the inguinal canal
Anterior: Aponeurosis of external oblique + internal oblique for lateral third
Posterior: Tranversalis fascia + conjoint tendon for medial third
Roof: Internal oblique and transversus abdominis
Floor: Inguinal ligament

Stations 121 and 122: Groin examination and groin swellings

• *Please examine this man's groin*
• *This patient has noticed some discomfort in her groin, please examine and discuss your findings with the examiner*

Possible cases in an OSCE
• Inguinal hernia (direct/indirect)
• Inguinal lymphadenopathy
• Saphena varix
• Femoral artery aneurysm

Unlikely cases in an OSCE
Repair of a femoral hernia is a surgical priority so is less likely to appear in an OSCE but you may be asked to discuss it.

Examination routine
• Listen carefully to the instruction given at the station. An instruction to examine the groin could cover pathology in both the groin and scrotum
• Introduction/consent/ask about pain
• *Exposure*: the patient should have their trousers and underwear removed and be covered with a sheet
• *Position*:
  • the position depends on the instruction
  • there is confusion about whether you should examine the patient lying down or standing up – it does not really matter on the order, but you must do both
  • it is probably easier to start with the patient lying down whilst you perform the inspection and then ask them to stand for palpation
  • herniae and varicoceles are sometimes only seen when the patient is standing up
  • try not to have the patient standing up and lying down several times!
• *General inspection*: general features of systemic disease. Are they well/unwell?
• *Screening test*: ask the patient to cough
• *System-specific inspection*: are any of the following visible?
  • obvious swelling
  • scars/sinuses
  • abnormal position or lie of the testis
  • discoloration, e.g. saphena varix
  • oedema
  • ulceration
  • lymph nodes
• If not already done, ask the patient to cough to see if this reveals any herniae
• *Palpation*:
  • examine from the side
  • initially demonstrate the anatomy (pubic tubercle, anterior iliac spine, inguinal ligament)
  • feel for any herniae, lumps or abnormalities and assess:

site	temperature
size	composition
surface	cough impulse
shape	reducibility
tenderness	controllability

  • if allowed, ask the patient if they can reduce the lump

• *Completion*:
  • also examine or ask to examine the contralateral groin and/or scrotum
  • consider a complete abdominal examination
  • cardiovascular and respiratory examinations may be necessary if considering operation
  • a full lymph node and abdominal examination would also be required if lymph nodes were the finding

Discussion points
• What is the difference between a direct and indirect hernia?
• What are the boundaries of the inguinal canal/rings?
• What are the boundaries of the femoral canal/ring?
• What are the complications of herniorrhaphy?
• Classify your differential of a groin lump

Inguinal hernia (direct/indirect): hints and tips
This is the most common groin lump in the OSCE. Knowledge of groin anatomy is key to this examination.
• Inspect first – is there an obvious hernia?
• If it is in the scrotum it must be indirect
• If no hernia is immediately visible then ask the patient to cough and also examine the patient standing up
• If there is a hernia present ask the patient if it 'goes back' (reduces), if it does ask them to reduce it (without causing discomfort) and then demonstrate whether it is indirect or direct by controlling the deep inguinal ring at the mid-point of the inguinal ligament
• If it can be controlled (i.e. an indirect inguinal hernia), the hernia will not reappear when, with your fingers over the deep ring, you ask them to cough or strain
• Remember you cannot 'get above' a hernia – a discrete mass in the scrotum is not a hernia!

Causes of a groin lump

Soft tissue	Lipoma
	Lymphadenopathy
Hernias	Inguinal
	Femoral
Vascular	Saphena varix
	Femoral artery aneurysm
Genitourinary system	Undescended testis
	Renal transplant

Principles of repair
• Because of the lower risk of complication and strangulation, an asymptomatic direct inguinal hernia does not have to be repaired, depending on the patient's wishes
• Femoral hernias have the highest risk of strangulation, and as such these will commonly be repaired as scheduled elective cases (i.e. as a priority)
• Recurrent hernias may now be repaired laparoscopically, as open surgery is difficult due to the presence of scar tissue

Station 123: Neck examination

Examination hints

- Remember the basics and define as for any lump:
  - Site
  - Size
  - Surface
  - Shape

- Associated features, e.g. pulsatility, lymph nodes, etc.
- Special examinations, e.g. tongue protrusion, swallowing

Anatomical regions in the neck

The anatomical triangles of the neck are useful clinically as different lumps can arise in each (see diagrams)

Anterior triangle borders
Midline of neck - anterior border of sternocleidomastoid ramus of mandible

Posterior triangle borders
Posterior border sternocleidomastoid clavicle - trapezius

General neck examination

1. Introduction and permission
- Position – neck and upper chest exposed, sitting upright away from wall, table, etc.
- Any pain in the neck?

2. Inspect
- Swelling (describe fully as above, including which triangle it is in)
- Scars esp. thyroid or parotid?
- Asymmetry of neck or face

3. Special tests
'Please take a sip from this glass of water and hold it in your mouth until I say swallow'. Get into clear viewing position. 'Now swallow for me'. Does mass rise upwards with swallowing? 'Now stick your tongue out at me'. Does lump rise with tongue protrusion?

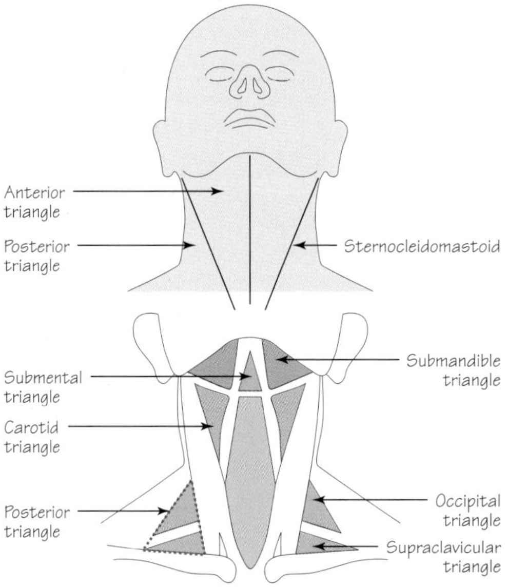

4. Palpation of the lump
- Repeat special tests, this time palpating the neck
- Further characterise lump on palpation, e.g. fluctuant, tender, tethered to skin

5. Palpate surrounding structures
- Lymph nodes (be able to name the different groups in the neck)
- Always look inside mouth (+ offer to examine ears if appropriate)
- Carotid pulses present/normal?
- Trachea midline?
- Offer to examine remainder of face and scalp if appropriate

6. Decision as to likely nature of lump

Diagram labels: Anterior triangle, Posterior triangle, Sternocleidomastoid, Submental triangle, Carotid triangle, Posterior triangle, Submandibular triangle, Occipital triangle, Supraclavicular triangle

If suspecting thyroid origin:
- Percuss sternum (retrosternal extension?)
- Auscultation of lump for bruit
- Offer to examine thyroid status (see Chapter 41)

If suspecting parotid origin:
- Note unilateral or bilateral
- Bimanual palpation of the gland
- Examine divisions of the facial nerve

If suspecting cystic hygroma:
- Seen in infants
- Transilluminates brightly

Station 124: Neck lumps

Thyroid swellings (goitre)
See Chapter 42 for thyroid disease
Solitary nodules need investigation to exclude carcinoma:
- Papillary carcinoma (60% of cases)
- Follicular carcinoma (25% of cases)
- Anaplastic carcinoma (10% of cases)
- Medullary carcinoma (5% of cases)

Parotid swellings
Consider:
- Stone or infection (may be secondary to stone)
- Malignancy (80% of salivary tumours in parotid gland; 80% of these are pleomorphic adenomas)

Location of neck lumps

Anterior triangle
- Thyroid lump
- Branchial cyst
- Cystic hydroma
- Carotid body tumours
- Salivary gland pathology (including parotid)

Posterior triangle
- Cervical rib

Midline
- Thyroglossal cyst
- Dermoid cyst

Anywhere
- Lymph nodes
- Note multiple lumps most likely to be lymph nodes
- Remember general causes of lymphadenopathy!

Station 123: Neck examination

The history is as for any other lump (see Ch. 50). Also refer to the endocrine and ENT chapters.

- *Please examine this woman's neck*
- *You may be directed towards the swelling (e.g. 'examine the parotid') or you may have to decide where to direct the examination yourself on the basis of initial findings*

Possible cases in an OCSE

- Lymphadenopathy
- Thyroid lumps
- Parotid swellings
- Other causes of neck swellings are much rarer in exams

Hints and tips

- *Do not start with peripheral signs of thyroid disease in a surgical OSCE station.* This is a common mistake – you must examine the lump first – it may not be thyroid in origin!
- Follow the basic line of examination shown opposite. Some important points of the neck examination are specific to different abnormalities
- *Thyroid lumps*:
  - rise on swallowing
  - do not rise with tongue protrusion
  - may extend into the chest behind the sternum
  - may have an overlying bruit (= likely Grave's)
  - know the thyroid state examination including relevant points in the history
- *Thyroglossal cysts*:
  - rise with tongue protrusion
  - also rise with swallowing!
- *Parotid lumps*:
  - may extend inside the mouth
  - it is important to visualise the internal salivary duct opening
  - an invasion of facial nerves means a malignant cause is more likely
  - bimanual palpation – is there a stone?
- *Cystic hygroma*: fluid filled and transilluminates brightly

Station 124: Neck lumps

Follow the basic line of examination shown opposite. To work out the aetiology consider the following.

Thyroid swellings

What is the nature of the swelling – diffuse, single or multinodular?

1 *Diffuse goitre*:
- Is the patient toxic? (likely Graves')
- Other causes:
  - physiological (e.g. puberty, pregnancy)
  - iodine deficiency
  - thyroiditis (frequently tender)
  - autoimmune (Hashimoto's)

2 *Single nodule*:
- May be single palpable nodule of multi-nodular goitre!
- Carcinoma always needs excluding
- Other causes:
  - adenoma
  - cyst

3 *Multinodular goitre*: can be due to benign hyperplasia/Grave's disease

Discussion points

- What is your differential diagnosis?
- What are the indications for thyroid surgery?
- What different operations are available?
- What are the complication of thyroid surgery?

Ix   *Bloods*   Thyroid function tests
                    Consider thyroid antibodies
    Imaging   Ultrasound
    Histology Fine needle aspiration cytology (with US guidance for solitary nodule)

Parotid swellings

Are they bilateral or unilateral?

1 *Bilateral causes include*:
- Viral infection (mumps)
- Bacterial infection (ascending sialadenitis)
- Inflammatory conditions (e.g. sarcoid, Wegener's)

2 *Unilateral causes include*:
- Salivary duct obstruction
- Salivary gland/duct stone
- Mucocele
- Neoplasm

Discussion points

- What is your differential diagnosis?
- What are the complications of parotid surgery?

Ix   *Bloods*   Thyroid function tests
    Imaging   Sialogram if appropriate (?stone)
                    CT/MRI head if appropriate
    Histology Fine needle aspiration cytology (US guided) if biopsy is required

Differential diagnosis of a neck lump

- *Thyroid*:
  - goitre
  - cyst
  - neoplasm
- *Neoplastic*:
  - primary lymphoma
  - secondary metastasis
  - salivary gland tumour
  - sternocleidomastoid tumour
  - carotid body tumour
- *Inflammatory*:
  - viral/bacterial lymphadenopathy
  - parotitis
- *Congenital*:
  - branchial cyst
  - cystic hydroma
  - dermoid cyst
- *Vascular*:
  - subclavian aneurysm
  - subclavian ectasia
  - carotid ectasia
  - carotid body tumour

Station 125: Breast history

History hints

- Is there a lump or pain in the breast?
- Location: quadrants, proximity to nipple, unilateral vs bilateral
- Tenderness (inflammatory, e.g. abscess)
- Are there any changes in the nipple?
- Discharge/bleeding from the nipple?
- Timing: how long has the change or lump been present?
- Timing: mid-cycle tenderness (fibrocystic change)
- ?Currently breast feeding (mastitis)
- Establish presence of any risk factors for breast cancer

Risk factors for breast cancer

Living in a developed country
Familial breast cancer (5% cases)
Previous proliferative breast disease
Early menarche: age 10 vs 15 years = 3x risk
Late first child: 5 vs 20 years post menarche = 3x risk
Late menopause: age 55 vs 45 years = 3x risk
Others:
- Nulliparity
- Exogenous hormones (HRT)
- Smoking

Station 126: Breast examination

ESSENTIALS CHECKLIST (WINCER)

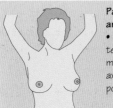

Patient sits with arms by side
- Inspect breasts, skin and nipples for abnormalities

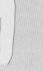

Patient raises arms in the air
- Look for any tethering or masses. Inspect axillae in this position

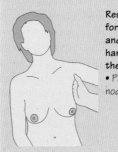

Patient presses hands into hips (to tense pectoralis major muscles)
- This will reveal any dimpling of the skin or fixation to underlying muscle

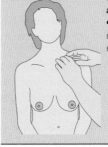

Rest the patient's forearm on yours and use the other hand to examine the axilla
- Palpate for any nodes

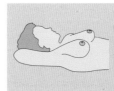

Patient sits with arms by side
- Examine for supraclavicular nodes

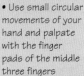

Lie the patient flat with one hand behind her head and examine each breast in turn

- Use small circular movements of your hand and palpate with the finger pads of the middle three fingers
- Work systematically over the breast
- Remember to examine the axillary tail

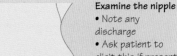
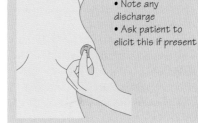

Examine the nipple
- Note any discharge
- Ask patient to elicit this if present

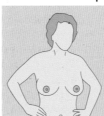

Station 125: Breast history

Student info: *This woman presents with a lump in her right breast. Please take a history from her*

Patient info: *You are Miss KL, a 32-year-old woman. Your PC is a lump in the right breast which was first noticed as a non-tender lump whilst in the shower 10 days ago. There are no changes in the skin and no nipple discharge. You are mid menstrual cycle. Your menarche was at 13 years. PMH: nil; drugs: oral contraceptive pill (OCP); allergies: nil. You are married with no children. You are a non-smoker and occasionally drink alcohol. Your mother and aunt both have had surgery for breast cancer*

Hints and tips

- See the history hints box opposite
- As with any surgical lump, obtain as much information about it from the patient in the history as possible: site, size, shape, tenderness, when it was first noticed, is it enlarging or shrinking, cycling in size, etc.
- Address patient concerns: this patient is likely to be particularly worried due to her family history

Discussion points

- What are the risk factors for breast cancer identified in this history?
- In which quadrant of the breast are cancers found most commonly?
- What are the benign causes of breast lumps?
- How do we stage breast cancer?

Possible causes of a breast lump	Cyst – usual onset around menopause
	Carcinoma – typically older patients
	Fat necrosis – related to trauma
	Fibroadenoma – younger patients, mobile lump
Causes of breast pain	Breast pain is an uncommon symptom of breast cancer
	Cyclical mastalgia
	Non-cyclical, e.g. usually musculoskeletal chest wall
Nipple discharge	Physiological or pathological:
	Lactation
	Hyperprolactinaemia
	Galactorrhoea
	Duct ectasia/papilloma
	Breast cancer
Ix	Triple assessment:
	clinical history and examination
	radiological assessment (mammogram or US)
	pathological assessment (biopsy or cytology)

Station 126: Breast examination

- *Please examine this woman's right breast*
- *Using the mannequin provided, please demonstrate examination of the right breast*

Common cases in an OCSE

- Normal breasts
- Carcinoma
- Cyst
- Fibroadenoma/fibroadenosis

Examination routine

- Introduction/consent/ask about pain
- *Exposure and position*:
  - patient removes upper body clothing, in gown, sitting up on edge of couch
  - briefly describe examination to them and obtain permission
  - patient removes gown and sits with arms by side
- *Inspection*:
  - overview of the breasts: symmetry or obvious masses
  - skin: scars, dimpling, peau d'orange, retraction
  - nipples: position, inversion, retraction, erythema, bleeding (Paget's disease of nipple), discharge
- *Manoeuvres*: examine both breasts whilst asking the patient to perform these manoeuvres:
  - patient raises arms above head. Look for: change in the relative position of the mass; nipple or skin tethering; look in axillae while patient's arms are raised
  - patient pushes hands down on hips, tensing pectoralis muscles. Look for: dimpling or fixation
- *Palpation of breasts*:
  - the patient now lies back at 45° with hands placed behind their head
  - using the fingerpads of your hand, gently press the breast against the chest wall by rolling fingers in small, circular motions. Work systematically over the breast
  - palpate the tail of the breast (the part extending towards the axilla) between fingers and thumb
- *Palpation of the nipples*:
  - palpate around the areola
  - palpate depression under nipple
  - note any discharge (ask patient to elicit as appropriate): if present, note unilateral or bilateral, colour, blood staining, single or multiple ducts
- *Palpation of nodes*:
  - examine the axillary and supraclavicular nodes
  - to examine axillary nodes, rest the patient's forearm on yours to relax the muscles and palpate the four walls and roof of the axillae
- Repeat the examination on the other side
- *Completion*:
  - offer to examine the abdomen, palpating for a liver (?metastases)
  - offer to examine the chest for a pleural effusion
  - ensure the patient is comfortable and appropriately covered up after your examination

Discussion points

- What are the risk factors for breast cancer?
- Breast screening: who, when, how?
- What are the features of a cancer on a mammogram?
- What are the treatment options for a patient with breast cancer?

Station 127: Examination of a lump

Key characteristic of any lump:
Site = Describe this anatomically, with reference to a fixed bony landmark if possible
Size = Estimate or use a tape measure
Surface = Describe the surface appearance
Shape = What does it look like? Ovoid? Hemispherical?

Other points to describe as appropriate to the lump (not all will be required every time):
Colour = Is it black and necrotic? Is it red and inflamed?
Consistency = Hard, firm or soft?
Tethering = Fixed to skin? Fixed to muscle?
Transilluminance = Shine a torch through it
Tenderness = Be gentle when assessing this
Temperature = Use back of hand to assess
Fluctuance = Place fingers of one hand either side. Pressing on a fluctuant lump with a finger from the other hand displaces the fingers either side of it
Pulsatility = As for an abdominal aortic aneurysm, is the mass expansile?
Origin = Where did the lump arise from?
Reducibility = Can it be pushed back in (hernia)?
Local lymph nodes = Never forget to assess these

Station 128: Lipoma

Benign fatty growths
Mostly subcutaneous, though GI or intramuscular forms arise
Slow growing in nature
Most common soft tissue tumour
Important to differentiate from malignant soft tissue tumours
Surgically excised (usually under local anaesthetic) for cosmesis if patient wishes, or for histopathology
Local recurrence can occur

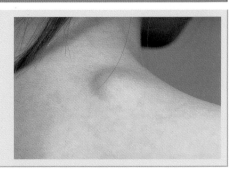

Station 129: Epidermoid cyst

aka sebaceous cyst
Do not have sebaceous origin!
Slow growing in nature
Can become inflamed and infected with associated discharge
Very rarely malignancy may arise from within them
Commonly found on the trunk, neck, scalp, limbs, face and scrotum
May be surgically excised (usually under local anaesthetic) for cosmesis or infections
Local recurrence can occur

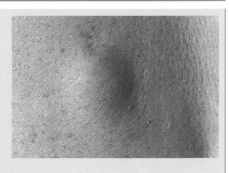

Station 128: Lipoma

• *Please examine the lump on this woman's shoulder*

Examination routine

• Listen carefully to the instruction: if asked to inspect, do not touch
• Introduce yourself to the patient and ask their permission to describe your findings and/or examine the lump
• Establish what concerns the patient has regarding this lump
• *Inspection*: describe the key characteristics as listed above
  • the absence of a punctum (see next station) is an important negative finding on inspection
• *Palpation*: ensure there is no tenderness prior to examining
  • lipomas may be fluctuant due to the contained fat being liquid at body temperature
  • they may feel lobulated
  • the 'slip sign' is classic for a lipoma – as it is not tethered to the skin, the lump slips away from you as you press it; lipomas are separate from the overlying skin
• *Completion*: thank the patient. Ensure they are covered up
ΔΔ   Lipoma, epidermoid cyst, liposarcoma
Ix   Usually the diagnosis is obvious and made clinically and no specific investigations are required
      If liposarcoma is suspected then specialist referral is required for imaging and tissue biopsy

Station 129: Epidermoid cyst

• *Please examine this woman's neck. Tell me what you see*

Examination routine

Proceed as with the case above. A sebaceous cyst is the main differential for a lipoma, but has several key differences on examination.
• *Inspection*: epidermoid cysts are typically hemispherical in shape
  • there may be associated erythema if the contents have become infected
  • having outlined the key points as for any lump, specifically look at the surface of the lump for a punctum
  • a cheese-like material may discharge through this
• *Palpation*: epidermoid cysts arise within the skin, such that the overlying skin cannot be 'pinched' over it. However, they are mobile over the tissues underlying this
  • the patient may be able to express the contents of the cyst through the punctum on squeezing
  • the consistency is usually firm
• *Completion*: thank the patient. Ensure they are covered up

ΔΔ   Epidermoid cyst, lipoma (malignancy can arise in rare cases)
Ix   Usually a clinical diagnosis
      If malignancy is suspected then specialist referral is required for imaging and tissue biopsy

Station 130: Preoperative assessment

A patient must be assessed for fitness to undergo the planned surgery in order to minimise potentially avoidable morbidity, mortality and cancelled operations. It encompasses:
• Medical optimisation preoperatively for both the anaesthetic and the surgery
• Obtaining relevant investigations to allow this
• Informed consent – make sure the patient knows what is being considered and why
• Plan for the particular operation and patient, e.g. ensure cross-matched blood will be available for an abdominal aortic aneurysm repair, bowel prep prescribed for colonic surgery or ITU booked for a high risk operation

Previous medical history
This will guide your functional enquiry and choice of investigations. Try to think what tests an anaesthetist might want before the operation. For example:
• CVS: ECG, echocardiography, exercise tolerance test
• Respiratory system: lung function tests, optimising asthma/COPD
• Is further specialist assessment of these systems required?

Medications
The effects of many drugs need to be considered before an anaesthetic/surgery. For example:
• Antibiotics – does the patient need preoperative antibiotics?
• Anticoagulants – what is the indication? Do they need stopping? Check clotting
• Antiplatelets – do they need stopping?
• Steroids – may need extra perioperatively
• Diuretics – check U&Es
• Insulin and other medications for diabetes – think about sliding scale and optimising control
• Digoxin – check K+

Allergies
Drugs e.g. antibiotics
Other substances, e.g.:
• Latex (most theatre gloves are latex)
• Iodine (often used as skin prep)
• Plaster (used in orthopaedics)
• Elastoplast

Family history
Important because:
• Patient may have specific concerns due to family members' experiences
• Patient may have an inherited condition that affects the surgery or anaesthetic (e.g. sickle cell anaemia)

Social history
• Smoker - more likely to have cardiorespiratory problems and post-op problems, e.g. chest infection, poor wound healing, etc.
• Alcohol consumption – altered liver function (clotting, drug metabolism); may have post-op withdrawl
• Is the patient going to be able to cope postoperatively?
  – Who's at home?
  – What is their performance status pre-op?
• Religious/cultural beliefs, e.g. Jehovah's Witnesses cannot receive blood transfusions.

Remember...
Cancelled operations due to avoidable problems (e.g. warfarin not stopped, blood not available) costs time and money and causes distress to the patient
Morbidity or mortality due to avoidable medical complications cost even more
If in doubt, ask the anaesthetist who is covering that operating list

Station 130: Preoperative assessment

Student info: *This patient is coming in for an anterior resection in 2 weeks time. You are the FY1 in the pre-assessment clinic. Please take and present a preoperative history*

Patient info: *You are Mr BW and are 69 years old. PC: rectal tumour; HPC: presented with PR bleeding. You were investigated with sigmoidoscopy plus biopsy and CT scan. PMH: hypertension, myocardial infarction 5 years ago; meds: aspirin, atenolol, bendroflumethiazide, simvastatin; allergies: penicillin. You have no significant family history. You live alone as your wife died of breast cancer 6 years ago. Systems review: patient gets chest pain on climbing stairs*

Hints and tips
• Remember that the history may contain more than one issue for discussion
• Work systematically through each area of the history
• Do not miss any areas out – if you do not ask the patient they may not volunteer the information (e.g. allergies)
• Focus on any potential problems in the systems review – try and quantify how significant a problem might be (e.g. with ischaemic heart disease, what is their exercise tolerance?)

Discussion points
• Ischaemic heart disease:
  • is the patient fit for anaesthetic?
  • are further investigations needed? ECG, echo, exercise tolerance test?
  • discuss with cardiologist/anaesthetist?
• Drugs:
  • ?stop aspirin pre-op
  • bendroflumethiazide – check U&Es
• Penicillin allergy: how severe was the reaction – rash or anaphylaxis?
• Social: living alone may cause problems with discharge and rehabilitation. Death of wife from cancer may exacerbate concerns

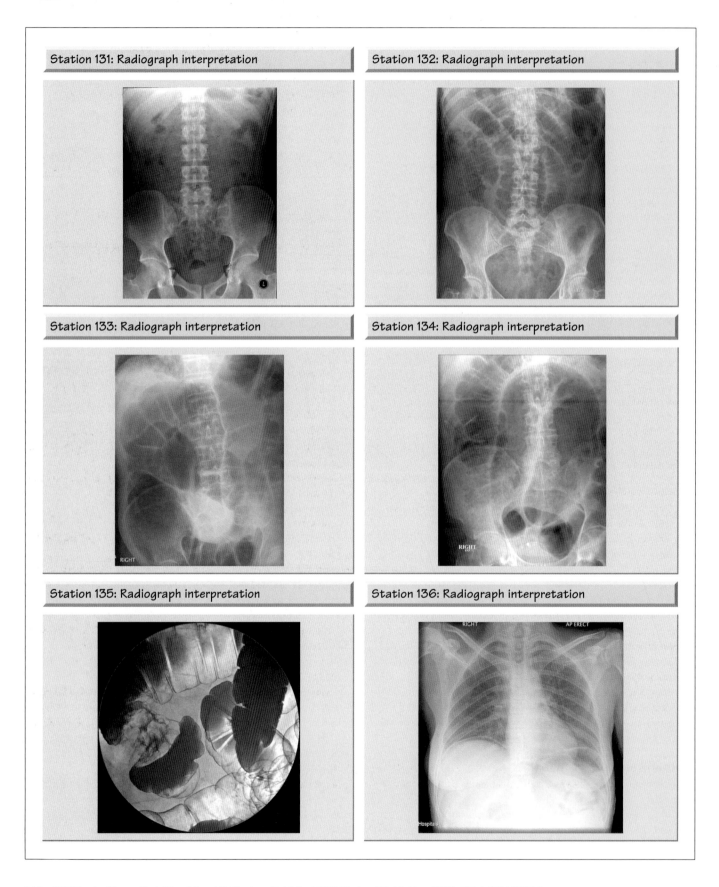

Station 131: Radiograph interpretation

Station 132: Radiograph interpretation

Station 133: Radiograph interpretation

Station 134: Radiograph interpretation

Station 135: Radiograph interpretation

Station 136: Radiograph interpretation

Station 131: Abdominal X-ray interpretation

• *This patient presented with abdominal pain and had an X-ray performed. Please examine the image carefully (see opposite) and report your findings*

Hints and tips

• Follow a pre-rehearsed system for reporting abdominal X-rays (AXRs)
• Start with the basics
• State type of image (plain radiograph, usually AP supine)
• Site (e.g. abdomen)
• Demographic details available (name, age, date taken)
• Note any markings (e.g. L/R or control). Comment on the adequacy of the film (hemidiaphragms to groins visible) and any features that may make interpretation difficult
• Work systematically through the features of the radiograph:
  • intraluminal gas distribution from rectum to stomach
  • extraluminal gas present?
  • soft tissues – examine organs from top to bottom
  • calcification – abnormal opacities, e.g. renal stones?
  • bone – including pelvis and vertebrae
  • note drains and lines visible
• Remember that there may be more than one abnormality
• State to the examiner that you would want to assess the patient clinically, including full history and examination

Station 132: Small bowel obstruction

• *This patient presented with nausea and vomiting. Please examine this image carefully (see opposite) and report your findings*

Hints and tips

• Follow the system described in Station 131
• This is a plain AP radiograph of the abdomen
• Demographic details are missing
• The important finding to note is the abnormal small bowel gas pattern indicating dilated small bowel. No intraluminal gas is visible in the distal large bowel or rectum
• Differences between small and large bowel:
  • size
  • position
  • quantity
  • mucosal markings
• Soft tissues are obscured by bowel gas and there is no abnormal calcification. No drains or lines are present
• Summarise your findings and present the diagnosis

Discussion points

• How can you tell this is small bowel rather than large?
• What are the causes of small bowel obstruction?
• As the FY1 on the ward, how would you treat this patient?

Station 133: Large bowel obstruction

• *This patient presented with abdominal pain and weight loss. Please examine this image carefully (see opposite) and report your findings*

Hints and tips

• Follow the system described in Station 131
• The important finding to note is the abnormal large bowel gas pattern indicating a dilated colon
• No drains and lines are visible
• Summarise your findings and present the diagnosis

Discussion points

• How can you tell this is large bowel rather than small?
• What are the causes of large bowel obstruction?

Station 134: Sigmoid volvulus

• *This patient presented with abdominal pain and absolute constipation. Please examine this image carefully (see opposite) and report your findings*

Hints and tips

• Follow the system described in Station 131
• The important finding to note is the large bean-shaped loop of dilated large bowel in the centre of the film

Discussion points

• What is a volvulus?
• Where else might they occur?

Station 135: Barium enema

• *This patient presented with abdominal pain and weight loss. Please examine this image carefully (see opposite) and report your findings*

Hints and tips

• This image is a double-contrast barium enema of the colon
• Comment on the different parts of large bowel anatomy (transverse colon, sigmoid colon)
• It shows an irregular circumferential filling defect in the caecum (a carcinoma)

Discussion points

• How do colon cancers in the sigmoid and descending colon usually present?
• What proportion of colon cancers occur in each of the parts of the large bowel?

Station 136: Erect chest radiograph

• *This patient presented with acute abdominal pain. Please examine this image carefully (see opposite) and report your findings*

Hints and tips

• Follow a method with which you are familiar (see Ch. 23 for interpretation of the chest radiograph)
• This CXR shows free extraluminal air present under both diaphragms, i.e. a pneumoperitoneum

Discussion point

• What are the causes of pneumoperitoneum?

Station 137: Intermittent claudication

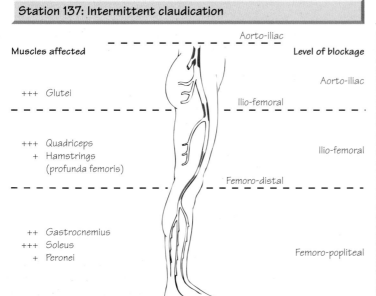

Muscles affected

+++ Glutei

+++ Quadriceps
  + Hamstrings
    (profunda femoris)

 ++ Gastrocnemius
+++ Soleus
  + Peronei

Level of blockage

Aorto-iliac

Ilio-femoral

Femoro-distal

Aorto-iliac

Ilio-femoral

Femoro-popliteal

Patients describe intermittent claudication as an aching pain in the leg, precipitated by exercise (typically walking) and relieved by rest.
The majority of patients will have other underlying vascular diseases, such as coronary atherosclerosis or cerebrovascular disease
*The level of vascular stenosis lies one arterial level above the most proximal symptomatic muscle group

Station 138: Acute pulseless leg

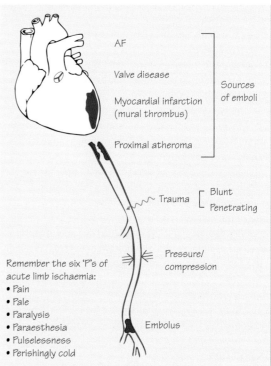

AF

Valve disease

Myocardial infarction
(mural thrombus)

Proximal atheroma

Sources of emboli

Trauma — Blunt
       — Penetrating

Pressure/compression

Embolus

Remember the six 'P's of acute limb ischaemia:
• Pain
• Pale
• Paralysis
• Paraesthesia
• Pulselessness
• Perishingly cold

Station 139: Abdominal aortic aneurysm

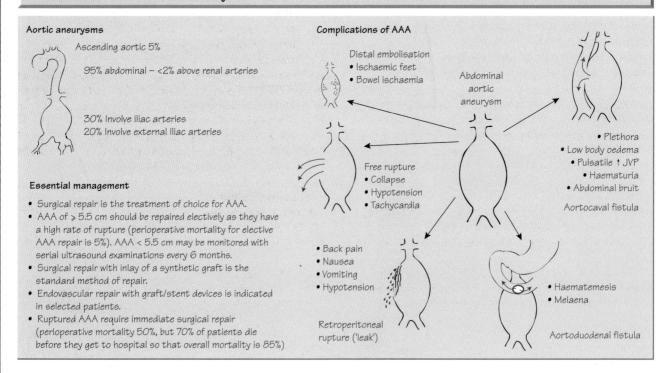

Aortic aneurysms

Ascending aortic 5%

95% abdominal – <2% above renal arteries

30% Involve iliac arteries
20% Involve external iliac arteries

Essential management

• Surgical repair is the treatment of choice for AAA.
• AAA of ≥ 5.5 cm should be repaired electively as they have a high rate of rupture (perioperative mortality for elective AAA repair is 5%). AAA < 5.5 cm may be monitored with serial ultrasound examinations every 6 months.
• Surgical repair with inlay of a synthetic graft is the standard method of repair.
• Endovascular repair with graft/stent devices is indicated in selected patients.
• Ruptured AAA require immediate surgical repair (perioperative mortality 50%, but 70% of patients die before they get to hospital so that overall mortality is 85%)

Complications of AAA

Distal embolisation
• Ischaemic feet
• Bowel ischaemia

Abdominal aortic aneurysm

Free rupture
• Collapse
• Hypotension
• Tachycardia

• Back pain
• Nausea
• Vomiting
• Hypotension

Retroperitoneal rupture ('leak')

• Plethora
• Low body oedema
• Pulsatile ↑ JVP
• Haematuria
• Abdominal bruit

Aortocaval fistula

• Haematemesis
• Melaena

Aortoduodenal fistula

Station 137: Intermittent claudication

Student info: *Mr JWS has been referred by his GP to the hospital out-patient clinic. He complains of pain in his right calf on walking and climbing stairs. Please take a history and present your differential diagnosis and initial management plan*

Patient info: *You are Mr JWS, a 65-year-old male with a 2-month history of worsening right calf pain on exertion. This typically comes on after walking to the local corner shop but is relieved by rest. You previously suffered a myocardial infarction 2 years ago and take a statin and aspirin. You have no other health problems*

Hints and tips

• Ascertain patient's understanding of the reason the GP has referred him to hospital
• Take a full pain history
• Establish how far he walks before the pain occurs (this is usually a fixed distance with intermittent claudication)
• Which muscles are affected?
• Does the pain resolve? Intermittent claudication pain is reversible on resting
• Are there symptoms suggesting neurological cause (chronic back pain and paraesthesia can be seen in cauda equina)?
• Determine the cardiovascular risk factors
• Assess impact of the surgery on the patient's life
• Address any concerns and fears the patient has

Discussion points

• What is your differential diagnosis?
• At what level might the occlusion be?
• What investigations would you request?

ΔΔ Atheromatous disease of the limb's arterial supply
      Cauda equnia (chronic due to osteoarthritis)
Ix *Bloods*   FBC – exclude polycythaemia
                Glucose – exclude diabetes
                Lipids – hyperlipidaemia?
    ECG
    Other   Ankle brachial pressure index (see Ch. 54)
    Imaging   Digital subtraction angiography
                Duplex US
Mx: mild symptoms   Lifestyle changes (stop smoking)
                         Consider aspirin/statin
Mx: severe symptoms/limb threatened   Angioplasty
                                           Stenting
                                           Surgery (bypass grafting)

Station 138: Acute pulseless leg

Student info: *Miss SG has been referred to hospital as an emergency with a painful, pulseless, cold leg. Please take a history*

Patient info: *You are Miss SG and are 80 years old. You are a resident in a nursing home and have been complaining of worsening pain in the left leg and an inability to move it. Your GP visited and was unable to find any pulses below the femoral artery, so called an ambulance to transfer you to hospital. PMH: AF. DH: digoxin, aspirin, statin*

Hints and tips

• Ascertain the patient's understanding of the current situation
• Establish the time course over which this has happened
• Take a history of the pain

• Enquire about the six Ps of an ischaemic limb
• Is there a source of emboli (e.g. AF, valvular disease, known aneurysm, previous atheromatous disease)?
• Are there risk factors for thrombosis (e.g. trauma, immobility)?
• Ask general cardiovascular history questions, including peripheral vascular disease
• Elicit relevant PMH and establish fitness for surgery
• Indicate this is an emergency and you would immediately inform your seniors of her admission for consideration of surgical intervention

Discussion points

• What is your differential diagnosis?
• What investigations would you request?
• What treatments are available?

ΔΔ Arterial embolus
      Thrombosis in situ
Ix *Bloods*   FBC, U&E, clotting, G&S
    ECG
    Other   Angiography

Station 139: Abdominal aortic aneurysm

Student info: *Mr FG is 76 and has attended A&E complaining of back pain. Please take a focused history. It is not necessary to examine him.*

Patient info: *You are Mr FG and are 76 years old. Your PMH: is one of controlled hypertension, raised cholesterol and a previous myocardial infarction 2 years earlier. Your pain started with back ache following breakfast. You have no urinary or bowel symptoms and no history of trauma. You were feeling well until this pain came on*

Hints and tips

• Ascertain the patient's understanding of the current situation
• Establish the time course over which this has happened
• Take a history of the back ache and ascertain there has been no trauma
• Establish vascular risk factors
• Establish negative urinary or bowel symptoms
• Elicit relevant past medical history
• A diagnosis of abdominal aortic aneurysm (AAA) should be considered in a patient of this age complaining of back pain. The multiple vascular risk factors would also support this, as would a negative history for urinary or bowel symptoms
• Differential diagnosis includes renal and musculoskeletal causes
• A leaking AAA is a surgical emergency and if this diagnosis is considered, it would be necessary to inform the examiners of your concerns

Discussion points

• What is your differential diagnosis?
• What investigations would you request?
• What treatments are available?

ΔΔ AAA ± leakage
      Renal tract pathology, e.g. kidney stone, infection
      Musculoskeletal
Ix *Bloods*   FBC, U&E, clotting, LFT
                Cross-match 6 units
    ECG
    Imaging   CXR, US abdomen, CT abdomen
Mx See opposite

Station 140: Peripheral vascular examination

Hints and tips
- For pulses remember to comment on:
- Presence/absence
- Rate
- Rhythm

1. Introduction and permission
- Patients will usually be positioned on a bed for peripheral vascular examination
- Feet and legs must be fully exposed to the groins
- Any pain in the limbs or feet?

2. Inspect
- Colour: pale from vascular insufficiency or pink from reactive hyperaemia? Any discoloration suggestive of ischaemia or gangrene?
- Trophic changes: hair loss? Skin loss? Asymmetry? Loss of muscle bulk?
- Ulceration: take particular care to inspect the key sites for ischaemic ulcers – lateral aspect of the foot and over malleoli. Look in places where they might be easily missed – heel of the foot and between the toes
- Scars from previous surgery
- Amputation of toes or distal limb

3. Feel
- Starting at the groin, feel down the legs with the back of your hands checking for a change in temperature. Compare both sides
- When you reach the feet examine the toes, checking capillary refill time (normal < 2 seconds)

Take time to inspect the patient. Many of your examination findings will be based on the initial observation

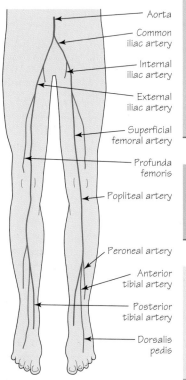

- Aorta
- Common iliac artery
- Internal iliac artery
- External iliac artery
- Superficial femoral artery
- Profunda femoris
- Popliteal artery
- Peroneal artery
- Anterior tibial artery
- Posterior tibial artery
- Dorsalis pedis

4. Palpation of peripheral pulses
- Start with the radial pulse first in order to note the rate and rhythm. This will help you establish what you are palpating for in the limbs
- Ensure you are familiar with the anatomical landmarks for the peripheral pulses together with techniques for palpation
- Compare each side as you move distally
- Begin in the lower limb with the femoral pulses
- Move down to the popliteal arteries
- Move onto the posterior tibial arteries. These may be palpated together at the same time standing at the foot of the patient's bed. Likewise for the dorsalis pedis

5. Listen
- Auscultate over the femoral pulse and the distal subsartorial canal (over the superficial femoral artery) for bruit. These are common areas of atherosclerosis

6. Completion
Tell the examiner you would like to:
- Perform Buerger's test (see opposite)
- Palpate the abdomen for an aortic aneurysm
- Measure the ankle brachial pressure index in both legs (see opposite)
- Examine the remainder of the cardiovascular system

Station 141: Ankle brachial pressure index measurement

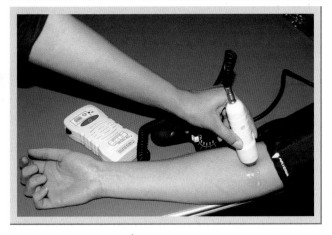

Station 143: Amputations

Amputations used in diabetes

Digital

Lisfranc/ transmetatarsal

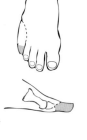

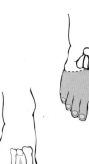

Ray

Syme's

Station 140: Peripheral vascular examination

See Chapter 55 for key findings on examination for different types of ulcers.

• *Mr SI is a 65-year-old gentleman with pain in his right leg and foot. These keep him awake at night and improve when he hangs his legs out of the bed. He previously had an MI 7 years ago and has high blood pressure. He smokes 10 cigarettes per day. Please examine the man's legs*

Buerger's test

The underlying principle is based on arterial insufficiency to the extent gravity may compromise arterial blood flow.

• With the patient reclined, ask if they have pain in their hip or leg
• Holding the leg gently at the ankle, raise the patient's leg slowly off the bed upwards
• In the presence of arterial insufficiency a point will be reached against gravity where the pressure of arterial blood supply cannot maintain perfusion and the leg turns white. This is *Buerger's angle*
• In a normal patient the leg can be raised to 90° without compromising arterial circulation
• Venous guttering may be seen when the leg is raised, as veins empty but are not refilled with blood due to the arterial insufficiency
• The second part of Buerger's test is to then lower the pale limb back down over the edge of the bed
• A reactive hyperaemia occurs as the arterial supply returns
• This leads to a characteristic pink-purple coloration of the skin

Discussion points

• Where is the level of vascular occlusion?
• What are the different causes of vascular occlusion?
• How would you tell whether this limb is viable?
• What investigations would you like to request?
• How would you manage this patient?

Station 141: Ankle brachial pressure index measurement

• *This patient has been experiencing pain in their calves on walking, which is relieved by rest. Please examine them and perform an ankle brachial pressure index (ABPI) measurement*

Hints and tips

• Make sure you've practised this before demonstrating it!
• Start with the basics: introduction/consent/any pain in legs?
• Perform with the patient lying supine in bed
• Ensure adequate exposure of the arms and calves
• Use a hand-held Doppler ultrasound probe to first locate the brachial artery. Do not forget to apply the jelly first
• Using a normal blood pressure cuff, perform routine syphygmomanometry using the Doppler probe instead of a stethoscope to determine systolic blood pressure
• Use the hand-held Doppler probe to locate the dorsalis pedis artery or the posterior tibial artery
• Place the BP cuff at a fixed point around the mid-calf
• Inflate and again determine the systolic BP using Doppler probe
• Repeat for other side if required (both brachial and ankle, placing the cuff at the same points as used for the other limb)
• Thank the patient (and wipe the jelly off them!)
• Calculate the ABPI (systolic BP at the ankle divided by the systolic BP in the arm to give a ratio)

• It is necessary at each point to warn the patient that the cuff is going to be inflated as this can be uncomfortable

How to interpret the findings

• Normal: ~1
• Claudication: ~0.9–0.6
• Rest pain: ~0.3–0.6
• Critical ischaemia: <0.3

Discussion points

• When would you perform an ABPI?
• What treatment is indicated by a given ABPI result?
• What may cause a falsely reassuring ABPI result?

Station 142: Abdominal aortic aneurysm

• *You are the surgical F1 on call. Mr OL is a 75-year-old gentleman with a swelling in his abdomen. This is non-tender and was noticed incidentally on examination by his GP, who sent him to you for assessment. Please examine his abdomen and describe your findings*

Examination routine

• *Inspection*: check the general appearance of the patient. Is there evidence of smoking (nicotine staining), tissue perfusion or trophic changes?
• *Palpation*:
  • start by assessing the radial pulse
  • move onto the abdomen and palpate superficially and deep
  • an abdominal aortic aneurysm (AAA) will be palpable in the epigastric region. Palpate in this area using the finger tips of both hands, gently pushing into the abdomen. Be careful not to cause any pain, as this may be uncomfortable even in a normal individual. Do not examine these patients too vigorously!
  • the key finding is that of a pulsatile, expansile mass pushing your fingertips apart. However, the aorta will also be palpable in a normal slim individual
  • try to estimate the diameter of the AAA
• *Auscultation*: listen to the abdomen for an audible bruit, particularly that of renal artery stenosis
• *Completion*: tell the examiner that you would continue to examine the rest of the cardiovascular system, particularly the legs and feet for distal complications of an AAA, and perform ABPI assessment

Discussion points

• What is an aneurysm?
• How would you investigate this swelling?
• How would you manage this patient?

Station 143: Amputations

• *Mr AS is a 55-year-old gentleman. He has recently had an amputation of his left leg. Please examine his legs and describe your findings*

Hints and tips

• Describe the level of the amputation (e.g. above knee)
• Comment on the overlying skin and any wounds or scars
• Look carefully for any evidence of skin grafting
• Note a prosthesis or walking aid
• Continue your examination as for Station 140
• On completion also add that you would want to observe the patient mobilising with their prosthesis, if appropriate

Discussion points

• What are the reasons for performing an amputation?
• What are the possible complications?

Station 144: Varicose veins

Anatomy

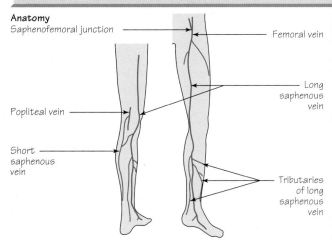

Saphenofemoral junction
Femoral vein
Long saphenous vein
Popliteal vein
Short saphenous vein
Tributaries of long saphenous vein

- Blood is normally restricted to flowing from superficial to deep and from distal to proximal via one-way valves
- When the valves are disrupted this leads to varicose veins
- Varicose veins are most common at the saphenofemoral junction and long saphenous vein

History hints

Aching leg pain	Swelling
Venous claudication	Previous ulceration
Skin changes	Cosmetic appearance
Previous treatments	Itch/eczema

Consider: pelvic masses, trauma, and previous DVT

- The long saphenous vein originates from the dorsal arch
- It passes anterior to the medial malleolus (a site for cut down)
- It then passes up the medial aspect of the leg where it passes a hand's breadth posterior to the patella
- It then passes up the medial aspect of the thigh to enter the (deep) femoral vein at the saphenofemoral junction
- Below the knee the vein is accompanied by the saphenous nerve, which provides sensation to the medial aspect of the foot

- The short saphenous vein passes posteriorly to the lateral malleolus
- It then ascends vertically, on the posterior surface of the calf, where it is adherent to the sural nerve (a sensory nerve that provides sensation to the lateral aspect of the foot)

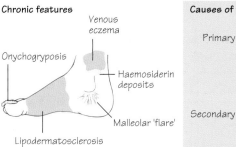

Skin and fat
Perforator
Muscle
Fascia

Chronic effects

Varicose (or venous) eczema
Skin pigmentation
Lipodermatosclerosis
Onychogryposis (toenails)
Ulcers: usually on medial aspect of ankle(gaitor area) and shallow

Chronic features

Venous eczema
Onychogryposis
Haemosiderin deposits
Malleolar 'flare'
Lipodermatosclerosis

Causes of varicose veins

Primary →
- Idiopathic, often familial
- Congenital e.g. Klippel-Trenaunay syndrome

Secondary →
- Obstruction to venous flow e.g. pregnancy, fibroids, lymphadenopathy, pelvic neoplasia
- Valve destruction e.g. DVT

Station 145: Leg ulcers

The term ulcer is defined as a discontinuity in a normal epithelial surface
The differential diagnosis for leg ulcers is broad and includes both medical and surgical causes:

Common sites of leg ulcers

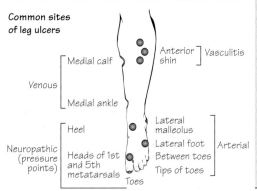

Venous
- Medial calf
- Medial ankle

Anterior shin] Vasculitis

Neuropathic (pressure points)
- Heel
- Heads of 1st and 5th metatarsals
- Toes

Lateral malleolus
Lateral foot] Arterial
Between toes
Tips of toes

Venous ulcers
- Secondary to venous hypertension
- Typically found in 'gaitor area' of medial ankle/leg
- Shallow, sloping edges, granulation tissue at base

Arterial ulcers
- Secondary to arterial insufficiency
- Painful, associated with signs of ischaemia in limb
- Typically found on lateral ankle, toe tips and heel

Neuropathic ulcers
- Classically associated with diabetes
- Painless, punched-out ulcers
- Found in pressure areas on sole of foot

Malignant ulcers
- May arise from malignant change in a chronic ulcer or from new malignancy

Traumatic, vasculitic and infectious ulcers may also occur

Station 144: Varicose veins

- *This man is coming in for surgery next week. Please examine his legs*
- *What features of chronic varicose veins are present in this patient?*
- *How would you determine the level of venous incompetency in this patient's legs?*

Examination routine

- Introduction/consent/ask about pain
- *Exposure*: the patient needs to be adequately exposed
- *Position*: standing, you should crouch down to examine the legs
- *General inspection*: look for general features of systemic disease. Is the patient well/unwell?
- *System-specific inspection*:
  - inspect from the front and behind
  - ask the patient to 'turn out' their leg to examine the medial aspect
  - look for distribution of varicose veins, scars (both legs, in groin and popliteal creases), venous flare, oedema, lipodermatosclerosis, varicose eczema, pigmentation and ulceration
- *Palpation*:
  - check with the patient first (painful?)
  - feel the veins – they might not be visible
  - feel for a cough impulse just below the SFJ
- *Percussion*:
  - gently feel over the saphenous opening whilst tapping the varicosities distally
  - if you can feel the impulse transmitted it implies incompetent valves = Chevrier's tap sign

Trendelenburg's test

Although a historical exam favourite this is seldom used in clinic today as it has been replaced with Doppler velocitometry and duplex scanning.
- With the patient lying supine, lift the leg and milk it proximally to empty it of venous blood
- Occlude the SFJ with your fingers
- Keeping pressure on the SFJ, ask the patient to stand
- If there is no venous filling, saphenofemoral valvular incompetence is demonstrated
- If there is filling of the veins, the incompetence must be lower down the limb
- The test can then be repeated at lower levels in the leg with a tourniquet to demonstrate the level of incompetence

Discussion points

- What are the causes of varicose veins?
- What types of management are available for a patient with varicose veins?
- What is the pathophysiology?

Rx *Medical* Properly fitted compression stockings
Losing weight (if appropriate)
Surgery 'High tie, strip and avulsion'

The most common operation is a 'high tie, strip and avulsion'. This involves the following:
- Dissect out the saphenous vein at the SFJ and tie off all the tributaries
- The saphenous vein is tied off and then a 'pin-stripper' is passed down the length of the long saphenous vein to the level of the knee (not below as it increases the risk of damage to the saphenous nerve)

- The vein in the thigh is then stripped out
- Small 'stab incisions' are made in the calf at pre-marked sites and the veins are 'avulsed' with a hook

Complications of surgery

- General: e.g. bleeding, DVT, infection, anaesthetic problems
- Specific: bruising, nerve damage (saphenous, sural) and recurrence. Skin changes will not be reversed by surgery!

Station 145: Leg ulcers

Student info: *Mrs SB is 71 and has come to see you in your GP practice complaining of a sore ulcerated area above her medial ankle in her left leg. You are the FY1 doctor in the GP surgery. Please take a history and tell us your differential diagnosis and initial investigations*

Patient info: *You are a 71-year-old female with a 1-month history of skin breakdown and ulceration. This has been weeping slightly and causing some discomfort. You have a history of eczema in this area that you have been applying steroid creams to. Otherwise you are well for your age and you maintain regular exercise. You have a PMH of DVT in the right leg following a long-haul flight to see family in Australia 10 years previously. You are not taking any regular medications. You are a non-smoker and drink no alcohol*

Hints and tips

- Ascertain the patient's prior knowledge of why the GP has referred them
- Let the patient explain their symptoms to you
- Establish what troubles the patient the most
- Take a full history relating to the ulcer: is there any pain, bleeding, infection, trauma, change in sensation?
- Ask about related symptoms that may suggest a cause:
  - diabetes
  - varicose veins (and symptoms thereof, e.g. venous eczema, itching, limb oedema)
  - note history of DVT
- General cardiovascular history questions
- Determine impact of symptoms on quality of life
- Establish past medical history and current medications
- Determine social history
- Address any concerns the patient may have

Discussion points

- What is your differential diagnosis?
- What do you think is the most likely cause?
- What treatment options are available?

ΔΔ See opposite for full list
In this case a venous ulcer secondary to venous hypertension (post-phlebetic) is most likely; however you must rule out the underlying arterial contribution
Ix *Bloods* FBC, blood glucose, U&E
Micro Swab ulcer site, ?infection
Other Ankle brachial pressure index
Mx A four-layer compression bandaging for uncomplicated post-phlebetic ulcers with no arterial contribution
Refer for hospital opinion and venography/angiography if symptoms persist

Station 146: Haematuria

Haematuria is a potentially serious symptom that always warrants further investigation

Renal
Pyelonephritis
Tuberculosis
Renal cell carcinoma
Renal adenoma
Renal cyst
Renal infarction
Arteriovenous malformation
Trauma
Glomerulonephritis

Ureteral
TCC
Stone *
Appendicitis

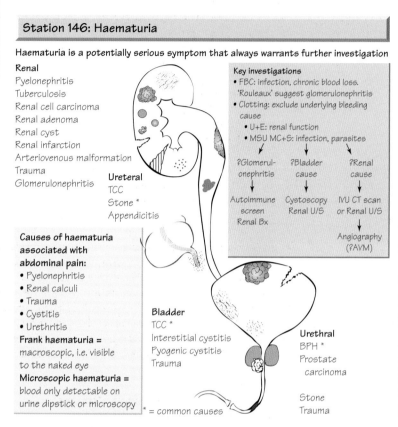

Key investigations
• FBC: infection, chronic blood loss. 'Rouleaux' suggest glomerulonephritis
• Clotting: exclude underlying bleeding cause
  • U+E: renal function
  • MSU MC+S: infection, parasites

?Glomerulonephritis → Autoimmune screen Renal Bx

?Bladder cause → Cystoscopy Renal U/S

?Renal cause → IVU CT scan or Renal U/S → Angiography (?AVM)

Causes of haematuria associated with abdominal pain:
• Pyelonephritis
• Renal calculi
• Trauma
• Cystitis
• Urethritis

Frank haematuria = macroscopic, i.e. visible to the naked eye

Microscopic haematuria = blood only detectable on urine dipstick or microscopy

Bladder
TCC *
Interstitial cystitis
Pyogenic cystitis
Trauma

Urethral
BPH *
Prostate carcinoma

Stone
Trauma

* = common causes

Station 147: Benign prostatic hypertrophy

Benign prostatic hypertrophy (BPH) is a common condition in males, present in 50% of 70-year-olds

Key lower urinary tract symptoms are divided into:

Outflow symptoms
Hypertrophy of the prostate obstructs urinary outflow:
• Hesitancy initiating flow
• Straining to micturate
• Poor stream
• Terminal dribbling
• Acute urinary retention

Detrusor instability
Subsequent hypertrophy of the bladder from chronic retention of urine leads to symptoms of voiding or irritability resulting from detrusor instability:
• Frequency
• Nocturia
• Urgency
• Urge incontinence

Bladder failure
Chronic urinary retention eventually leads to pathological dilation of the bladder and symptoms of bladder failure:
• Painless urinary retention
• Incontinence from overflow
• Recurrent infection from urinary stasis

Station 148: Renal calculi

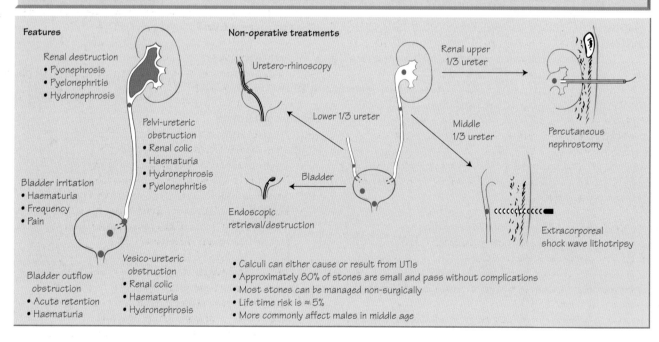

Features

Renal destruction
• Pyonephrosis
• Pyelonephritis
• Hydronephrosis

Pelvi-ureteric obstruction
• Renal colic
• Haematuria
• Hydronephrosis
• Pyelonephritis

Bladder irritation
• Haematuria
• Frequency
• Pain

Bladder outflow obstruction
• Acute retention
• Haematuria

Vesico-ureteric obstruction
• Renal colic
• Haematuria
• Hydronephrosis

Non-operative treatments

Uretero-rhinoscopy

Lower 1/3 ureter

Endoscopic retrieval/destruction

Bladder

Renal upper 1/3 ureter

Middle 1/3 ureter

Percutaneous nephrostomy

Extracorporeal shock wave lithotripsy

• Calculi can either cause or result from UTIs
• Approximately 80% of stones are small and pass without complications
• Most stones can be managed non-surgically
• Life time risk is ≈ 5%
• More commonly affect males in middle age

Station 146: Haematuria

Student info: *Mr JP has been referred by his GP to the hospital clinic with haematuria. There is a palpable mass on the right side of the abdomen. Please take a history and present your differential diagnosis*

Patient info: *You are Mr JP, a 55-year-old male who is normally fit and well. Over the past week you have noticed some blood in your urine. You have experienced some pains in your right flank over the past few months. You seem to have lost a little weight and are pale.*

Hints and tips

• Take a full history of his symptoms
• Initial haematuria at the onset of micturition suggests a more distal urethral cause; terminal haematuria at the end of micturition suggests a more proximal bladder or prostate cause
• The passage of clots in urine suggests a ureteric or pelvic cause
• Quantify the amount and frequency of blood loss
• Are there any other symptoms related to micturition (pain, etc.)?
• Establish the patient's normal pattern of micturition
• Does the patient have any symptoms suggestive of outflow problems, bladder instability or failure? (See Station 147)
• Is there any associated abdominal pain? This is a key symptom in helping distinguish the cause. Take a focussed history and include the following: pneumaturia, previous/recurrent UTI, anaemia, weight loss, trauma, previous/recurrent renal stones, pyrexia, bleeding disorders, liver disorders, anticoagulant therapy
• Establish risk factors for renal stones or urological malignancy
• Assess impact of the symptoms on the patient's life
• Address any concerns the patient has (i.e. his fears)

ΔΔ   The patient's symptoms suggest renal cell carcinoma
      Other possible causes are listed opposite

Ix   *Bloods*   FBC – exclude anaemia
                    Clotting – bleeding abnormality?
                    U&Es – abnormal renal function?
                    LFTs – liver metastases?
    Micro   Urine dipstick; urine MC&S – UTI?
    Imaging   Imaging for haematuria is dependent on level of the suspected cause, as indicated in the diagram opposite

Station 147: Benign prostatic hypertrophy

Student info: *Mr TF is 61 and has come to see you in your GP practice complaining of difficulty urinating. Please take a history and discuss a differential diagnosis*

Patient info: *You are a 61-year-old male with a 3-month history of difficulty voiding urine. You have to stand and wait a long time before flow starts and strain to aid this.*

Hints and tips

• Ascertain the patient's current knowledge of the situation
• Take a full history relating to the urinary symptoms: hesitancy, poor flow, terminal dribble, urge, incontinence
• Establish the patient's normal pattern of micturition and the presence of frequency and nocturia
• Ask about related symptoms that may suggest cause: haematuria, urinary tract infections
• Are any concerning systemic symptoms present?
• Determine impact of symptoms on quality of life

Discussion points

• What are the complications of untreated BPH?
• What treatment options are available?

ΔΔ   Benign prostatic hypertrophy
      Urinary tract infections (though these may also be secondary to BPH)
      Neuromuscular disorders

Ix   *Bloods*   FBC – evidence of infection?
                    U&Es – abnormal renal function?
    Micro   Urine dipstick; urine MC&S – UTI?
    Other   Uroflowmetry + residual volumes
                    US of kidneys and bladder
                    Intravenous urogram
                    Cystoscopy

Rx   *Medical*   Classic 'watchful waiting'
                    α-adrenergic blockers; 5α-reductase inhibitors
                    Long-term catheter (if not fit for surgery)
    Surgical   TURP; open prostatectomy

Station 148: Renal calculi

Student info: *Mr RB has been referred to hospital as an emergency with a painful abdomen. You are the FY1 doctor in the surgical assessment unit. Assess and advise the patient on your management plan*

Patient info: *You are Mr RB and are 45 and live at home with your wife. You experienced a sudden onset of severe pain in your right flank 2 hours ago and your wife called an ambulance. The pain is the worst you have ever experienced and radiates down into your right groin and scrotum. Your health is normally good and you take no medications*

Hints and tips

• Take a history of the pain; clarify the precise time course
• Any symptoms of outflow obstruction?
• Previous history of stones (high risk of recurrence)
• Presence of pre-existing urinary symptoms
• Establish the presence of any risk factors for renal calculi (e.g. dehydration, hypercalcaemia, gout, malignancy)

Discussion points

• What are the three points within the renal tract where stones may commonly become lodged?
• What treatments are available?

ΔΔ   Renal colic
      Appendicitis (if right sided)
      Abdominal aortic aneurysm (a classic catch)
      In women of reproductive age you must also consider
      gynaecological emergencies, e.g. ectopic pregnancy

Ix   *Bloods*   FBC – evidence of infection?
                    U&Es – abnormal renal function?
    Micro   Urine dipstick; urine MC&S
    ECG
    Imaging   Kidney, ureter and bladder X-ray (90% of renal stones are opaque); intravenous urogram

Rx   NSAIDs are indicated for pain relief; IV fluids
      80% of stones will pass without intervention
      If the stone fails to pass or there is associated infection or obstruction, then the appropriate intervention depends on the level of the stone within the renal tracts (see opposite)

Station 149: Examination of the external genitalia/scrotal swellings

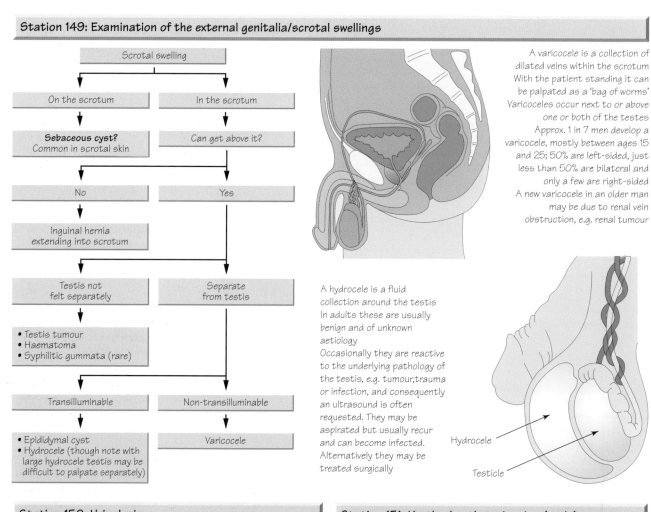

Scrotal swelling

↓ ↓

On the scrotum → In the scrotum

Sebaceous cyst? Common in scrotal skin → Can get above it?

↓ ↓

No → Yes

↓

Inguinal hernia extending into scrotum

↓ ↓

Testis not felt separately → Separate from testis

↓ ↓

- Testis tumour
- Haematoma
- Syphilitic gummata (rare)

↓ ↓

Transilluminable → Non-transilluminable

↓ ↓

- Epididymal cyst
- Hydrocele (though note with large hydrocele testis may be difficult to palpate separately) → Varicocele

A varicocele is a collection of dilated veins within the scrotum With the patient standing it can be palpated as a 'bag of worms' Varicoceles occur next to or above one or both of the testes Approx. 1 in 7 men develop a varicocele, mostly between ages 15 and 25; 50% are left-sided, just less than 50% are bilateral and only a few are right-sided A new varicocele in an older man may be due to renal vein obstruction, e.g. renal tumour

A hydrocele is a fluid collection around the testis In adults these are usually benign and of unknown aetiology Occasionally they are reactive to the underlying pathology of the testis, e.g. tumour, trauma or infection, and consequently an ultrasound is often requested. They may be aspirated but usually recur and can become infected. Alternatively they may be treated surgically

Hydrocele

Testicle

Station 150: Urinalysis

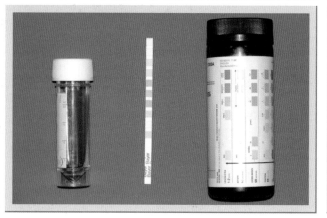

Station 151: Urethral catheterisation (male)

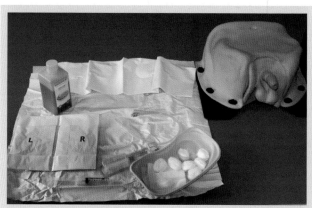

Station 149: Examination of the male external genitalia/scrotal swellings

• *Please examine this man's external genitalia*

Possible cases in an OSCE
• Hydrocele; varicocele; epididymal cyst

Unlikely cases in an OSCE
• Testicular tumour; infections

Examination routine
• Introduction/consent
• *Exposure*: the patient should have their trousers and underwear removed and be covered with a sheet
• *Position*: if the patient is lying supine, examine on the couch first but ask him to stand at the end to check for a varicocele
• *General inspection*: general features of systemic disease. Are they well/unwell?
• *Screening test*: ask the patient to cough
• *System-specific inspection*:
  • inspect groin and scrotum looking for scars
  • ask the patient if they have any pain
  • palpate each testis in turn while observing the patient's face
  • place your fingers behind the testis as a support while palpating very gently with the flat of your thumb
  • try and identify the epididymis
  • note any lumps or irregularity
• *Completion*: state that you would complete your examination by performing a full abdominal examination

Discussion points
• What are the causes of a scrotal lump and how can you differentiate them?
• What types of hydrocele are you aware of and what management strategies are available?

Hints and tips: epididymal cyst
• Commonly found in men over 40
• Occur uni- or bilaterally
• May vary in size (unless large, not always obvious on inspection). They are discrete from the testis
• May be loculated
• May transilluminate
• Usually they can be managed conservatively unless they are causing pain

Hints and tips: hydrocele
• There is fluid surrounding the testis so it is not distinguishable on palpation, i.e. it will appear like a large testis
• A hydrocele will transilluminate with a pen-torch
• Can 'get above' it to distinguish it from a hernia

Hints and tips: varicocele
• Scrotum usually looks normal
• Usually not obvious until patient is standing
• Separate from the testis
• Non-transilluminable
• Can 'get above' it
• May have cough impulse
• Feels like 'a bag of worms'

Station 150: Urinalysis

• *Mrs PM has experienced symptoms of colicky abdominal pains. She has provided you with the following urine sample. Please test it and report your findings*

Hints and tips
• Check you have the right sample (name, DOB, etc.). Wear gloves
• Inspect sample (colour, turbidity, macroscopic haematuria)
• Familiarise yourself with the interpretation chart, e.g. how long to wait before reading colours of the various reagents. A stopwatch may be provided for this
• Dip into urine, ensuring that all reagent strips are covered
• Remove immediately and tap off excess urine
• Interpret the colour changes by comparing each reagent to the chart provided at the appropriate time point. Document the results
• Offer to send to microbiology depending on results and patient's symptoms
• Safely dispose of the urine and test strip as appropriate

Discussion points
• When might you perform urinalysis?
• What conditions can be diagnosed by urinalysis?
• What results might indicate a UTI?

Station 15: Urethral catheterisation

• *Using the equipment on this tray and the mannequin provided, show me how you would insert a urinary catheter in a male patient*

Hints and tips
• You must pretend that there is a real patient in front of you. Say that you would *introduce* yourself (explain who you are, what you are going to do and why), *position* the patient (flat) and *expose* them correctly
• Check correct patient
• Explanation of reason for carrying out procedure
• Check equipment (catheter, 10 ml syringe, 10 ml of water for balloon, lubricating anaesthetic gel, sterile cleaning solution and swabs, sterile drape, sterile gloves, catheter bag and stand)
• Arrange equipment aseptically
• Wash hands aseptically/sterile gloves/consider apron
• Try to keep a 'clean' right hand (R) and a 'dirty' left hand (L) throughout the procedure ('no touch' technique)
• Lay the drape over the 'patient' and retract the foreskin (L)
• Clean penis with swabs and solution
• Hold penis vertically (L) and squirt lubricating gel down urethra (R)
• Pass catheter down the urethra (R) until up to the 'hilt' and urine is coming through
• Inflate the balloon with 10 ml of water *only when urine is passed* (R)
• Attach catheter bag
• Reduce foreskin (L)
• Tidy up and wash hands
• Record the procedure in notes and document residual urine volume
NB. An alternative technique is to wear two pairs of sterile gloves and take one off following the cleaning step.

Discussion points
• What are the indications for inserting a catheter?
• If you are unable to insert a catheter first time, what are your options?
• What are the complications of urinary catheter insertion?

Key points in any musculoskeletal history

Affected joint/acute or chronic/pattern of involvement
Pain (site, severity, frequency, analgesia)
Stiffness (?early morning)
Swelling and deformity
Functional impairment
Systemic symptoms
PMH/previous trauma/FH

Station 152: Swollen knee

Acutely swollen	Chronically swollen
Septic arthritis	Osteoarthritis
Gout/pseudogout	Rheumatoid arthritis
Reactive arthritis	Other inflammatory arthritis
Recent trauma	Previous trauma

Chronic knee swelling

Left/right	Physiotherapy ?Any relief
Duration of symptoms	Walking aids
Pain (see above)	Activities of daily living
Stiffness – when	House/flat - stairs
Swelling and deformity	Independent?
Analgesic requirements	Who is at home?

Management of acutely swollen joint

An acutely swollen joint is septic arthritis until proven otherwise and should be dealt with urgently
ABCDE: patient may have systemic sepsis and require resuscitation
Adequate analgesia: if truly septic there will be considerable pain and the patient will be reluctant to move the joint, which will be hot, red, swollen and tender
Investigations:
• FBC, U&Es, CRP/ESR, blood cultures
• X-ray of joint (AP and lateral)
• Aseptic joint aspiration and send fluid urgently to lab for Gram stain and crystals
• Broad-spectrum IV antibiotics (flucloxacillin; a cephalosporin if <4 years old)
• Keep NBM and inform senior colleague as patient may need urgent joint washout

Station 153: Gout

Typical patient   Male in his thirties
Obese and hypertensive
Fond of alcohol

Acute attack: sudden onset pain lasting ~ 2 weeks, often follows minor trauma/alcohol excess/unaccustomed exercise. Usually metatarsophalangeal joints of the first toe, ankle or fingers

Chronic gout: recurrent attacks ➡ joint damage with chronic pain, stiffness and deformity. May have tophi.
? on allopurinol/diuretics/other medications.

Station 154: Rheumatoid arthritis

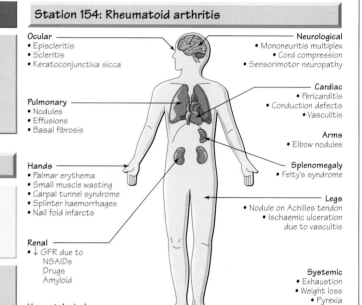

Ocular
• Episcleritis
• Scleritis
• Keratoconjunctiva sicca

Neurological
• Mononeuritis multiplex
• Cord compression
• Sensorimotor neuropathy

Pulmonary
• Nodules
• Effusions
• Basal fibrosis

Cardiac
• Pericarditis
• Conduction defects
• Vasculitis

Arms
• Elbow nodules

Hands
• Palmar erythema
• Small muscle wasting
• Carpal tunnel syndrome
• Splinter haemorrhages
• Nail fold infarcts

Splenomegaly
• Felty's syndrome

Legs
• Nodule on Achilles tendon
• Ischaemic ulceration due to vasculitis

Renal
• ↓ GFR due to NSAIDs
 Drugs
 Amyloid

Systemic
• Exhaustion
• Weight loss
• Pyrexia
• Muscle wasting
• Evidence of steroid use (thin skin, Cushingoid)

Haematological
• Thrombocytosis
Anaemia: chronic disease, GI blood loss due to NSAID therapy, bone marrow suppression due to DMARDs, pernicious anaemia

Early vs late features of RA
Early features
Insidious onset, ↓ weight, fatigue, weakness
Polyarthritis (proximal finger joints > wrists > feet > knees > shoulders), tenosynovitis (wrist/fingers)
Later features
Progressive deformity esp. ulnar deviation of fingers, radial and volar deviation of wrist, valgus deformity of knees. Pain becomes a constant ache. ↓ ROM and function. Neck pain and stiffness

Associations with rheumatological disease

Symptom	Association
Face	Dry eyes, dry mouth, mouth ulcers
Cardiovascular	Pericarditis, Raynaud's phenomenon, thromboembolic disease
Dermatology	Rashes, nail changes
Gastroenterology	Diarrhoea, jaundice, dysphagia
Genitourinary	Rashes, ulcers, STD
Haematology	Anaemia, splenomegaly
Neurology	Mononeuritis multiplex, peripheral neuropathy, cervical myelopathy
Respiratory	Interstitial lung disease, pleural effusions

Station 152: Swollen knee

Student info: *Mrs RF is an 84-year-old female referred by her GP to the orthopaedic clinic with a 4-year history of worsening left knee pain. You are the orthopaedic FY1. Please take a history*

Patient info: *You are Mrs RF (84 years old) with a 4-year history of left knee pain. The pain had a gradual onset and has progressively worsened; it is worse with exercise, and relieved by rest. Your walking distance is limited to half a mile. You struggle with the stairs following a period of inactivity and also getting out of a chair/car seat. You are occasionally woken by pain at night, and there is intermittent knee swelling. PMH: diet-controlled diabetes; DH: paracetamol. Your mother and older sister both had knee problems as they got older; your sister had a knee replacement. You are widowed and live in a house with the only toilet upstairs*

Hints and tips
- Determine what the patient's expectations are from her hospital visit, i.e. tablets/knee replacement/other?
- The history has two key components:
  - what are her symptoms?
  - how do her symptoms affect her quality of life and ADLs?

Discussion points
- How would you manage this patient?
- This woman is placed on the waiting list for a knee replacement. Two weeks prior to the operation you see her in the preoperative assessment clinic. What investigations do you arrange?

△△   Osteoarthritis; a first presentation of an inflammatory arthritis is unlikely in a patient of this age

Ix   *Imaging*   Knee X-ray (standing AP and lateral views)

Mx   Depends on severity of symptoms, X-ray appearances, patient co-morbidities, previous management and patient expectations

   Medical   Analgesia (PRN or regular); load reduction (↓ weight, use of stick); physiotherapy to maintain movement and strength; modification of ADLs

   Surgical   Joint replacement surgery

Pre-op work-up

   Bloods   FBC, U&Es, glucose, clotting, G&S

   Urine   UTI (if any) needs treating prior to surgery

   ECG   If >50 years/PMH of heart disease/↑ BP/smoker

   Imaging   If knee X-rays greater than 6 months old then repeat them; CXR only if clinical indication

The painful hip

In an elderly patient complaining of hip pain, the key issues in the history and subsequent management plan are the same as for the knee.

Station 153 Gout

Student info: *Mr BB is a 35-year-old male who has been sent to hospital by his GP with a 1-week history of severe pain in his left great toe. You are the FY1 doctor in A&E. Please take a history*

Patient info: *You are Mr BB, aged 35 years and a wine taster. One week ago, you experienced sudden-onset severe pain in the middle of the night following a day of heavy drinking. The pain is constant and worse on weight bearing. You were given diclofenac by your GP, giving some relief. The toe is red, shiny, hot, swollen and tender. It causes pain but you can still move it. You have no history of trauma, no other joint problems and are systemically well. You have had this pain before – but never this severe. This is the first time you have sought help. You are overweight and already seeing your GP for BP monitoring*

Hints and tips
- Determine Sx. How severe is the pain? Can he move his toe? Previous episodes? Is he systemically unwell?
- Is he on any treatment?
- What does the patient think is causing the pain?

Discussion points
- What is your differential diagnosis?
- What investigations would you consider for this patient, and how do you distinguish gout from septic arthritis?
- Can you discuss the management of acute gout and how it differs from that of chronic gout?

△△   Acute attack of gout, with a history of chronic gout

   With any acutely painful joint, you must exclude a septic arthritis as this can result in rapid joint destruction

Ix   *Bloods*   FBC, CRP/ESR, uric acid

   Micro   Aspirate joint; urgent Gram stain and crystals (a negative Gram stain and the presence of negatively birefringent urate crystals confirms diagnosis)

   Imaging   X-ray of joint (chronic gout → joint erosion)

Mx   Acute attack: NSAIDs, colchicine, IM corticosteroid

   Chronic gout: ↓ weight, ↓ alcohol, allopurinol

   Lifestyle changes (↓ alcohol, ↓ weight, ↑ exercise)

   Optimise vascular RF

Station 154: Rheumatoid arthritis

Student info: *Mrs AE is a 38-year-old female referred by her GP to the rheumatology out-patients with painful hands. You are the FY1 doctor. Take a history to be presented to the consultant*

Patient info: *You are Mrs AE, a 38-year-old, left-handed female. You are a self-employed dress maker with a 3-year history of slowly worsening pain in the MCP joints, especially in the morning. There is now also pain in the wrists. Your fingers are swollen and you have recently noticed some deformity. You are struggling with work, writing and dressing (especially doing buttons up). You also have occasional knee pain. PMH: fatigue; you have not felt yourself for the last couple of years. You have no current medications. Your mother has RA*

Hints and tips
- Determine patient's reason for coming to hospital
- Determine Sx and their effect on her ADLs. A functional history is essential with hand problems
- Is there a FH of joint problems?

Discussion points
- What investigations would you consider?
- What is rheumatoid factor? Is it always present in RA?
- What are the principles of managing RA?
- Describe the classic hand deformities seen in RA

Ix   *Bloods*   FBC, U&Es, CRP/ESR, rheumatoid factor, antinuclear factor

   Imaging   X-rays of both hands (AP and lateral views)

Mx

Onset   NSAIDs; physiotherapy to preserve movement; psychological support

Early phase   NSAIDs and low-dose steroids; second-line drugs – disease-modifying agents, e.g. methotrexate; physiotherapy; rest + joint injections when flare ups

Progressive   Second-line drugs; consider anti-TNFα agents; splintage/orthoses; soft tissue releases/osteotomies

Late disease   Arthrodesis/arthroplasty

Station 155: Musculoskeletal examination

*Essentials checklist - WINCER
General inspection/observation
± screening test (**function**)
System specific inspection (**look**)
Palpation (**feel**)
Move – active and passive
Measure
Special tests
Completion

Station 156: GALS screen [1]

GALS screening questions

'Do you have any pain or stiffness in your muscles, joints or back?'
'Can you dress yourself completely without any difficulty?'
'Can you walk up and down stairs without any difficulty?'

Station 157: Spine examination

- Introduction/consent/ask about pain
- Exposure/position
- **Look:**   General condition and systemic features
              From the back: scoliosis, scars, pigmentation, hair, café au lait spots
              From the side: kyphosis, lumbar lordosis
- **Feel:** Tenderness
- **Move:** Flexion / extension / lateral flexion / rotation
- **Special tests:** Screen for prolapsed intervertebral disc and perform Schober's test
- **Completion:**   Examine the abdomen
              Vascular and neurological examination of lower limb
              Thoracic and lumbar spine X-rays

Schober's test

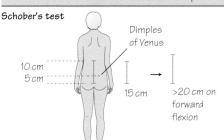

Dimples of Venus

10 cm
5 cm

15 cm

>20 cm on forward flexion

Mark the skin 10 cm above and 5 cm below the dimples of Venus (posterior superior iliac spines)

Ask patient to bend forward with straight legs
Distance between marks should increase to >20 cm

GALS screening examination

Gait
'Please walk over to the door, turn round and walk back'
Look for: symmetry, arm swing, stride length, heel strike, stance and toe off
Ability to turn normally

Arms
'Put your hands behind your head' (**A**)
Tests shoulder abduction, external rotation and elbow flexion
'Put your arms straight'
Tests elbow extension
'Put your hands out in front, palms down and fingers outstretched'
Tests finger extension. Inspect for joint swelling or deformity
'Now turn your hands over'
Tests supination. Inspect for muscle wasting, erythema or deformity
'Make a fist and squeeze my fingers'
Tests finger flexion. Tests for grip
'Touch each finger with your thumb' (**B**)
Tests opposition. Access precision pinch
Squeeze across the MCP joints (**C**)
Check for signs of tenderness

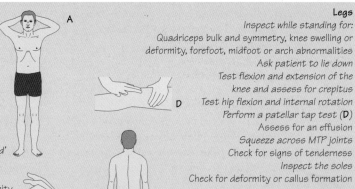
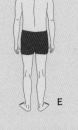
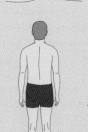
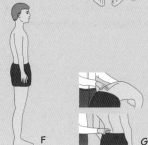
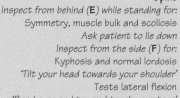

Legs
Inspect while standing for:
Quadriceps bulk and symmetry, knee swelling or deformity, forefoot, midfoot or arch abnormalities
Ask patient to lie down
Test flexion and extension of the knee and assess for crepitus
Test hip flexion and internal rotation
Perform a patellar tap test (**D**)
Assess for an effusion
Squeeze across MTP joints
Check for signs of tenderness
Inspect the soles
Check for deformity or callus formation

Spine
Inspect from behind (**E**) while standing for:
Symmetry, muscle bulk and scoliosis
Ask patient to lie down
Inspect from the side (**F**) for:
Kyphosis and normal lordosis
'Tilt your head towards your shoulder'
Tests lateral flexion
'Bend over and try and touch your toes'
Tests lumbar spine flexion
Assess this while palpating the spine.
Place 2 fingers on the lumbar vertebrae and watch for increased space between them on flexion (**G**)
Press over the midpoint of supraspinatus
Checking for fibromyalgia

Documentation

	Appearance	Movement
Gait	✓	
Arms	✓	✓
Legs	✓	✓
Spine	✓	✓

A tick means normal
If an abnormality is found, place a cross in the box and write summary of the clinical problem under the chart

Station 155: Musculoskeletal examination

Musculoskeletal OSCE stations will be a combination of rheumatological and orthopaedic cases that may also involve neurological components. The candidate may be required to examine the whole of a joint, several joints or just demonstrate certain aspects (e.g. special tests).

Examination routine

- Introduction/consent/ask about pain. It is particularly important to ask about pain because you are likely to be moving the patient's joints
- *Exposure*: remember adequate exposure includes the opposite limb (to allow comparison) and the joints above and below
- *Position*: this will depend on the joint, but usually standing or lying on the couch
- *General inspection*:
  - general condition of the patient and functional ability
  - general inspection for system-specific disease (e.g. Cushingoid features might suggest steroid treatment for RA; ↑ RR in a patient with autoimmune-associated interstitial lung disease, telangiectasia and sclerodactyly would suggest scleroderma)
- ± *Screening test* (i.e. *function*): this might include a GALS screen (see opposite) or a joint-specific screening test (e.g. hand grip)
- *Look* (*system-specific inspection*):
  - skin (erythema, atrophy, scars, rashes, wounds, nail changes)
  - soft tissues (swelling, muscle wasting)
  - bone (deformity, e.g. valgus; abnormal bone alignment, e.g. ulnar deviation)
- *Feel* (*palpation*):
  - skin (temperature)
  - soft tissue (swelling, tenderness, effusion)
  - bone (swelling, tenderness)
- *Move*:
  - passive (the examiner moves the relaxed joint)
  - active (the patient moves the joint)
- *Measure*: leg length, range of movement and muscle bulk
- *Special tests*: see each individual joint station for examples
- *Completion*:
  - examine the joint above and below
  - examine the neurovascular status
  - consider examination of other systems depending on your diagnosis, e.g. respiratory system if the patient has RA
  - request some suitable imaging

A note on swelling

- Soft tissue swelling: boggy swelling (synovitis), fluctuant swelling (effusion)
- Bone swelling: hard, immobile (e.g. osteophytes)

Station 156: GALS screen

- *Please perform a GALS (gait, arms, legs and spine) locomotor screening examination on this patient*

Hints and tips

The routine is summarised opposite. It has been broken down into each relevant area but in reality it is easier to start with the gait and then complete the weight-bearing aspects of the routine, including inspection from the front, side and back before lying the patient down. This avoids moving the patient from the couch to standing too many times. Ask the screening questions first.

- Introduction/consent/ask about pain
- *Exposure*: down to underwear
- *Position*: initially standing
- *Routine*: as opposite
- *Completion*: if an abnormality is detected, then a full history and regional examination of the affected joints would need to be performed

Station 157: Spine examination

- *This 22-year-old male has been referred by his GP with a spinal deformity. Please examine his back*

Hints and tips

- Introduction/consent/ask about pain
- *Exposure*: remove top
- *Position*: stand the patient with their back to you
- *General inspection*: see above
- *Look* (*system-specific inspection*):
  - look from the back: scoliosis, swellings, scars, abnormal pigmentation, hair, café au lait spots
  - look from the side: kyphosis, abnormal lumbar curvature
- *Feel*: feel the spinous processes – start at the prominent spinous process of T1 and work down. Then palpate the paraspinal muscles and the sacroiliac joints
- *Move*:
  - forward flexion: ask the patient to lean forward as far as they can whilst keeping their legs straight. They should be able to get their finger tips within 7 cm of the floor
  - extension: place hands on buttocks and lean back as far as they can – normally about 30°
  - lateral flexion: stand up straight with hands on thighs and lean to each side in turn – normally about 30° each side
  - rotation: sit in a chair with arms crossed, and twist shoulders round to both sides – normally about 40°
- *Special tests*:
  - straight leg test: screen for a prolapsed intervertebral disc. Lie the patient flat on their back and get them to straight leg raise. If there is pain in the back it could be a central disc prolapse. If there is pain in the leg which worsens on passive dorsiflexion of the foot there could be nerve root irritation from a prolapsed lateral disc
  - Schober's test: assessment of spinal mobility (see opposite)
- *Completion*:
  - neurological examination of the legs
  - check femoral pulses (back, buttock and leg pain can be due to iliac artery stenosis)
  - examine abdomen (?pain radiating from large abdominal malignancy)
  - AP and lateral X-rays of the thoracic and lumbar spine

Station 158: Hip examination

- ESSENTIALS CHECKLIST
- Introduction/consent/ask about pain
- Exposure/position
- **Look:**
  General condition, discomfort, walking aids
  Skin discoloration, scars, sinuses, fixed flexion deformity, muscle wasting, leg length discrepancy
- **Feel:** skin temperature, tenderness
- **Move:**
  Flexion and extension
  Abduction and adduction (AB 40° and AD 25°)
  Internal and external rotation (IR/ER 45° from midline)
- **Special tests:** Thomas' test
- **Ask the patient to stand:**
  Trendelenberg test
  Assess gait
- **Completion:**
  Examine the back and the knee
  Vascular and neurological examination of the lower limb
  Consider completing musculoskeletal system exam
  Hip X-rays

Modified Thomas' test for flexion/extension

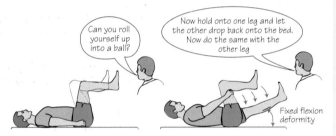

Trendelenburg's test

Assesses the hip abductors
Stand in front of the patient, put your arms out in front of you and get the patient to rest their hands on your forearms
Ask the patient to lift the foot of their bad leg off the floor and hold it for 30 seconds. Then repeat with the good leg
If they are unable to hold their pelvis horizontal and it drops to one side then the test is positive. You will see them lurch slightly to the side and feel them push down onto your forearm. As they are supporting themselves on your forearms they should not fall

Patient with an abnormality of the left hip - findings
A. Standing normally
B. Standing on right leg with normal hip abductors so pelvis remains stable
C. Standing on abnormal left hip with weak abductors so pelvis drops and shoulder moves in compensation

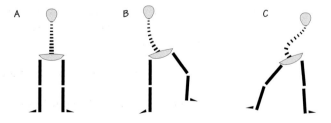

Station 159: Knee examination

- ESSENTIALS CHECKLIST
- Introduction/consent/ask about pain
- Exposure/position
- **Look:**
  General condition, discomfort, walking aids
  Deformity, skin discoloration, scars, swelling, sinuses, muscle wasting
- **Feel:** skin temperature, effusion, tenderness
- **Move:** flexion/extension (-5° → 135°)
- **Special tests:**
  Collateral ligaments
  Cruciate ligaments
  Menisci
- **Ask the patient to stand:** assess gait
- **Completion:**
  Examine the hip and ankle
  Vascular and neurological examination of the lower limb
  Consider completing musculoskeletal system exam
  Knee X-rays

Cruciate ligament tests

1. Flex both knees to 90° and look at them side on for a posterior sag (indicates a tear of the posterior cruciate ligament)
Now sit on the patient's feet – warn them first – and put both of your hands around their knee joint. With your fingers push up on the hamstring tendons (to counteract them pulling the tibia backwards relative to the femur) and place your thumbs anteriorly on the joint line. Gently lean back, pulling on the tibia to see if it can be drawn forwards – anterior drawer test. +ve test = anterior cruciate ligament tear
2. Lachman's test

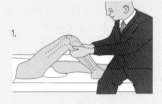
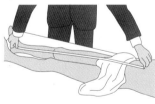

Leg length

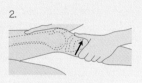
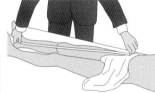

Apparent leg length – measure xiphisternum to medial malleolus of each ankle in turn while the patient is lying supine with their legs parallel
Fixed flexion deformity - apparent leg length will be shorter on the affected side
Fixed abduction deformity - apparent leg length will be greater
True leg length – check the pelvis is perpendicular to the long axis of the body and the legs are placed symmetrically. Measure ASIS to medial malleolus of the ipsilateral ankle. If there is a difference between the two legs, then it is due to a 'true' difference in the length of the bones. By flexing the knee to 90° and observing from the side you can determine whether the shortening is in the femur or the tibia

Station 158: Hip examination

- *This 70-year-old female has been referred by her GP with a painful right hip. Please examine this patient's hips*
- *Please perform Thomas' and Trendelenberg's tests on this patient*

Hints and tips

Explain clearly to the patient what you are going to do *before you do it*. This is particularly important in a musculoskeletal examination when you are going to move the patient's limbs around. Do *not* hurt the patient. Ask if they have any pain before you touch the patient, and throughout your examination be watchful of their face to see if you are causing them any discomfort.

- *Never* examine a joint in isolation; always examine both sides so you can compare
- Introduction/consent/ask about pain
- *Exposure*: remove shoes, socks and trousers. Pull top up above hip joints. At all times maintain the patient's dignity.
- *Position*: lying as flat as possible
- *General inspection*: see Chapter 59
- *Screening test*: gait
- *Look (system-specific inspection)*:
  - when inspecting the hip, get the patient to roll slightly away from you so as not to miss any posterior scars/sinuses
  - leg length discrepancy – measure the true and apparent leg length (good leg first; see opposite)
- *Feel*: check for any skin temperature discrepancy, and then feel for tenderness. Tenderness over the greater trochanter can be caused by trochanteric bursitis (= inflammation of the bursa that overlies the greater trochanter); this is not uncommon in patients with hip osteoarthritis
- *Move*: assessment of movement should ideally be an active rather than a passive process (the patient moving their joint rather than the examining doctor):
  - assess flexion and extension
  - assess abduction and adduction on each side. Stabilise the pelvis by putting some gentle pressure on the anterior superior iliac spine (ASIS) whilst assessing the range movement
  - assess internal and external rotation with the hip and knee flexed.
- *Special tests*: these are part of the routine hip examination
  - *Thomas' test*: this assesses flexion of the hip joint as well as any loss of extension (fixed flexion deformity). Place your hand under the lumbar lordosis. Get the patient to fully flex their good hip and knee, observing with your hand that the lumbar curvature is fully flattened. With their good hip fully flexed, look to see whether or not the other leg has remained flat on the bed. If the other leg has become slightly flexed then that indicates a fixed flexion deformity of that hip. Then get the patient to fully flex their bad hip, before straightening the good hip and looking for a fixed flexion deformity on that side
  - *Trendelenburg's test*: ask the patient to stand. Assess gait and perform test (see opposite)
- *Completion*:
  - examine the joint above and below, and assess the neurovascular status of the limb
  - consider other aspects of the musculoskeletal system
  - request appropriate X-rays

Station 159: Knee examination

- *This 64-year-old male has been referred by his GP with a painful left knee. Please examine him*

Hints and tips

- Always examine both knees so you can compare
- Introduction/consent/ask about pain
- *Exposure*: remove shoes, socks and trousers. Maintain dignity
- *Position*: lying as flat as possible
- *Look*:
  - overall impression of the patient as for Station 158
  - is there any varus/valgus/fixed flexion deformity?
  - look for any scars, in particular for arthroscopy portal scars (which can be difficult to see) and previous joint replacement scars
  - is the knee swollen? If so is it a joint effusion?
- If the knee is swollen, perform the following tests:
  - *patella tap* (for large effusions): slide your hand firmly from 15 cm above the knee joint to the level of the upper pole of the patella. Tap the patella firmly with three fingers and listen and feel for a click
  - *bulge test* (for smaller quantities of fluid): empty the medial compartment by pressing on that side of the joint, then sharply swipe across the lateral side of the joint and observe for a ripple or bulge to appear on the medial aspect of the knee. Also look for a swelling in the popliteal fossa – it could be a Baker's cyst (a posterior herniation of the knee joint capsule containing synovial fluid)
- If you suspect muscle wasting then measure the thigh circumference at a set distance (e.g. 15 cm) above the superior pole of the patella and compare with the other side
- *Feel*: check for any skin temperature discrepancy, and then feel systematically around the joint for tenderness. Start with the knee in extension and then feel around the patella:
  - *grind test*: move the patella up and down while pressing it gently against the femur. Painful grating is suggestive of osteoarthritis in the patellofemoral joint
  - *apprehension test*: move the patella from side to side and see if it makes the patient feel as if their patella might dislocate (especially if a young female patient)
  - flex the knee to 90° and feel around the joint line, and along the course of the medial and lateral collateral ligaments (MCL, LCL)
- *Move*: as with the hip joint, assessment of movement should be an active rather than a passive process:
  - straight leg raise – this assesses the extensor mechanism
  - assess joint flexion. Normally the knee flexes until the calf meets the hamstring. During this movement place your hand over the front of the knee and feel for any clicks or crepitus
- *Special tests*: these are part of the routine knee examination and should be carried out unless the examiner stops you:
  - *cruciate ligament tests* – see opposite
  - *collateral ligament test*: tuck the patient's foot under your arm and flex the knee to 20–30°. Then apply valgus and varus stresses to the knee alternatively whilst feeling the joint line for opening. Opening of the medial joint on valgus stress signifies a MCL injury, while opening of the lateral joint on varus stress signifies a LCL injury
  - *menisci test*: you should know about McMurray's test, but do not perform it unless asked to as it can hurt the patient if positive
- Ask the patient to stand and assess gait
- *Completion*:
  - examine the hip and ankle, and assess the neurovascular status of the leg
  - request standing AP X-ray of the knees and a lateral of the affected knee

Station 160: Hand examination

- ESSENTIALS CHECKLIST
- Introduction/consent/ask about pain
- Exposure/position
- **Look:**
  General condition/specific facies/general signs
  Swelling/deformity/muscle wasting/skin quality/scars/nail changes
- **Feel:** skin temperature/tenderness/nodules/effusions/crepitus/swelling
- **Move:** wrist/finger
- **Special tests:** Phalen's test, Tinel's test
- **Completion:**
  Check sensation
  Examine the elbow
  Examine other joints if involved

  Consider examining for extra-articular manifestations of disease
  Hand X-rays

A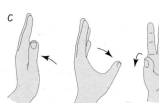

B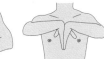

C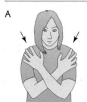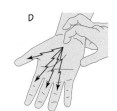

D

Hand signs in RA
Radial deviation at the wrist
Ulnar deviation of the fingers (MCP joint subluxation and dislocation)
Swan neck deformity of the fingers (hyperextension of PIP joints with fixed flexion of MCP and DIP joints)
Boutonnière deformity of the fingers (flexion of PIP joint with extension contracture of DIP and MCP joints)
Z-shaped thumb

Early rheumatoid hand

Fusiform symmetrical MCP + PIP swelling

Extensor tenosynovitis

Wrist tenderness/ swelling
Prominent ulnar styloid

Late rheumatoid hands

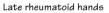

MCP destruction causing subluxation and ulnar deviation of the fingers

Swan-neck deformity of the fingers

Hand signs in OA
Heberden's nodes (DIP joints)
Bouchard's nodes (PIP joints)
NB. RA tends to affect the proximal small joints of the hand, and OA the distal joints

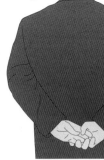

Station 161: Shoulder examination

- ESSENTIALS CHECKLIST
- Introduction/consent/ask about pain
- Exposure/position
- **Look:**
  General condition/systemic features
  Asymmetry and obvious deformity
  Scars
- **Feel:** Skin temperature, tenderness
- **Move:**
  Abduction/forward flexion/internal rotation/external rotation
  (Do the movements yourself to encourage the patient)
- **Special tests:** rotator cuff
- **Completion:**
  Examine the elbow and neck
  Vascular and neurological examination of upper limb
  Shoulder X-rays

Shoulder movements

Internal rotation

External rotation

Extension

Flexion

Abduction

Adduction

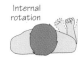

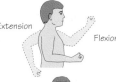

Scratch test

E

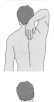
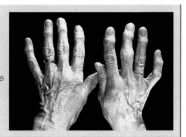

Station 160: Hand examination

• *This 46-year-old female has been attending the rheumatology clinic for the past 5 years. Please examine her hands*

Hints and tips

• Introduction/consent/ask about pain
• *Exposure*: ask the patient to roll their sleeves up to above the elbow
• *Position*: with the patient sitting up, place a pillow on their lap and ask them to place their hands on the pillow, with palms facing downwards
• *General inspection*: see Chapter 59
• *Screening test and function*:
  • ask the patient to cross their arms across their chest (Fig. A, see opposite) and look for evidence of rheumatoid nodules or psoriatic plaques and make a brief assessment of function
  • grip strength – 'squeeze my fingers'
  • pincer strength – 'touch your thumb to your index finger'
  • 'please pick up this object'
  • 'can you undo your top button?'
• *Look* (*system-specific inspection*): inspection is the key component of any hand examination:
  • inspect the dorsal surface and then the palmar, looking for swelling, deformity, muscle wasting, erythema, scars and atrophy. Also check for any nail changes (e.g. vasculitic lesions)
  • look for specific changes associated with rheumatoid arthritis (RA) and osteoarthritis (OA) (see opposite)
• *Feel with the palms up*: feel the peripheral pulses and bulk of the thenar and hypothenar eminences
• *Feel with the palms down*:
  • assess for any skin temperature discrepancy
  • squeeze across the MCPs (see Ch. 59)
  • next gently bimanually palpate each joint in the hand and the wrist in a systematic way looking for swelling and tenderness
• *Move*:
  • passive – this can be performed during palpation but be careful not to hurt the patient and watch their face during the movements
  • active – do the movements yourself and get the patient to copy
  • assess wrist flexion and extension (Fig. B)
  • 'make a fist' – finger flexion
  • 'extend your fingers'
  • 'spread your fingers' – ulnar nerve
  • 'thumb abduction' – median nerve (Fig. C)
• *Special tests*:
  • Phalen's test – for suspected carpal tunnel syndrome (CTS). Get the patient to flex their wrists for 30 seconds – they will develop parasthesiae in the median nerve distribution if positive
  • Tinel's test (Fig. D) – tap the anterior surface of the patient's wrist with your finger. A positive test is if tingling is reproduced (?CTS)
• *Completion*:
  • check sensation in distribution of median, ulnar and radial nerves
  • if you suspect a tendon rupture, test the superficial and profundus flexor tendons
  • examine elbows for skin changes or nodules if not already done
  • look for extra-articular manifestations of RA
  • ask to view any radiographs of the hands

Station 161: Shoulder examination

• *This 73-year-old male has been referred by his GP with a painful left shoulder. Please examine this patient's shoulders*

Hints and tips

• Introduction/consent/ask about pain
• *Exposure*: ask the patient to remove their top
• *Position*: sitting on a chair, away from a wall
• *General inspection*: see Chapter 59
• *Screening test and function*:
  • ask the patient to 'put your hands behind your head' (see Fig. A, Ch. 59)
  • then to 'put your hands behind your back' (Fig. E)
• *Look* (*system-specific inspection*):
  • inspect from the front, side, back and above the patient
  • look for any asymmetry or obvious deformity
  • start from the middle and work out: prominent sternoclavicular joint → deformed clavicles → prominent acromioclavicular joint → wasted deltoid
  • ask the patient to stand up and push their hands against the wall, looking for winging of the scapula due to weakness of the serratus anterior (see Ch. 64)
• *Feel*: check for any skin temperature discrepancy, and then palpate for tenderness:
  • ask the patient to lift their arm to enable palpation of the humeral shaft and head via the axilla
  • glenohumeral joint (anterior, posterior and lateral aspects)
  • sternoclavicular joint, clavicle and acromioclavicular joint
• *Move*:
  • abduct all the way up. Look for difficulty initiating movement, pain during movement and inability to hold arm fully abducted. If the patient is unable to actively perform this movement, then see if their arm can be moved/held passively (see Ch. 63)
  • forward flex all the way up above head, and then swing back into extension
  • external rotation: 'bend your elbows and tuck them into your side and then externally rotate' (60°)
• *Special tests*:
  • scratch test: if the three movements are possible (see opposite), the pathology is unlikely to be of shoulder joint or tendon in origin
  • assessment of the rotator cuff (SITS): (i) **s**upraspinatus – resisted initiation of abduction; (ii) **i**nfraspinatus/**t**eres minor – resisted external rotation; and (iii) **s**ubscapularis – hand on buttock with palm facing away from body. Get the patient to push their hand away from their buttock against resistance
• *Completion*:
  • examine neck and elbow
  • neurovascular examination of the upper limb
  • shoulder X-rays

Station 162: Osteoarthritis of the hip

History hints

Osteoarthritis in the elderly

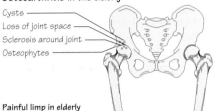

Cysts
Loss of joint space
Sclerosis around joint
Osteophytes

Gradual onset
Slowly worsened
Pain on exertion
Relieved by rest
Difficulty getting
 out of chair

Painful limp in elderly

Examination hints

Limp/walking aid
Fixed flexion deformity
Leg length
Abduction/adduction
Internal/external rotation – remember which is which
Gait and Trendelenberg's test
Examine back and knee
Neurological examination
Peripheral pulses
X-rays: AP hips and lateral of the affected side

Signs in right-sided OA of the hip

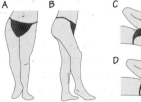

A – Apparent shortening
B – Flexion deformity
C – Thomas' test demonstrating a fixed
 flexion deformity
D – Limitation of flexion
E – Limitation of internal rotation
F – Limitation of abduction

Frequency of articular involvement in RA

Temporomandibular 30%
Cervical spine 40%
Acromioclavicular 50%
Crico arytenoid 10%
Sternoclavicular 30%
Shoulder 60%
Elbow 50%
Hip 50%
Wrist 80% (early)
Metacarpophalangeal, proximal interphalangeal 90% (early)
Knee 80%
Ankle, subtalar 80%
Metatarsophalangeal 90% (early)

Station 163: Ruptured anterior cruciate ligament

History hints

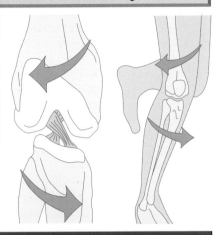

Sustained whilst
 bearing weight
 on a flexed knee
Immediate swelling
Unable to bear weight
Continues to give way
Work/hobbies

Examination hints

Walking aids
Swelling/bruising
Limited range of movement
Positive anterior drawer test and Lachmann's test
Examine hip and ankle
Neurological examination
Peripheral pulses
X-rays: standing AP of both knees and lateral of affected side
 Would expect them to be normal

Station 164: Rheumatoid knee

History hints

Pain
Swelling
Deformity
Giving way
What previous treatment – any benefit?
Other joints affected
Family history
Current medications

Examination hints

Deformity/muscle wasting
Skin changes: thin skin
Range of movement: limited and stiff
Instability
Examine hip and ankle
Neurological examination
Peripheral pulses
X-rays: standing AP of both knees and lateral of affected side

Station 162: Osteoarthritis of the hip

• *Please examine this patient's right hip*
• *Please take a history from this 78-year-old man who has been having pain in his hip when walking*

Example scenario

• *History*: 78-year-old man. Retired gardener. PC: right hip pain; gradual onset 2 years ago. Progressively worsened since. Pain comes on with exertion (e.g. after 3 km walk) and is relieved by rest. Occasional pain getting out of a chair/out of the car. His pain does not stop him partaking in any ADLs. Not taking any analgesia. No previous history of hip problems. Normally fit and well
• *On examination*: patient appears well and is walking with no apparent discomfort or stiffness. No fixed flexion deformity or leg length discrepancy. Flexion to 100°; abduction 30°; adduction 10°; internal rotation 15°; external roation 20°. Trendelenberg's test is negative. Examination of back and knee unremarkable. Good peripheral pulses and no neurological deficit in the lower limb
• *X-rays*: AP and lateral X-rays of the hips show mild sclerosis and osteophyte formation. There is minimal loss of joint space

Discussion

This gentleman has hip pain but with only minimal disturbance to his quality of life. There is a reasonable preservation of range of movement and no deformity.

Management of OA

• *Medical*:
  simple analgesia, physiotherapy, lifestyle modification
• *Surgical*: joint replacement
In most cases, unless the patient presents with advanced disease, you would consider a trial of non-operative management first.

Station 163: Ruptured anterior cruciate ligament

• *Please examine this patient's left knee*
• *Please demonstrate the anterior draw test on this patient*

Example scenario

• *History*: 22-year-old man. Window cleaner and keen rugby player. Presents with left knee problems. Tackled playing rugby 3 months ago. At the time of the tackle he was bearing weight on his left leg, which was slightly flexed. He felt as if something 'popped' inside his knee and it swelled up immediately. He was unable to bear weight and had to be helped from the pitch. He attended A&E and was given a splint and some crutches. He has seen the physiotherapists. The swelling and pain have improved. He is normally fit and well
• *On examination*: patient appears well and is walking with the aid of crutches. There is some evidence of bruising around the knee and mild swelling. Patella tap is negative but the bulge test is positive. There is no tenderness. He is able to straighten his leg but experiences discomfort with the straight leg raise. Knee flexion is limited to 100°. There is a positive anterior drawer test, but no posterior sag. His collateral ligaments appear to be intact
• *X-rays*: Standing AP and lateral X-rays of his knee appear normal

Discussion

The patient has a ruptured left anterior cruciate ligament (ACL) and the injury was sustained whilst bearing weight through a flexed knee. The knee became immediately swollen (meniscal injuries swell gradually). Subsequently, he experienced his knee giving way and on examination, there were signs of a resolving haemarthrosis (blood in the joint) and a positive anterior drawer test.

In the acute setting it would have been difficult to assess the knee due to swelling and pain. A splint and crutches provide support whilst the acute injury settles down. This gentleman would be a candidate for having his ACL repaired – he is young, works up a ladder and is a keen sportsman. Prior to reconstruction further assessment of the internal derangement of his knee is required (using MRI scan or an arthroscopy). This may also reveal an injury to one of the menisci.

Mx   Continue with physiotherapy whilst awaiting a MRI scan
      Plan to reconstruct ACL if scan confirms clinical findings.

Station 164: Rheumatoid knee

• *Please examine this patient's right knee and discuss other aspects of the musculoskeletal system that you would like to examine*

Example scenario

• *History*: 68-year-old female. Retired housewife. Recently widowed and lives alone in a house. PC: right knee pain. Long history of joint problems starting in her mid thirties. Hands affected first, initially with pain and swelling at the MCP joints. Hands and wrists became progressively more deformed with time. MCP joints replaced in her mid forties. She no longer has pain in her hands, but they are very stiff. She struggles with most activities of daily living such as dressing and picking up a cup. Occupational therapists have provided numerous aides, enabling her to manage on her own and maintain her independence. Since her early forties she has also had problems with her knees. Initially they were swollen and very painful. Over the years despite lots of physiotherapy her knees have become progressively more deformed. The pain is much less these days but she is now troubled by her right knee giving way. She has been on numerous medications for her joints in the past, but she is no longer on anything and has been told that her RA 'has run its course'. She has no hip problems and reports that she is otherwise fit and well and wants to have 'something done'
• *On examination*: extensive rheumatoid disease affecting hands, wrists and knees. Looking at the knees, there are gross bilateral fixed flexion valgus deformities, which are worse on the right. There is considerable wasting of the quadriceps muscle. The joints are stiff but not swollen, red or hot. There is marked instability of the right knee. There is a good pain free movement of the hips
• *X-rays*: standing AP and a lateral X-rays show significant joint destruction and deformity

Discussion

Occasionally RA first presents as a monoarthropathy in the knee, but it is more often the case that the knee is affected as part of a polyarthropathy. An elderly patient with 'burnt out' RA is much more likely to be found for an exam than someone with an acute exacerbation. With advanced disease the management options are limited.

Mx   *Non-operative*   Physiotherapy, a walking stick/frame plus some form of supportive knee brace
      Operative   Knee replacement (a knee replacement in this woman would be technically challenging, with a higher than usual risk of an unsatisfactory outcome)

Station 165: Painful shoulder

History hints

Right/left handed
Pain
Trauma/trigger factor
When does it hurt: with what movement/activity?
Ability to do normal activites/hobbies
Previous episodes
Neck problems

Examination hints

Appearance – would expect it to be normal
Tenderness
Range of movement:

        Flexion/extension
        Abduction
        Internal/external rotation

If unable to perform active movement, is passive tolerated?
If difficulty abducting – what part of arc is problematic?

0°	Rotator cuff tear
60–120°	Painful arc syndrome
140-180°	OA

Neck and upper limb neurovascular examination
X-rays: AP and lateral of the shoulder joint

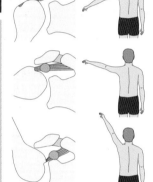

Painful arc/impingement syndrome

Station 166: Ankylosing spondylitis

History hints

Age at onset (< 40 years, male)
Back pain + morning stiffness
Improves with activity
Associated features
(e.g. red eye)
Impact on life
FH of spinal disease

Examination hints

Question mark posture
Wall – occiput test
Observe from the side:
  Cervical hyperextension
  Thoracic kyphosis
  Loss of lumbar lordosis
  Flexed knees and hips
Signs of extra-articular disease

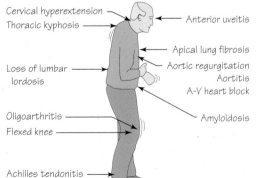

Articular features

Cervical hyperextension
Thoracic kyphosis
Loss of lumbar lordosis
Oligoarthritis
Flexed knee
Achilles tendonitis

Associations (the 'A's)
Anterior uveitis
Apical lung fibrosis
Aortic regurgitation
Aortitis
A-V heart block
Amyloidosis

Vertebrae
Squaring and syndesmophytes
Fibrosis/ossification of ligaments
→ 'Bamboo spine'
→ Rigid ↓ mobility
→ Risk of fracture

Station 167: Hallux valgus

History hints

Congenital/acquired
Uni/bilateral
Pain
Deformity
History of pointy shoes
Any treatment:
• Changing shoes, insoles, padding
• Surgery

Examination hints

It is all about observation
'Marked hallux valgus with prominence of the 1st MT head, worse on the the left. There is an overlying inflamed bunion with crowding and deformity of the lesser toes' (NB. A bunion = protective bursa)

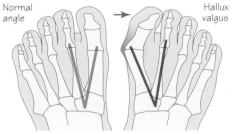

Normal angle

Hallux valgus

Station 168: Charcot joint

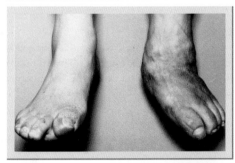

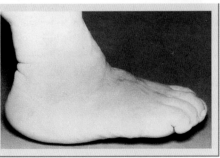

Station 165: Painful shoulder

- *History*: 60-year-old right-handed man. Office worker and keen tennis player. Presents with right shoulder pain that has been troubling him for the last month. It started following a weekend spent decorating his spare bedroom. He gets pain with most movements of his shoulder, but particularly on abduction. He is currently unable to play tennis
- *On examination*:
  - inspection: shoulder appears normal
  - palpation: significant tenderness along the anterior edge of the acromium
  - move: discomfort on abduction moving through the range 60–120°. As the arm passes beyond 120° the pain eases. Other movements are normal. He has a good range of pain-free neck movement.
  - neurovascular examination of the upper limb is normal
- *X-rays*: appear normal

Discussion

His history is suggestive of a painful arc syndrome (subacute supraspinatus tendonitis) caused by repetitive irritation of the supraspinatus tendon where it passes beneath the coracoacromial ligament (see opposite). The space beneath the ligament is tightest when the shoulder is abducting between 60° and 120°.

Mx

Medical	Short course of NSAIDs; physiotherapy
	Consider steroid injection into subacromial space if symptoms persist > 1 month
Surgical	Consider arthroscopic subacromial decompression if symptoms persist > 3 months

Other 'arc problems'

- An inability to initiate abduction suggests a rotator cuff tear. These patients will tolerate passive abduction, and can hold their arm up in the air using their deltoid muscle
- A high painful arc (140–180°) is more likely to be due to osteoarthritis of the acromioclavicular joint

Station 166: Ankylosing spondylitis

- *History*: 19-year-old male student. Four-year history of worsening back pain and stiffness. Gradual onset with no history of preceding back problems or trauma. It started as an occasional ache in his lower back. His pain is worse first thing in the morning and after any period of inactivity. Over the last 18 months he has found it increasingly difficult to stand up straight. Other than being permanently tired he is fit and well
- *On examination*: patient appears well, but walks with a slightly stooped posture. On inspection there is exaggerated thoracic kyphosis with flattening of his lumbar lordosis. As he stands looking forwards both his hips and knees are slightly flexed. Asking the patient to stand with his heels, buttocks and back against a wall, he is unable to get the back of his head to touch the wall. No neurovascular abnormality
- *X-rays*: AP and lateral X-rays of the thoracolumbar spine are taken. On the AP view there is the characteristic appearance of a 'bamboo' spine. On the lateral view the vertebral bodies look abnormally square, with a loss of their anterior concavity

Discussion

The history and examination are typical for ankylosing spondylitis (AS), though the symptoms could theoretically be caused by one of the other seronegative arthropathies.

AS presents with a history of progressive back ache and pain prior to the detection of the kyphosis. The patient compensates for the kyphosis with flexion of the hips and knees, and also by exaggerating the cervical lordosis. However, he is unable to compensate when asked to stand straight with his heels, buttocks and head against the wall (the wall test). The HLA B27 is positive in 90% of patients with AS.

Mx	*Early stages*	Physiotherapy to maintain posture and function
		NSAIDs to try to prevent pain and stiffness
	Later stages	Corrective spinal fusion

Scoliosis is a spinal deformity observed from behind the patient rather than from the side. It can be congenital or idiopathic, becoming apparent during one of the growth spurts, or in later life in the presence of osteoporosis. Treatment may be non-operative or operative depending on the severity of the curve.

Spondyloarthropathies

Ankylosing spondylitis; psoriatic arthritis; reactive arthritis, e.g. Reiter's syndrome; enteropathic arthritis

Station 167: Hallux valgus

- *History*: 50-year-old woman. Presents with bilateral forefoot pain and deformity. This has been getting worse for several years. She now finds that it is causing significant problems with her quality of life. She is also embarrassed to take her shoes off. She has tried insoles and padding, but with no symptom relief
- *On examination*: the patient walks with a little discomfort wearing soft, comfortable shoes. Bilaterally there is a prominence of the 1st metatarsal head, with the great toe angled laterally and frequently rotated. The lesser toes appear slightly crowded. On the medial aspect of the 1st metatarsal head there is a large inflamed bunion

Discussion

This is the commonest of the foot deformities. Remember that a bunion is a protective bursa formed in pressure areas, and is secondary to the underlying deformity.

Mx	*Non-operative*	Footwear modification, insoles and padding
	Operative	Corrective osteotomy – depending on the severity of the bony deformity on X-ray
Causes	*Primary*	Congenital
	Secondary	RA
		Poor muscle tone in old age
		Poor shoes

Station 168: Charcot joints

Charcot's disease is a rapidly progressive neuropathic arthritis, with considerable joint destruction. As seen in the photographs opposite the joint is deformed and swollen, but has a surprisingly good and painless range of movement.

- Patients complain of weakness, instability, swelling and deformity, but *not* pain
- The joint lacks position sense and pain sensation
- X-rays show gross destruction of the bony anatomy
- There is no treatment, and management usually involves splintage
- Occasionally the joints require surgical fusion

Upper limb nerve injuries: general

History hints

History of trauma
Sensory disturbance
Motor disturbance
Functional limitation

Examination hints

Examination of all nerve injuries relies on anatomical knowledge
Injuries can be broadly divided into nerve root injuries and peripheral nerve injuries

For each nerve root of the brachial plexus and each major peripheral nerve you should know:
• Common mechanisms of damage
• Motor distribution
• Sensory distribution
• Clinical assessment of the nerve

Myotomes	Shoulder	Elbow	Wrist	Fingers	Reflex
C5	Abduction and external rotation	Flexion			Biceps
C6		Flexion, pronation/supination	Flexion/extension		Supinator
C7	Adduction and internal rotation	Extension	Flexion/extension	Flexion/extension	Triceps
C8		Extension		Flexion/extension	Finger
T1				Abduction/adduction	

Station 169: Radial nerve lesion

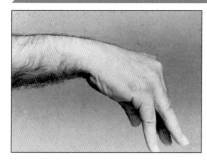

Patterns of sensory loss

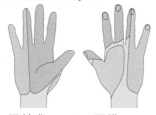

■ Median nerve   ■ Ulnar nerve
■ Radial nerve

Station 170: Median nerve lesion

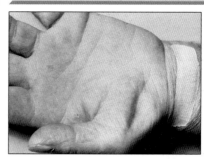

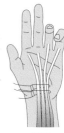

FDP

Station 171: Ulnar nerve lesion

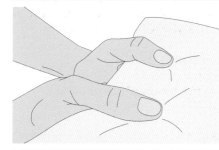

Froment's test
Right = normal thumb adduction
Left = loss of ulnar nerve and hence thumb flexion (median)

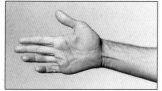
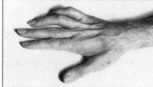

Station 172: Long thoracic nerve lesion

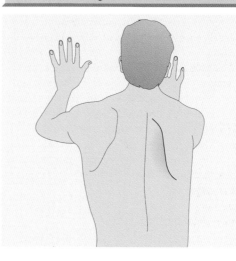

Winging of scapula: occurs following injury to the long thoracic nerve

NB. For dermatomal distribution see Chapter 32

Upper limb nerve injuries

- *Please examine this patient's hands*
- *Please check the neurology in this patient's arms*
- *This patient has had previous surgery on their neck, please examine their upper limbs*

Hints and tips

- Listen carefully to the instruction and follow the most appropriate examination routine as described in the neurology or musculoskeletal chapters
- Introduction/consent/ask about pain
- *Exposure*: expose the whole upper limb, neck and thorax (have a look at the cervical spine as well)
- *Position*: sitting up
- *General inspection*: as described in Chapter 59. For example:
  - signs of acromegaly – ? carpal tunnel syndrome
  - cachexia and Horner's – ?wasting of the small muscles of the hand due to a brachial plexus lesion, i.e. Pancoast's tumour
- *Routine*: as per relevant chapter
- *Completion*: consider examining the rest of the neurological and musculoskeletal systems and also think about other systems that could be relevant, e.g. respiratory system if considering a Pancoast's tumour

Root injuries

Brachial plexus nerve root injuries can occur with neck trauma. Classically, lower brachial plexus root injuries (C8, T1) occur with traction to the abducted arm (e.g. grabbing onto something when falling or during a breech delivery). This leads to wasting of the intrinsic muscles of the hand and sensory loss to the ulnar border of the hand.

Damage to the upper roots C5/C6 occurs in Erb–Duchenne palsy, which was originally described as a result of shoulder trauma during delivery. It results in a limp shoulder (paralysis of abductors), internally rotated shoulder (paralysis of lateral rotators) and pronated forearm (paralysis of biceps). It may also involve a flexed wrist if there is C7 involvement – 'waiter's tip position'.

Station 169: Radial nerve lesion
Classic causes of injury
- Fractures of the shaft of the humerus
- Pressure in axilla from a crutch or chair

Motor loss
- Loss of triceps action only with very high injuries (muscle innervated proximally)
- Wrist drop (loss of forearm extensors) (opposite)
- Loss of finger extension

Sensory loss
- Dorsal radial $3^1/2$ digits
- Autonomous area = 1st dorsal webspace of hand

Station 170: Median nerve lesion
Classic causes of injury
- Carpal tunnel compression
- Supracondylar fractures of humerus in children
- Pentrating injuries
- Dislocation of the lunate

Motor loss
- *Wrist level*:
  - loss of function and later wasting of the thenar eminence (LOAF – two radial **l**umbricals, **o**pponens pollicis, **a**bductor pollicis brevis and **f**lexor pollicis brevis)
  - inability to abduct thumb (test by asking the patient, with the palm up, to point thumb to ceiling against resistance)
  - loss of true opposition
- *Above cubital fossa*:
  - wasting of forearm and thenar eminence (opposite)
  - loss of flexors to thumb and index finger
  - chronically the hand forms 'Benediction' position (opposite)

Sensory loss
- Palmar radial 3.5 digits
- Autonomous area = pulp of index finger

Station 171: Ulnar nerve lesion
Classic causes of injury
- Compression at the elbow
- Fracture at the medial epicondyle
- Penetrating injuries
- Marked cubitus valgus
- Lacerations at the wrist

Motor loss
- *Wrist lesion*:
  - hyperextension at MCP joint and flexion at interphalangeal joint of the little and ring fingers due to loss of the ulnar two lumbricals
  - wasting of intrinsic muscles of the hand – 'guttering' of dorsum of the hand
  - inability to adduct thumb = basis of Froment's test (see below)
- *Elbow (high) lesion*:
  - flexor carpi ulnaris is also lost
  - less flexion of the ring and little fingers
  - deformity is less severe = 'ulnar paradox'

Sensory loss
- Ulnar 1.5 fingers

Froment's test
Loss of the ulnar nerve results in the loss of the adductor pollicis, which means that the patient 'cheats' and flexes the thumb (median nerve) to grip a piece of paper between the thumb and index finger.

Station 172: Long thoracic nerve lesion
Classic cause of injury
- Iatrogenic – during axillary dissection for breast cancer

Motor loss
- Serratus anterior (C5–C7)

Examination
- Look for evidence of surgery or injury to lateral thoracic wall, e.g. surgery
- Ask the patient to push against a wall whilst standing
- Look for 'winging' of the scapula – the medial aspect will stick out. This is due to the unopposed action of the pectoralis minor

Station 173: Management of major injuries

Primary survey

A	Airway maintenance with cervical spine control
B	Breathing and oxygenation
C	Circulation and control of bleeding
D	Disability (neurological status)
E	Exposure

Adjuncts to the primary survey

Adjuncts are used to aid the primary survey.
- The monitoring of pulse, BP, ECG trace and oxygen saturations
- The insertion of urinary and gastric catheters should be considered as part of the resuscitation phase
- X-rays: AP CXR, AP pelvis and a lateral c-spine
- Do not allow X-rays to slow down the primary survey

Secondary survey

Head-to-toe evaluation of the patient with 'AMPLE' history and thorough physical examination

A	Allergies
M	Medication
P	Past medical history/?pregnant
L	Last meal
E	Event relating to the injury

Management of an open fracture

An open fracture represents a communication between the external environment and the bone, often associated with soft tissue damage and is susceptible to bacterial contamination. Open fractures are therefore prone to problems with infection and healing

Clinical assessment (history, examination, analgesia, X-rays):
- Where and how did the injury occur – on a farm or in an office? This is important when considering which antibiotics are appropriate
- Where is the wound? If it is near a joint it should be assumed that it communicates with the joint
- Assess distal neurovascular status

Management:
- Prompt recognition
- Debridement and gentle lavage
- Photograph
- Betadine-soaked dressing
- Splint (POP backslab)
- Antibiotics ± tetanus
- Keep NBM and D/W senior colleague as patient requires urgent formal wound debridement and fracture stabilisation in theatre

Glasgow Coma Scale

Eye opening		Verbal response	
Spontaneous	4	Orientated	5
On command	3	Confused	4
On pain	2	Words	3
Nil	1	Sounds	2
		Nil	1

Motor response	
Obeys	6
Localises pain	5
Normal flexion	4
Abnormal flexion	3
Extension	2
Nil	1

Life-threatening breathing injuries

Tension pneumothorax
SOB, ↑RR, asymmetrical chest movement, deviation of trachea away from affected side, ↓air entry, hyper-resonance
Mx: urgent needle decompression and chest drain
Flail chest ± pulmonary contusion
Serious hypoxia may result from injury to underlying lung
Mx: oxygen ± ventilation
Massive haemothorax: see below
Open pneumothorax
Sucking chest wound, through which air passes in preferentially to the trachea
Mx: an occlusive dressing taped securely on three sides followed by a chest drain

Life-threatening circulatory problems

Massive haemothorax
SOB, ↓mvt of chest wall, ↓air entry, dull percussion note
Mx: chest drain. If there is > 1500 ml of blood in the chest, or there is a rate of blood loss > 200 ml/h for 2-4 hours then it is likely that the patient will require a thoracotomy
Cardiac tamponade
↑pulse, ↓BP, ↑JVP, muffled heart sounds
Mx: pericardiocentesis. Will require thoracotomy
Abdominal injuries
Shock can result from occult haemorrhage in the abdomen and pelvis. Assess the abdomen by inspection, auscultation, percussion and palpitation. Suspicion of an abdominal injury necessitates further investigation (US/CT/DPL/laparotomy)
Musculoskeletal trauma
Shock can result from a femoral or pelvic fracture
Mx: splint the limb enabling clot formation, pain control and prevention of further damage. Always assess the distal neurovascular status first

Station 173: Management of major injuries

- *This 42-year-old male has been brought to A&E following a road traffic accident. You are the first doctor to arrive in resuscitation, please begin your assessment*

Hints and tips

This station could be run as a moulage, with an actor having been 'made up' to have an injury, or could utilise a mannequin (see Ch. 11). Trauma is the commonest cause of death in people under 40 years of age.
- Most deaths occur within the first hour of injury, often before the patient arrives in hospital; the cause of death in these patients is usually

severe brain or cardiovascular injury for which resuscitation would have little effect
• A second, and much smaller, peak of trauma deaths occurs between 1 and 4 hours after injury. These deaths usually result from hypoxia or uncompensated blood loss and are usually preventable. The period during which lives can be saved by prompt and efficient treatment is called the *golden hour*
• A third peak of deaths occurs days or weeks later when patients die of late complications of trauma and multiple organ failure
• The Advanced Trauma Life Support (ATLS) program has become the standard for emergency trauma care. The ATLS consists of four inter-related stages:
  • a rapid *primary survey with simultaneous resuscitation*
  • a detailed *secondary survey*
  • constant *re-evaluation*
  • initiation of *definitive care*

Primary survey

The most important principle in the management of the trauma patient is to treat the greatest threat to life first, and not wait for a detailed history prior to the evaluation of an acutely injured patient. However, gathering information from pre-hospital personnel will provide useful information that may guide you in your resuscitation, including mechanism of injury.

The most immediate threat to life is loss of an airway. This is followed by the inability to breathe, the loss of circulating blood volume and, finally, the presence of an expanding intracranial mass lesion. The pneumonic *ABCDE* (see opposite) defines the specific, ordered evaluations and interventions that should be followed in all injured patients.

The management and resuscitation of a trauma patient can be carried out by one person using the principles of ATLS. In reality, management of the injured patient is a team effort, with doctors with special skills and expertise providing care simultaneously.

Airway with cervical spine control
• *Causes* of compromised airway include:
  • decreased level of consciousness
  • facial or neck trauma
  • severe burns causing airway oedema
  • inhalation of vomit or teeth
• *Clinical assessment*: 'Hello, my name is James. I am one of the doctors looking after you. Can you tell me your name and what happened?' The patient who responds clearly can be assumed to have a patent airway. Patients who are unconscious, agitated or cyanosed may have airway obstruction. (*Stridor* is the sound of an obstructed airway)
• *Management*:
  • maintain airway control with a cervical spine control; always assume that the patient has a neck injury until proven otherwise. Therefore, the neck requires inline immobilisation throughout, either manually or with a hard collar and sandbags
  • high-flow oxygen with a reservoir bag
  • check for foreign bodies and clear if present
  • in managing the compromised airway, adjuncts include jaw thrust, naso/oropharyngeal airways or a definitive airway with a cuffed endotracheal tube

Breathing and oxygenation
Even if the airway is clear, the peripheral tissues will not be adequately oxygenated unless the patient can breathe.
• *Clinical assessment*:
  • expose the chest
  • look for external injuries, and check respiratory rate and symmetrical chest movement
  • check for deviation of the trachea
  • percuss and auscultate the chest
  • monitor oxygen saturations
  • life-threatening injuries must be identified and managed

Circulation and haemorrhage control
Shock is defined as inadequate tissue perfusion and oxygenation. Hypotension (shock) following injury must be considered to be hypovolaemic in origin until proven otherwise. Other types of shock encountered in the severely injured patient are cardiogenic, neurogenic and septic shock.
• *Clinical assessment*:
  • level of consciousness
  • skin colour
  • pulse/BP/capillary return
  • urine output
• *Management*:
  • sites of external haemorrhage should be identified and the bleeding controlled with direct pressure
  • insert two wide-bore IV cannulae
  • resuscitate with 2 L of warm Hartmann's solution
  • the reponse to this initial resuscitation then guides the subsequent circulatory resuscitation
  • life-threatening injuries must be identified and managed

Disability
A rapid neurological evaluation is performed at the end of the primary survey. The GCS is a quick, simple method for determining the level of consciousness (see opposite). Check the pupil size and reaction and look for any evidence of a spinal cord injury. Remember that hypoglycaemia, alcohol and other drugs can alter a patient's level of consciousness (do not forget glucose).

Exposure
The patient should be exposed, cutting off clothing if necessary. Caution must be taken to prevent the patient becoming hypothermic.

Re-evaluation
Throughout the primary survey the patient should be undergoing continual resuscitation and re-evaluation. Aggressive resuscitation and the management of life-threatening injuries, *as they are identified*, are essential to optimise patient survival. If there is any change in the patient's condition, or following any intervention, you should reassess the patient and return to 'A'. The patient is likely to be frightened and in pain, so do not forget to give appropriate analgesia (usually morphine).

Transfer to definitive care
If it becomes apparent during the primary survey that the patient's needs exceed the local capabilities, then transfer to an appropriate facility should be arranged via a senior doctor to senior doctor referral.

Secondary survey
The secondary survey does not begin until the primary survey has been completed, resuscitation is established and the patient is showing normalisation of their vital signs. The secondary survey involves a head-to-toe evaluation of the patient including a full history and a complete, whole body examination. The AMPLE pneumonic (see opposite) is a useful aide memoir for this purpose.

Station 174: MSK imaging interpretation – hips and pelvis

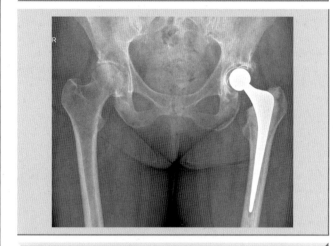

Station 175: MSK imaging interpretation – knee

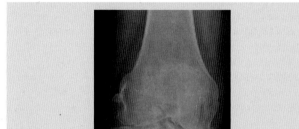
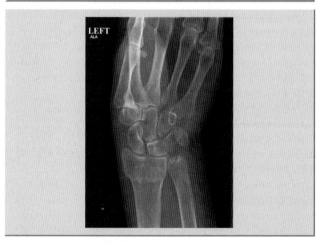

Station 176: MSK imaging interpretation – hands

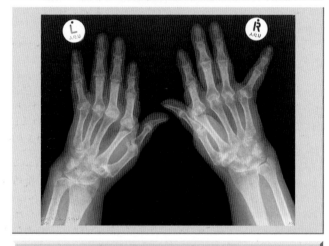

Station 177: MSK imaging interpretation – wrist

Station 178: MSK imaging interpretation – hip

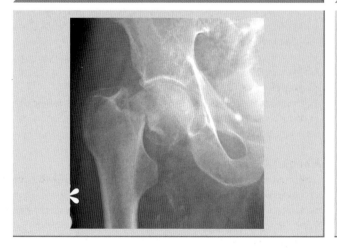

Station 179: MSK imaging interpretation – pelvis

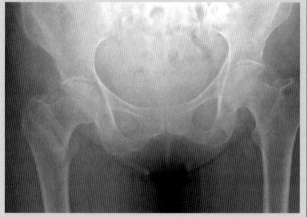

Musculoskeletal (MSK) imaging

Plain X-rays are good for assessing bone. They are frequently the first-line investigation in the assessment of musculoskeletal disorders. However, it is important to remember that X-rays are not sensitive to subtle changes and can be difficult to interpret in areas of complex anatomy.

When taking a plain X-ray of a bone or joint it is customary to take two differing projections. This gives the interpreter an appreciation of the orientation, and minimises the chance of missing subtle abnormalities, e.g. a small hairline fracture. X-rays should always be reviewed with the clinical picture in mind.

When interpreting an X-ray it is important to have a system:
- Check it is the right film of the right patient
- Check that you have two views
- Check that the X-ray is adequate, e.g. if you are concerned about a fracture in a long bone you need to see the entirety of that bone as well as the joints above and below
- Look at the bones, the joints and the surrounding soft tissues

Station 174: MSK imaging interpretation – hips and pelvis
- This is a plain radiograph of Mr X, taken on the date Y
- It is an AP view showing his hips and pelvis
- On the left side there is a total hip replacement
- On the right side, the hip joint does not appear normal with a loss of joint space, sclerosis, subchondral cysts and osteophytes
- This is consistent with a diagnosis of osteoarthritis
- For completeness, request a lateral view

Hints and tips
- Check the name and date. If you feel that it is the wrong way round then turn it, but this would be unusual in an exam
- Ideally you should have two views; if you are only given one view then make a point of telling the examiner that you would like a second view. In this case you would like a lateral view of the affected hip
- When looking at a normal hip X-ray you see the smooth contours of the ball and socket joint, with a well-preserved joint space. The X-ray characteristics of osteoarthritis can be remembered by the pneumonic LOSS: loss of joint space; osteophytes; sclerosis; subchondral cysts

Station 175: MSK imaging interpretation – knee
- This is a plain radiograph of Mr X, taken on the date Y
- It is an AP view of his right knee
- These views would normally be taken with the patient weight bearing
- There is loss of joint space, osteophytes, sclerosis and subchondral cysts; there is a valgus deformity
- This is consistent with osteoarthritis
- Also request a lateral view and a standing AP of the other knee

Station 176: MSK imaging interpretation – hands
- This is a plain radiograph of Mrs X, taken on the date Y
- It is an AP view of both of this patient's hands and wrists
- There is marked articular destruction at the MCP joints, proximal interphalangeal (PIP) joints and at the wrist joint
- There is subluxation of the MCP joints
- There is also ulnar deviation at the MCP joints and radial deviation at the wrist joint
- A lateral view would provide more information, e.g. are there swan neck deformities?
- The bone around the joints appears to be osteopaenic
- These changes are consistent with this patient having RA

Station 177: MSK imaging interpretation – wrist
- This is a plain radiograph of Mr X, taken on the date Y
- This is an AP view of a wrist joint showing a transverse fracture of the distal radius with radial shortening and flattening
- Request a lateral view, which should show dorsal displacement and angulation of the distal fragment, with the characteristic 'dinner-fork' deformity of a Colles' type fracture

Hints and tips
- This type of injury was described by Abraham Colles in 1814
- When describing a fracture the things that you are looking for are:
  - location – where it is
  - fracture pattern – transverse, oblique, comminuted, butterfly fragment
  - direction of displacement of the distal fragment, and the extent of the displacement
  - rotation and shortening

Station 178: MSK imaging interpretation – hip
- This is a plain radiograph of Mr X, taken on the date Y
- This is an AP view of the right hip
- There is a fracture at the base of the neck of the femur (intracapsular)
- Request an AP of the other side and also a lateral

Hints and tips
- The hip capsule attaches just proximal to the inter-trochanteric line
- With an intracapsular fractured neck of femur we are concerned about the blood supply to the femoral head, which can develop avascular necrosis
- *Management*: either reduce the fracture and fix it with screws (this only tends to be done in younger patients as they must not weight bear for several weeks after surgery) or perform a hemi-arthroplasty (half a hip replacement). Some surgeons may consider a total hip replacement. Following a hemi-arthroplasty or total hip replacement, the patient can get out of bed and start walking the next day
- You should know the Garden classification

Station 179: MSK imaging interpretation – pelvis
- This is a plain radiograph of Mr X, taken on the date Y
- This is an AP view of the hips
- There is a fracture of the neck of the right femur
- This is an extracapsular hip fracture, running between the greater and lesser trochanters
- Request a lateral view

Hints and tips
- With an extracapsular fractured neck of femur we are not concerned about the blood supply to the femoral head
- *Management*: reduce the fracture and fix it with screws and a plate. The implant is called a dynamic hip screw
- The patient can get out of bed and start walking the next day

Paediatric history

General information
- Name, age and birth date, sex, race, referral source, relationship of the child and informant

Presenting complaint
- Presenting complaints
- Record the child's and mother's own words

History of present illness
- 'Why did you bring him/her?'
- 'What concerns you?'
- List symptoms in chronological order
- When did the present illness start?
- Enquire about developments, exacerbating and relieving factors, contacts and travel
- Current treatments and previous

Systems review
- Special emphasis needs to be on feeding and on growth
- Child's general health, e.g. acute weight change, fever, weakness or mood alterations
- Other key features: appetite and feeding, inputs and outputs, sleep, parental coping

Past medical history
More detail required than an adult PMH but the amount of detail will depend on the age of the child and their presenting complaint
Prenatal history
- Maternal infections during pregnancy, vaginal bleeding, toxaemia, obstetric investigations including fetal scans or procedures
Birth history
- Pregnancy duration, nature and type of labour and delivery, birth weight
Neonatal history
- Apgar scores and presence of cyanosis or respiratory distress ± resuscitation
- Jaundice, anaemia, convulsions, dysmorphic states or congenital anomalies
- Neonatal infections, hypoglycaemia, hypothermia
- Accidents

General considerations
- Rapport is everything. It is impossible to examine a screaming child, and the parent will not like you
- Think carefully about the environment, e.g. non-threatening, friendly, availability of toys
- The adult with the child is essential; the history may need to come from them
- Tailor the clinical encounter depending on the age of the child. Approach children at their own pace
- 90% of the examination can be done without touching the child, purely by observation
- Ask the parents about their hopes, fears and expectations about the illness

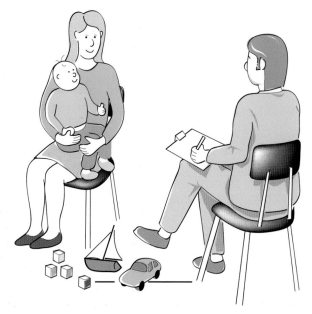

Social history
- Details of the family unit (number in the family, who lives at home, marital status of parents, main carer, family finances, occupations, smokers)
- Schooling
- Hobbies and habits
- Effect of the illness on the family

Family history
- Stillbirths, TB, jaundice, diabetes mellitus, renal diease, seizures, jaundice, malformations
- Are siblings and parents alive and well?
- Genetic chart may be helpful for inherited diseases
- Include any significant family

Drug history and allergies

Immunisation history
- Types, dates and reactions

Developmental history
- Ages of achievement of milestones, weights and positions on growth charts and comparison to siblings/peers
- School performance
Feeding history
- Breast or bottle and type of milk
- History of vomiting, regurgitation, colic, diarrhoea?
- Age of weaning
- Food intolerances, eating patterns
Behavioural history
- Sleep problems, use of alcohol or drugs, bad temper, hyperactivity, withdrawal, response to strangers, crying, nail biting

General hints and tips

Due to the unpredictable nature of dealing with babies and small children, many of the OSCE stations will involve older children, mannequins or data interpretation with photos or other clinical information. History stations for babies could involve a real life parent or an actor. Rather than an OSCE, some medical schools use a long case exam or Objective Structured Long Examination Record (OSLER), which is less demanding on the children, and all the examples which follow could easily fit into an exam of this sort. In the OSCE, the child will not be unwell and history taking should be tailored to the duration of the station and also the age of the patient.

Station 180: Bronchiolitis

Student info: *Mrs JG has brought her 11-month-old boy to see his GP. He has developed noisy breathing over the last 24 hours and she is concerned about him. Please take a full history from Mrs JG and be prepared to discuss the case with the examiner. You are not required to examine the baby*

Patient info: *You are a 31-year-old mother and have brought your 11-month-old boy, Robert, to see his GP. You have had no previous pregnancies and this one ran smoothly. Robert has had no medical problems since birth and has reached normal developmental milestones. He has been unwell for 3 days with initially a runny nose and then has developed problems with his breathing. He seems at times to be fighting for his breath although he has not had any episodes where he has stopped breathing. There has been no stridor or hoarse voice. He has a cough and has not been feeding well. You are concerned because several of his friends have also been struggling with what was thought to be a cold, but one of them required admission to hospital last week. He has had no previous episodes of difficulty breathing and there is no family history of childhood respiratory problems*

Hints and tips

• Ascertain the mother's current understanding of the situation including her reason for visiting the GP
• Determine symptomatology and timing
• Take a full respiratory history
• Determine negative history of atopy
• Establish history of poor feeding
• Confirm no past medical history or previous problems with breathing
• Determine if there have been any episodes of apnoea
• Establish a list of contacts who are unwell, including the history of the baby being admitted to hospital
• Address any concerns the mother has, in particular her worry about whether the child needs to be admitted

Discussion points

• What is your differential diagnosis?
• What features in the history point to each of these diagnoses?
• What features would you look for on examination?
• What is the cause of bronchiolitis?
• How might you investigate a patient with bronchioloitis?

• How do you treat bronchiolitis?
• When would you consider hospital admission?

△△　Bronchiolitis
　　Viral-induced wheeze
　　Upper respiratory tract infection – viral/bacterial
　　Pneumonia

Station 181: Failure to thrive

Student info: *Miss JK has brought her 9-month-old baby, Ruth, to see you on the advice of her health visitor. You are the GP and the concerns raised have been over Ruth's apparent lack of growth. Please take a full history and be prepared to discuss with the examiners a differential diagnosis. It is not necessary to examine the child. Her weight is now below the 2nd centile, despite being above the 25th at 5 months.*

Patient info: *You are a 25-year-old single mother who has brought Ruth, your 9-month-old, to see her GP because of concerns about her weight. Ruth is your first child and you are a single parent although you have supportive grandparents. You are concerned about Ruth's lack of weight gain. You had an unremarkable pregnancy and birth. There have been no problems with diarrhoea, vomiting, abdominal bloating or respiratory problems. Ruth just seems to have a problem eating enough, despite your best efforts. In fact if you are completely honest it has got to the stage where you find feeding time stressful which probably makes the situation worse. Ruth's father left when she was just 2 months old and you have been struggling and at times find yourself low in mood and lonely. Ruth has reached her normal developmental milestones. There is no family history of illness. If offered you would be happy for the health visitor to come around during feeding time*

Hints and tips

• Verify the reason for the mother attending
• Ascertain the problem in the mother's own words
• Conduct a full systems review in particular looking for gastrointestinal, respiratory or infective symptoms
• Establish the history of normal pregnancy and birth
• Establish the negative PMH and FH
• Establish a rapport with the mother and elicit her worries and concerns regarding the poor weight gain
• Elicit the low mood and stress that the mother finds during feeding
• Ask about developmental milestones
• Elicit the fact that the mother is a single parent and note the details of her partner and the grandparents
• Suggest the health visitor visits at feeding time to observe the process
• Address any other concerns
• Arrange further follow-up

Discussion points

• What does the term failure to thrive (FTT) mean?
• What are the causes of FTT?
• How would you investigate these possible causes?
• Discuss management options

Cardiovascular history hints

Breathing difficulties	Cyanosis	Failure to thrive	Associated syndromes, e.g. Down	FH of congenital heart disease
Exercise tolerance	Poor feeding	Episodes of fainting	History of murmur	

Station 182: Paediatric cardiovascular examination

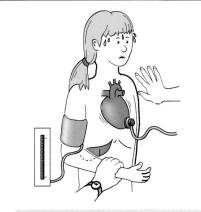

PALPATION
Pulse – Rate, rhythm, character
    Radiofemoral delay
    Peripheral pulses
Capillary refill
Apex beat   Hepatomegaly
Thrills/heaves   BP (appropriate cuff size)

AUSCULTATION
Appropriate size of stethoscope
Heart sounds
Murmurs

GENERAL INSPECTION
• Dysmorphic features, e.g. Down syndrome
• Central cyanosis
• Nutritional state
• Increased respiratory rate
• Pallor
• Scars – Midline sternotomy (ASD, VSD)
    Left thoracotomy (PDA closure)

← REMEMBER THE ESSENTIALS CHECKLIST

Age	Systolic BP	Pulse
<1	70–90	110–160
1–5	80–100	95–140
5–12	90–110	80–120
>12	100–120	60–100

Station 183: Congenital heart disease

Type of presentation		**Acyanotic**	**Cyanotic**
Heart failure	VSD (30% CHD)	L → R shunt	↑ pulmonary blood flow
Murmur	Pulmonary stenosis (8%), ASD (8%)	VSD, ASD, PDA	Tetralogy of Fallot
Shock	Coarctation of the aorta (6%)		
	Aortic stenosis (5%)	*Obstructive lesion*	↓ pulmonary blood flow
Cyanosis	Tetralogy of Fallot (6%)	Stenoses (aortic, pulmonary)	Transposition of the great arteries
	Transposition of the great arteries (5%)	Coarctation of aorta	Hypoplastic left heart syndrome

	VSD	PDA	ASD	Coarctation	ToF
Defect	Usually in the membranous part of the septum	Patent vessel between descending aorta and pulmonary artery	Three types: ostium secundum, ostium primum and sinus venosus	Narrowing of the aorta Often other associations	VSD Pulmonary stenosis Over-riding aorta Right ventricular hypertrophy
Clinical	Often asymptomatic Failure to thrive, heart failure if severe (Eisenmenger's syndrome – very rare and late) Parasternal thrill	Heart failure Displaced apex Collapsing pulse	Most children are free of any major symptoms Heart failure Chest infections Growth impaired	Collapse in newborn ↓ or absent femoral pulses Radial/femoral delay ↑ upper limb BP	There is a spectrum, which may include: hypoxic spells, pallor, cyanosis, dyspnoea, poor exercise tolerance, finger clubbing, growth retardation, polycythaemia
Auscultation	Harsh pansystolic murmur LLSE	Continuous murmur below left clavicle ('machinery murmur')	Fixed splitting of 2nd heart sound. Ejection systolic murmur in pulmonary area	May have murmur best heard on the back or no murmur	Ejection systolic murmur Loud S2
Ix	CXR: ↑ pulmonary vascular markings (pulmonary plethora)	CXR: pulmonary plethora ECG: left ventricular hypertrophy (LVH)	CXR: ↑ transverse cardiac diameter + pulmonary plethora	CXR: rib notching ECG, infants: RVH ECG, childhood: LVH	CXR: usually normal ECG → RVH Right axis deviation
Mx	Treat cardiac failure Antibiotic prophylaxis Surgical closure if still apparent at 1 year – many close spontaneously	Treat cardiac failure Prostaglandin synthetase inhibitors in the neonate Surgery if necessary	Closure if significant shunt Either surgery or via cardiac catheter by age of 5 years	IV prostaglandin E2 to keep duct open Surgical repair or balloon dilation of the narrowing	Relieve cyanotic spells by squatting Surgery dependent on severity

Station 187: Stridor

• *Please discuss with the examiner the different causes of stridor and how they can be managed*

Discussion points

• What is the cause of croup?
• Discuss the management of a child with croup
• Discuss the management of acute epiglottitis

Causes

• *Acute*: epiglottitis; inhaled foreign body; croup; tonsillar abscess; anaphylaxis
• *Chronic*: structural abnormalities, e.g. upper airway (micrognathia, pharyngeal cyst), larynx (vocal cord palsy, floppy larynx) or tracheal (stenosis, tracheomalacia)

Ix	Epiglottitis	*Do not investigate until the airway is secured*
		FBC and blood cultures
	Croup	None
	Foreign body	CXR (radio-opaque object)
		Bronchoscopy
	Chronic	Microlaryngoscopy
		Barium swallow
Mx	Croup	Supportive
		Pulse oximetry ± IV fluids
		Nebulised steroids
		Oral steroids
		Steam may improve symptoms
	Epiglottitis	*Acute emergency examination of the throat is contraindicated*
		Intubation and stabilisation
		IV antibiotics

Station 188: Cystic fibrosis

• *Please examine the respiratory system of John, who is 12*
• *Emma has a chronic respiratory problem. Please examine her hands and listen to her lungs at the back*

Hints and tips

• Check for a portacath or a Hickman line (chest wall) or other long-term venous access (percutaneously inserted central catheter (PICC) in the arm) – used for repeated courses of antibiotics. Also check the abdomen for a percutaneous endoscopic gastrostomy (PEG) tube.

Discussion points

• What is the genetic problem in cystic fibrosis (CF)?
• How do patients with CF present?
• What tests and monitoring are necessary for suspected CF?
• Discuss the management principles for a child with CF

Aetiology

Cystic fibrosis is an autosomal recessive condition that occurs in one in 2500 (one in 25 are carriers). A mutation with the cystic fibrosis transmembrane regulator protein (CTFR) on epithelial cells causes a problem with the chloride channel. This leads to viscid secretions that block bronchioles and exocrine pancreatic ducts.

Presentation		Recurrent chest infections (50%)
		FTT despite normal intake (30%)
		Meconium ileus (10%)
		Pancreatic insufficiency and malabsorption
		Rectal prolapse (rare)
		Some children are not diagnosed until they start school
Ix	Imaging	CXR
	Other	Sweat test – high concentrations of sodium and chloride are diagnostic
		Lung function tests
		Faecal elastase – low in CF
Mx		
Rx	Medical	Regular exercise
		Treatment of infections
		Oral, IV or nebulised antibiotics
		Consider prophylactic antibiotics
		Mucolytics
		Inhaled bronchodilators (± steroids) if airway reversibility on lung function testing
		Good nutritional intake – high calorie diet
		Pancreatic enzyme supplements
		Vitamin supplements
	Surgery	Consideration of heart/lung transplant
	Monitoring	Monitor for diabetes and liver problems
	MDT	Regular chest physiotherapy
		Specialist nurses, dietician, family unit
		GP, respiratory paediatrician
		Psychosocial counselling
	Education	For patient and family

Station 189: Chesty child

• *Please state the causes of pneumonia in a child and discuss the investigation and treatment*
• *Write short notes on bronchiolitis including diagnosis, investigation and management*

Hints and tips: bronchiolitis

• Acute respiratory distress
• Obstruction of the small airways
• Caused by RSV in about 80% of cases
NB. Not all that wheezes and crackles in winter is bronchiolitis (consider heart failure).

Ix	Nasopharyngeal aspirate for immunofluorescence
Mx	Supportive
	Humidified O_2 – aim for sats > 92%
	Adequate hydration and nutrition

Causes of pneumonia and bronchiolitis

• Bacterial: *Streptococcus pneumoniae, Haemophilus influenzae, Staphylococcus, Mycoplasma pneumoniae*
• Viral: respiratory synctial virus (RSV); influenza; parainfluenza; coxsackie; metapneumovirus

Indications for hospitalisation

Hypoxaemia; increasing respiratory distress; significant feeding problems; social problems

Gastroenterology history hints

Feeding habits	Vomiting	Urinary symptoms (including enuresis)	Weight gain	Bowel habit
Weaning	Posseting	FH of abdominal problems (e.g. coeliac, IBD)	Appetite	Abdominal pain

Station 190: Paediatric abdomen examination

FACE
Pallor   Jaundice
Mouth ulcers   Periorbital oedema

HANDS
Clubbing   Koilonychia
Pallor   Palmar erythema

GENERAL INSPECTION
• Well/unwell
• Nutritional state/muscle wasting
• Any sign of pain

REMEMBER THE ESSENTIALS CHECKLIST

TORSO INSPECTION
Abdominal distension   Masses
Hernias   Scars
Buttock wasting   Spider naevi

PALPATION/PERCUSSION
Warm hands
Be gentle
Observe carefully for any signs of discomfort
Do not hurt the child. Can they blow their
   tummy out or suck it in?
Examine as per adult routine (Chapter 26)

AUSCULTATION
Appropriate size of stethoscope
Bowel sounds
Renal bruit

COMPLETION
State you would:
• Examine external genitalia (undescended   • Examine for rectal fissures
   testes, hydroceles, hernias)   Never do a PR exam, or even offer to do

Station 191: Constipation

History and examination hints
Bowel habit (varies in children)
Breastfed babies tend to open their bowels
   less often
Stool frequency consistency and colour
Soiling or inappropriate defaecation
Pain on opening bowels
History of PR bleed or anal fissure
Age of onset (infancy may = Hirchsprung's)
Diet
Faeces may be palpable, esp. left iliac fossa
Observe nutritional status and growth chart

Station 192: Vomiting

History and examination hints
Timing and volume
Differentiate posseting from vomiting
Projectile vs non-projectile
Green vomit (bile) is always pathological
Weight gain/feeding history
Fever and systemic symptoms
Associated GI symptoms
Nutritional state/hydration
Palpable pyloric mass
Abdominal distension
High-pitched bowel sounds
Signs of infection

Station 193: Abdominal pain

History and examination hints
Acute/chronic
SOCRATES:
   Site
   Onset
   Character
   Radiation
   Alleviating factors
   Timing
   Exacerbating factors
   Severity
Associated GI, GUS or constitutional symptoms
Feeding history
Social history

Station 194: Lumps and bumps

Should	The	Child	Find	Lumps
Site	Tenderness	Colour	Fluctuation	Lymphatic drainage
Size	Temperature	Contour	Filling	Lumps elsewhere
Shape	Transition	Consistency	Emptying	
Shift	Thrill	Cough impulse	Bruit	

Station 191: Constipation

- *A young child with constipation is bought in by her mother. Please discuss the potential causes for a change in bowel habit like this and what investigations are necessary. Assuming no 'serious pathology', how would you manage this case?*

Causes

Acute	Dehydration, e.g. fever
	Bowel obstruction (rare)
Chronic	Functional
	Hirschsprung's disease
Ix	Rarely required
	Rectal biopsy needed for Hirschsrpung's
Mx	Diet (high fibre)
	Laxatives: lactulose, senna, Movicol
	Toilet training

Station 192: Vomiting

- *Sarah is 4 weeks old. Her mother is concerned because she has been having problems with vomiting. You are the foundation doctor in general practice. Please take a focused history from the mother regarding this problem. Be prepared to discuss a differential diagnosis and management plan with the examiner*

Hints and tips

- Ascertain the mother's reason for bringing Sarah to see you
- Take a focused history of the main symptoms using the checklist and hints opposite
- Establish the parent's ideas, concerns and expectations
- Answer any questions posed

Discussion points

- What would your differential for vomiting in the newborn period include?
- What characteristic features would be apparent if the diagnosis was pyloric stenosis?

Causes

Overfeeding	
Mechanical	Pyloric stenosis
	Gastro-oesophageal reflux
	Small bowel obstruction (emergency)
Infective	Post tussive (e.g. whooping cough)
	Meningitis
	UTI
	Gastroenteritis
Neurological	Raised intracranial pressure
Psychological	Bulimia (older child)
Toxins	Accidental ingestion of toxin

A note on pyloric stenosis

- Projectile vomiting
- Usually after a feed
- Gradually worsens, usually weeks 4–6 of life
- Child is keen to feed
- Failure to thrive ± dehydration
- Palpable pyloric mass
- Surgery required – Ramstedt's procedure or endoscopically

Ix	*Bloods*	U&E (dehydration)
		Chloride/bicarb (metabolic alkalosis, low K$^+$, Cl$^-$)
	Imaging	US abdomen
Mx	Treat the underlying cause	
	Maintain adequate hydration and nutrition	

Station 193: Abdominal pain

- *Please examine the abdomen of this 14-year-old male (simulated patient). He has been complaining of abdominal pain*

Hints and tips

A child with acute abdominal pain will not appear in your OSCE, although a simulated older patient could. The idea being that the examiners want you to demonstrate a competent examination routine, without causing any distress.

Causes	*GI*	Appendicitis
		Inflammatory bowel disease
		Intussusception
		Bowel obstruction
		Constipation
		Irritable bowel
	Renal	Pyelonephritis
		Renal stone (rare in a child)
	Endocrine	Diabetes
	Infection	Lower lobe pneumonia
		Gastroenteritis
		Mesenteric adenitis
		Parasites
	Gynaecological	Period pain
Ix	*Bloods*	FBC, U&E, LFT, amylase, ESR
	Imaging	AXR, US abdomen, barium enema
	Micro	Urine MC&S, stool for culture and ova

Station 194: Lumps and bumps

- *A 7-year-old boy, Peter, has been referred to the surgical clinic with a neck lump. You are the FY2 doctor in clinic. Please examine the lump and discuss a differential diagnosis*

Hints and tips

See Chapter 48 for neck examination.

Causes of a neck lump

Lateral	Lymph node
	Branchial cyst
	Cystic hygoma
	Sternomastoid tumour
	Submandibular gland
	Parotid gland neoplasm
Midline	Lymph node
	Submental lymph node
	Thyroglossal cyst
	Thyroid swelling
	Dermoid cyst

Infectious diseases history hints

Is the child well or unwell?	Main symptoms
Onset and timing of symptoms	Feeding
Associated systemic symptoms	Fever
Rash	Contacts
Previous episodes	Immunisation history

Investigation hints for infections

- Send specimen for microbiological investigation – i.e. microscopy, culture and sensitivity (MC&S)
- Measure antibody levels – two samples, one early on in the illness and the second after 2-3 weeks. A positive result is by demonstration of a rise in antibody levels
- Direct detection, e.g. immunofluorescense (pharyngeal secretions to identify respiratory syncytial virus) or polymerase chain reaction amplification, e.g. herpes

Station 195: Infectious diseases with rashes

MEASLES
- Very infectious
- Incubation period 10–14 days
- Sx of prodromal illness: fever, cough, coryza, conjunctivitis, lymphadenopathy, Koplik's spots
- Florid rash after 3-4 days

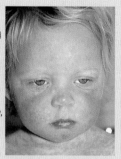

RUBELLA
- Incubation 14–21 days
- Sx: mild fever and malaise, pink macular rash for 3 days, general lymphadenopathy

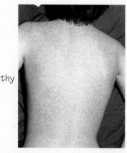

CHICKEN POX
- Incubation 14–16 days
- Symptoms: rash, low-grade fever, spots (in crops), macule → papule → vesicle → crusts
- Mouth ulcers

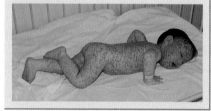

ERYTHEMA INFECTIOSUM
- Fifth disease
- Human parvovirus B19
- Mild fever
- Slapped cheek appearance of rash
- Usually no other symptoms

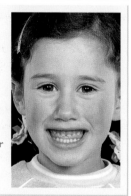

HERPES SIMPLEX
- HSV type 1
  Very common, usually asymptomatic, only 10% become ill
  Spread by infected saliva
  Infection of mouth, skin and eyes
- HSV type II
  Spread by genital infection
  Important in newborn and sexually abused children

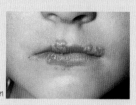

KAWASAKI DISEASE
- Mucocutaneous lymph node syndrome
- Usually < 5 years age
- Diagnostic criteria: fever for > 5 days and 4 of 5 of:
  Conjunctivitis
  Inflamed mouth and pharynx
  Polymorphous rash
  Red hand and feet with desquamation
  Cervical lymphadenopathy

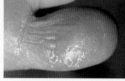

Station 196: Meningitis

History hints

Prodromal illness, e.g. flu-like	
Fever	Poor feeding
Irritable	Headache

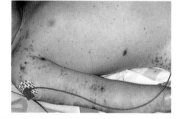

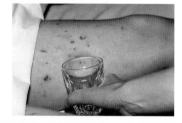

Examination hints

Neck stiffness	Crying
Bulging fontanelle	Rash
Kernig's sign (pain on leg extension)	
Brudzinski's sign (flex neck and the child flexes their knee)	

Bacterial meningitis

Child	Newborn
Neisseria meningitides	Group B streptococcus
Streptococcus pneumoniae	Escherichia coli
Haemophilus influenzae	Listeria

Viral meningitis

Enteroviruses	Arboviruses
Mumps	

General hints and tips

Unwell children with infectious diseases will not appear in person in an OSCE. The stations could be of a written variety with pictures or with an examiner guiding through a structured viva.

With regards to skin rashes, it will be necessary to describe the lesion before offering a differential diagnosis. Please review the dermatology section of this book for guidance on describing skin lesions (see Chapters 87–93).

Station 195: Infectious diseases with rashes

• *Please describe the rashes shown in the following pictures and discuss a differential diagnosis, investigations and treatment of each*

• *Please match the pictures shown to the most likely diagnosis*

• *Write short notes on each of the following infections, including where appropriate the complications of each: rubella, measles, herpes simplex and chicken pox*

Hints and tips: measles

Sx	Rash + 3 'Cs' (cough, coryza, conjunctivitis)
Δ	Immunofluorescence of nasopharyngeal aspirate
Complications	Otitis media
	Pneumonia
	Corneal ulcers
	Encephalitis (rare)
Rx	Supportive
	Antibiotics for secondary infection

Hints and tips: rubella

Sx	Mild illness in children
	Serious complications if developed during first trimester
Δ	Rise in antibody titre if required

Complications of congenital infection

• Death
• Cardiovascular system (CVS) – congenital heart disease
• Eyes – cataracts
• ENT – deafness
• GI – FTT, jaundice

Hints and tips: chickenpox (varicella)

Sx	Itching rash, mainly on the trunk
Δ	Mild illness unless immunocompromised
Complications	Secondary infection
	Pneumonia
	Encephalitis
Rx	Supportive
	Antibiotics for secondary infection
	Antihistamines
	Calamine lotion
	IV aciclovir and zoster immunoglobulin in immunocompromised

Hints and tips: herpes simplex

• Herpes simplex virus (HSV) 2 is a genital infection spread by sexual contact

• Neonates contract the virus during delivery
• Delivery should be via Caesarean section if the mother has active lesions

Complication	Meningoencephalitis
Rx	Aciclovir

NB. Children should not be kissed by people with cold sores.

Station 196: Meningitis

• *This photo is of a 7-year-old child who has arrived at A&E with a fever, non-blanching rash and history of a runny nose and poor feeding for 24 hours. Please discuss with the examiner how you would manage this case*

Hints and tips

This history suggests meningococcal septicaemia and is an emergency scenario. It could be tested in a station using a mannequin, a simulated patient with a 'painted on' purpuric rash or as a structured viva.

• Stick to the ABCDE approach (see Ch. 11)
• Meningococcal disease presents with signs of meningism, septicaemia or both
• If meningococcal disease is considered, it is essential to give intravenous antibiotics without delay (e.g. benzypenicillin)
• The definitive diagnosis is by blood culture or PCR. Do not do a lumbar puncture in the acute phase as this will not change management. Throat swabs can also be sent
• Viral meningitis will show a lymphocytic CSF, whereas a bacterial one will have polymorphs
• The prognosis for viral meningitis is better for survival but morbidity is high
• Remember to provide support for the parents who will be worried
• Household (kissing) contacts should receive prophylaxis

Discussion points

• What are the organisms causing meningitis in different age groups?
• Discuss the management of a patient with suspected meningitis
• What are the complications of meningitis?
• What clinical features may help suggest a diagnosis of meningitis?
• Discuss antibiotic treatment and the target organism for each

Complications	Death
	Septic shock
	Deafness
	Epilepsy
	Developmental delay
Mx	
Antibiotics	Newborn → double coverage – ampicillin (group B *Streptococcus* + *Listeria*) + aminoglycosides (gentamicin) (*Escherichia coli*)
	> 2 months: single coverage → third-generation cephalosporin (ceftriaxone) to cover *Haemophilus influenzae* + meningococcus + *Pneumococcus*
	Consider erythromycin for *Mycoplasma* or aciclovir for encephalitis, if the history or CSF examination indicates

Station 197: Immunisations

Immunisation schedule[1]

Age	
2 months	Diphtheria, tetanus, pertussis (DTaP) + polio (IPV) + Haemophilus influenzae (Hib) + pneumococcal (PCV)
3 months	DTaP + IPV + Hib + meningococcal C (Men C)
4 months	DTap + IPV + Hib + PCV + Men C
12 months	Hib + Men C
13 months	Mumps, measles, rubella (MMR) + PCV
31/2 to 5 yrs	DTaP + IPV + MMR
13–18 yrs	Diphtheria, tetanus (Td) + IPV

NB. The guidelines for BCG (bacilli Calmette-Guerin) vaccine have changed. Until recently it was offered to all school children. It is now given to at-risk neonates or adults who are at high risk of developing tuberculosis

Guidelines

General contraindications
Acute febrile illness
Previous anaphylactic reaction or serious local reaction

Live vaccines - contraindications
Immunocompromised children, e.g. chemotherapy, steroids

Also:
- Follow the age guidelines as suggested (even in premature babies)
- If an immunisation is missed, give at the next available opportunity (i.e. no need to start the course again)
- Live vaccines should be administered on the same day at different sites if possible. If not possible then allow a 3-week gap between injections

Station 198: Childhood infections

MUMPS
- Caused by paramyxovirus
- Incubation 16–21 days
- Sx: fever and malaise, enlargement of the parotid glands
- Tx: supportive

PERTUSSIS
- Bordetella pertussis: 7-day incubation
- Catarrhal stage: 1–2 weeks
- Cough: paroxysmal, with inspiratory whoop
- Cyanosis and apnoea can occur
- Lasts 4–6 weeks
- Serious illness in small babies

DIPTHERIA
- Corynebacteria diphtheria
- Rare in developed countries
- Incubation 2–7 days
- Sx: sore throat and inflammed tonsils
- Pharyngeal aspirate may spread to upper airway obstruction
- Exotoxin may cause myocarditis

Station 199: Skin lesions

A
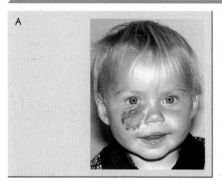

B
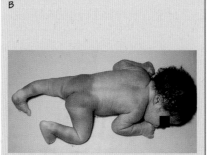

C
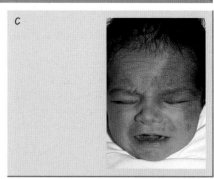

D
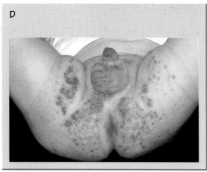

E
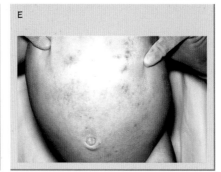

F
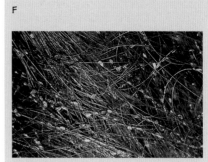

Station 197: Immunisations

This station could be presented in several ways. It could be a written station, asking for a brief description of the timing and types of immunisation offered, or could be included as part of a structured viva.

The most likely is that there will be a simulated or real parent who has come to see their GP to discuss immunisations. This discussion could be targeted at different levels, e.g. the station could merely be assessing your explanation of the immunisation schedule to a parent or could involve a more complex scenario where a parent is refusing to let their child have an immunisation.

• *Write short notes on the immunisation schedule for pre-school children*
• *Please discuss with the examiner the complications of immunisations and contraindications*

Student info: *You are a FY2 GP doctor. Mrs PK has brought her 13-month-old daughter Emma to see you after receiving a letter stating that Emma was due her next set of immunisations. Please discuss the situation with Mrs PK. You note from the computer record that Emma had a mild febrile illness following her 4-month immunisations which had concerned her mother*

Parent info: *You are a 28-year-old mother called Mrs PK. Your daughter Emma is just over 12 months old. You have received a letter from the GP surgery stating that Emma is due her next set of immunisations. She has had all her previous injections. After one set of injections she developed a fever which you were very concerned about although the doctor felt it was not related to the immunisation. You are concerned because Emma is due to have the MMR vaccination which you have read can cause autism. You are not willing to risk this and cannot see the point in this immunisation as you have seen children who have had measles, mumps and rubella and they never seem particularly unwell. You will need to be convinced by the doctor that this immunisation is in your child's best interests*

Hints and tips

• Establish rapport with the mother and child
• Review the previous immunisation history
• Clarify which immunisations are now due
• Establish the mother's concerns and reasons for that concern
• Appreciate that measles, mumps and rubella can be trivial illnesses but discuss the possible serious complications of each of the diseases
• Discuss the side effects of the immunisations
• Discuss the fact that there is *no* evidence for the association with autism
• Summarise that the small risk of side effects from the immunisation far outweighs the potentially serious risks of not being immunized

Station 198: Childhood infections

Hints and tips: measles

Sx	Febrile illness with enlargement of the parotid glands
Δ	Clinical rise in antibody titre
ΔΔ	Cervical adenitis
Complications	Meningitis
	Pancreatitis
	Epididymo-orchitis
Mx	Supportive

Hints and tips: pertussis

Sx	'Whooping cough'
Δ	Clinical nasal swab

Complications	Bronchopneumonia
	Convulsions due to asphyxia from spasms
	Subconjunctival haemorrhage
	Facial petechiae
	Death in a small baby

Station 199: Skin lesions

• *Please examine the skin of this child and describe the lesion*
• *Look at the following photographs and discuss a diagnosis of each condition and, where necessary, possible treatment*

Strawberry naevus (Fig. A)
• Capillary haemangioma
• Common
• Raised red lesion due to proliferation of blood vessels
• Usually regress after 2 years
• Usually require no treatment unless obstructing vision, or in a difficult location (e.g. nappy area); pulsed lasers aid regression

Mongolian spots (Fig. B)
• Blue/grey lesions (similar to a bruise)
• Usually sacral area
• Tend to fade with time
• Rare in Caucasians
• Can be mistaken for child abuse

Port-wine stain (Fig. C)
• Capillary haemangioma
• Flat compared to strawberry naevus
• Does not fade
• Association: Sturge–Weber syndrome (intracranial haemangioma)

Mx Laser; camouflage with cosmetics

Nappy rash (Fig. D)
• Common
• Erythematous rash with sparing of skin creases
• Prolonged contact of stale urine causes an ammonia dermatitis
• If left untreated, rash can become vesicles which can develop a superimposed bacterial or fungal infection

Mx Regular nappy changes with good washing; exposure to air; barrier creams; nystatin cream for superimposed fungal infection

Scabies (Fig. E)
• Itchy papulovesicular rash leading to excoriations
• Look carefully for burrows in the interdigital spaces in an older child
• Diagnosis by microscopy usually not necessary

Mx Malathion lotion; treat close contacts; wash bedding and clothes

Head lice (Fig. F)
• Also known as pediculosis
• Nits = the eggs
• Itchy scalp

Mx Anti-lice shampoo; treat all close contacts; fine comb

[1] www.immunisation.nhs.uk.

Station 200: Newborn baby check

General
Best conducted in a warm, well-lit room with the mother in attendance
REMEMBER THE ESSENTIALS CHECKLIST
Assess overall appearance, tone, maturity and rousability, and plot weight, length and head circumference on growth chart in the red book

Arms and hands
Normal shape and moving normally? Evidence of traction birth injury (e.g. Erb's palsy); count fingers and check for clinodactyly (incurving of fingers). Check palmar creases (single can be Down's)

Abdomen
Look at abdominal girth and shape; carefully check the umbilical stump for infection or surrounding hernia; gently palpate for organs (it is common to be able to feel a liver edge in healthy newborns) and any masses/herniae; check the external genitalia carefully (palpate for presence of testicles in boys) and visually inspect the anus for position and patency (has meconium been passed?)

Peripheral pulses
Check brachial and femoral pulses for rate, rhythm and volume
Hyperdynamic pulse - consider patent ductus arteriosus
Weak pulse – consider congenital cardiac anomaly impairing cardiac output (e.g. coarctation)
Radiofemoral delay - consider coarctation of the aorta

Head
General shape
Fontanelles: normal, sunken or bulging
Chignon from ventouse
Dysmorphic features

Hips
Barlow and Ortolani tests for congenital hip dislocation

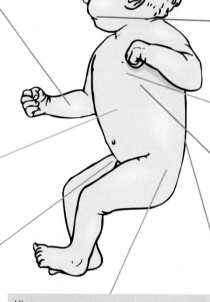

Eyes
Jaundice
Red reflex looking for cataracts or signs of ophthalmic infection

Ears
Shape and size: are they 'low set'? Any skin tags

Mouth
Colour of mucous membranes: are they cyanosed?
Cleft lip or palate
Natal teeth

Heart
Check cardiac position by palpation and feel for any thrill or heave; listen to the heart sounds carefully and for any added sounds or murmurs

Lungs
Watch respiratory pattern, rate and depth; look for any evidence of intercostal recession and listen for stridor; listen to the lung fields for added sounds

Back
Look carefully at skin over back and at spinal curvature/symmetry; is there any evidence of spina bifida occulta or sacral pit hidden by flesh creases or dimples? Palpate the spine gently

Station 201: Neonatal resuscitation[1]

Apgar score

Score	0	1	2
Colour	White	Blue periphery	Pink
Respiration	Absent	Weak cry, irregular	Strong cry and adequate breaths
Heart rate	Absent	<100	>100
Tone	Limp	Some flexion	Good flexion
Reflex to suction	No response	Grimace	Cough

Newborn life support

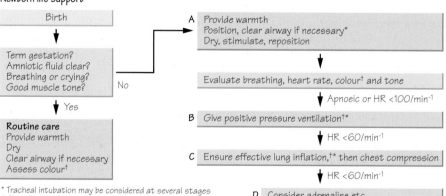

Birth
↓
Term gestation?
Amniotic fluid clear?
Breathing or crying?
Good muscle tone?

No →

A Provide warmth
Position, clear airway if necessary*
Dry, stimulate, reposition
↓
Evaluate breathing, heart rate, colour† and tone
↓ Apnoeic or HR <100/min⁻¹

↓ Yes

Routine care
Provide warmth
Dry
Clear airway if necessary
Assess colour†

B Give positive pressure ventilation†*
↓ HR <60/min⁻¹
C Ensure effective lung inflation,†* then chest compression
↓ HR <60/min⁻¹
D Consider adrenaline etc

* Tracheal intubation may be considered at several stages
† Consider supplemental oxygen at any stage if cyanosis persists

Station 200: Newborn baby check

• *Please demonstrate to the examiners how you would perform a new baby check on this child*

Hints and tips

• Perform a systematic 'head-to-toe' examination to detect structural abnormalities
• Consider BCG immunisation needed for at-risk babies

Abnormalities that may indicate a significant underlying cause

• Wide fontanelles: cranial abnormalities due to congenital syndromes or excessive CSF production
• Third fontanelle, between the anterior and posterior can indicate Down's syndrome
• Abnormally shaped or placed ears may indicate fetal alcohol syndrome, craniofacial abnormalities due to abnormal branchial arch development or conditions such as Edward's syndrome (trisomy 18) or congenital renal anomalies
• Single palmar crease can indicate Down's syndrome but is most often found in children who do not suffer from this condition
• Abnormalities of the face, jaw and ears are often associated with hearing dysfunction; hearing tests should be performed and ENT assessment requested

Common findings detected in the newborn screening examination

• Macular haemangioma 'stork marks': found around the eyes and nape of neck in 30–50% of babies. Those around the eyes normally disappear in the first year, but they persist on the nape of neck (NB. capillary haemangiomas generally appear later)
• Blue-black pigmented area (Mongolian blue spots): seen at base of back and on buttocks. They are common in dark-skinned parents but can occur in Caucasian infants, and normally disappear over the first year
• Erythema toxicum neonatorum: a fluctuating, widespread erythematous rash with a raised white/cream dot at the centre of a red flare, mostly apparent on the trunk; disappears spontaneously without treatment in the first 2 weeks
• Heat rash: also known as miliaria; it may appear as either red, macular patches or superficial, clear vesicles that are most marked on the forehead and around the neck. It is associated with warm, humid environments and will clear in cooler, drier conditions
• Breast enlargement: seen in both girls and boys, who may secrete small amount of milk. It is thought to be due to a response to circulating maternal hormones; no significance unless the condition persists/progresses
• White pimples: also known as milia; seen on the nose and cheeks and found in approximately 40% of newborns. They are due to blocked sebaceous glands, and clear spontaneously
• Oral cysts: found on the palate near the midline and on the gums (also known as Epstein's pearls); may be larger and on the floor of mouth. They usually resolve spontaneously
• Teeth: these can be present at birth; no action is required unless they are loose or abnormal, in which case they may have to be extracted as they may be inhaled
• Sacral dimples: common; examine carefully to detect underlying sinus or evidence of spina bifida occulta

Discussion points

• Discuss some abnormalities that you could find during a newborn baby check

Station 201: Neonatal resuscitation

• *You are the paediatrician on call and have been asked to attend a Caesarean section because the team are worried about the baby. You are standing by as the delivery occurs and the baby is blue and not breathing. Using the mannequin provided please manage this situation*

Resuscitation procedure

General

• Keep the baby warm and assess
• Make sure the cord is securely clamped
• Dry the baby, remove the wet towels and cover the baby
• Assess colour, tone, breathing and heart rate
• Get help

Airway

• Best position: on back with head in neutral position
• Chin lift or jaw thrust may be necessary

Breathing

• If not breathing by 90 seconds, give five inflation breaths, which clears fluid from the lungs
• If HR is < 100, this should rapidly increase as oxygenated blood reaches the heart; if HR increases, aeration was successful
• If HR increases but there is no spontaneous respiration, continue to provide regular breaths at a rate of about 40/min until spontaneous respiration starts
• If HR does not increase, lungs are not aerated; consider the following:
  • is the baby's head in the neutral position?
  • do you need jaw thrust?
  • do you need a longer inflation time?
  • do you need a second person's help with the airway?
  • obstruction in the oropharynx (laryngoscope and suction)?
  • consider a Guedel airway?
• If the heart rate remains slow (< 60/min) or absent following five inflation breaths, despite good passive chest movement, start chest compression

Chest compression

Almost all babies needing help at birth will respond to successful lung inflation with an increase in heart rate followed quickly by normal breathing. However, in some cases chest compression is necessary.

• Chest compression should be started only when you are sure that the lungs have been aerated successfully
• In babies, the most efficient method of delivering chest compression is to grip the chest in both hands in such a way that the two thumbs can press on the lower third of the sternum, just below an imaginary line joining the nipples, with the fingers over the spine at the back
• Compress the chest quickly and firmly, reducing the anteroposterior diameter of the chest by about one-third
• The ratio of compressions to inflations in newborn resuscitation is 3 : 1

Drugs

These are only needed if there is no significant cardiac output despite effective lung inflation and chest compression.

• Use adrenaline (1 : 10,000), sodium bicarbonate (4.2%) and dextrose (10%)
• Best delivered via an umbilical venous catheter

[1] Resuscitation Council UK. *Newborn life support algorithm*. Resuscitation Council UK, 2005. Available at www.resus.org.uk.

Station 202: Developmental assessment

Age	5 major categories of developmental milestones				
	Gross motor	Fine motor	Senses	Social	Educational
Birth	Absent head control Prone – flexed		Blinks to light Startled to noise		
6 weeks	Better head control Prone – hip extended		Cries/coos	Smiles	
3 months	Lifts head Prone - rests on forearms	Hands held open	Alert Watches movement of adult Turns to sound	Laugh	
6 months	Good head control Prone – press up Sit – self propping Stand – with support	Palmar grasp Transfers hand to hand	Double syllable sounds (da da)	Laugh Not shy	
9 months	Prone – crawls Sit – alone Stand – pulls to standing, or stands holding on	Early pincer grip Reaches for objects	Localisation of quiet sounds Babbles	Chews solids Stranger anxiety Peek a boo	
12 months	Stand – cruises, walks with hand held	Refined pincer grip Offers objects	Few words (daddy) Knows name Understands simple commands	Finger feeds Drinks from cup Waves bye Cooperates with dressing	
18 months	Walks and stoops to pick up toys	Builds tower of 3 cubes Scribbles	6–20 words, occasionally 2 together	Drinks from cup with 2 hands Uses spoon	Points to objects
2 years	Runs, kicks ball Stairs holding on	Tower of 6 bricks Draws vertical line	2–3 word sentences	Dry by day Temper tantrums	Points to several body parts Identifies pictures
3 years	Walks upstairs, one foot per step Pedals tricycle	Tower of 9 bricks Draws circle	Full sentences	Dresses self (except buttons, laces) Washes hands Eats with fork and spoon	Recognises and names colours
5 years	Hops and skips Walks on toes	Draws triangle, man	Fluent grammatical speech	Uses knife and fork Fully dresses and undresses self	Improved understanding, counting, reading, repeating and memorising

Station 203: Growth

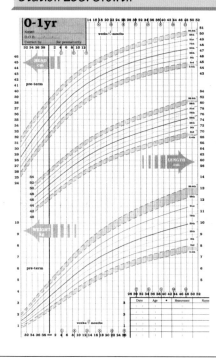

The growth chart
- The chart depicts nine equidistant centiles
- 50th centile = median for the population
- 98th centile = 2% children are taller or heavier
- Mark the measurement with a dot
- Correct for prematurity up to 2 years
- Any flattening of the growth warrants assessment

Occipitofrontal circumference (OFC), i.e. head circumference
- Inelastic tape
- Pass the tape from the occiput, over the ears to the forehead
- Take three measurements and record the largest
- Document the result on the chart

Height/length
Length should be used up to 2 years of age
Measure height barefoot with straight knees
Document the result on the chart

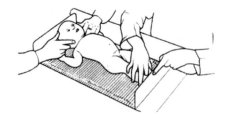

• *Please perform a developmental assessment on John and discuss with the examiner how old you think he is and why*

Hints and tips

From an organisational point, this is an easier station to include. The majority of patients will be children who have reached normal developmental milestones and you will be asked to assess this and discuss your reasons with the examiner. It also allows the examiners to assess your general approach to a well child. Alternatively, the station could be set up as a written question using photos to depict various stages of development or as a structured viva.

• Start by saying 'I will assess (child's name) in the five developmental domains of . . .' (see opposite)

• Then ask the parent if they have any concerns about the child's hearing or vision. If your patient is blind or deaf, everything changes!

• The parent can give you most of the information, but you probably will not be allowed to ask for it!

• Observe the child at play initially; once you approach they may become reluctant to take part in the activity. Keep talking

• Although the majority of subjects will be healthy, do not ignore any clues around the room or from general inspection of the child (e.g. hearing aid, glasses, walking aids, Down's syndrome)

• Have the categories at the back of your mind while observing

• Next formally test each category of milestone in turn (see table opposite) starting in the order that the skills are acquired (i.e. you have to be able to sit before you can walk)

• Discover a milestone the child can do and a more advanced one they cannot to help determine which stage they are at

• Present your findings as you go along

NB. Development is not always at the same stage in each category – this is normal. There is also a wide variation between children. Remember to correct for prematurity until 2 years old and that developmental testing before 6 months is less reliable. It may be necessary to assess development on separate occasions, especially if the parents' history differs from what is observed.

Discussion points

• What are the causes of developmental delay and how would you test for them?

• At what age would you expect a child to be crawling/walking/grasping/drawing a circle, etc?

• What are the primitive reflexes and how might you test for them? (Although this question has no clinical use, it is an exam favourite!)

Causes of developmental delay

• *Congenital* (75%):
  • chromosome abnormality, e.g. Down's syndrome, fragile X
  • endocrine, e.g. hypothyroidism
  • metabolic, e.g. phenylketonuria
  • neurological, e.g. hydrocephalus, neurodegenerative conditions
  • neurocutaneous syndromes, e.g. neurofibromatosis
  • idiopathic, e.g. autism
• *Acquired* (25%):
  • prenatal, e.g. fetal alcohol syndrome, infections (e.g. rubella)
  • perinatal, e.g. prematurity, hypoxia, birth injury
  • postnatal, e.g. infection, trauma, abuse, prolonged hospitalisation, acute illness

• *Please measure the head circumference of this toddler and plot the result on the chart provided*

• *Please measure the height of John who is 5. Plot the result on the growth chart*

• *Please discuss with the examiner the following growth charts (e.g. normal, premature baby, hydrocephalus, Turner's, etc.)*

• *Please measure the height and weight of this child, mark on the charts provided and calculate the BMI*

Hints and tips

All aspects of growth measurement could be assessed at an OSCE station although, due to the difficulty, measuring a baby's length would be less likely. As in Station 202, the children are likely to be well and have normal development. Abnormalities of growth could be depicted on charts that the examiners could hand to you.

• Remember the importance of inspection (dysmorphic features)
• Look for signs of chronic disease
• Assess weight and muscle bulk
• Try and make an assessment of pubertal development if appropriate (voice, body shape) (it will never be necessary to undress a child)
• Familiarise yourself with any measuring devices and the charts (preferably prior to the exam as the equipment used will be that used in your hospital!)
• If asked, mark the results clearly on the chart
• Avoid any possibly distressing terms (e.g. stunted growth, looks abnormal, etc.)

Discussion points

• What are the causes of short stature?
• How would you investigate a child with short stature?
• What are the causes of tall stature?
• What abnormalities of head growth are you aware of?

Causes of short stature

• Familial
• Constitutional delay of growth
• Intrauterine growth retardation
• Nutritional
• Chronic disease
• Emotional and psychological
• Endocrine, e.g. GH deficiency, hypothyroidism
• Chromosomal, e.g. Down's, Turner's
• Skeletal dysplasias, e.g. achondroplasia
• Iatrogenic, i.e. post steroids or post chemotherapy

Causes of tall stature

• Familial
• Endocrine, e.g. GH excess, thyrotoxicosis, congenital adrenal hyperplasia
• Chromosomal, e.g. Klinefelter's syndrome
• Connective tissue disease, e.g. Marfan's

Head growth

• 80% of head size is achieved before the age of 5 years
• Anterior fontanelle is usually closed by 12–18 months

Station 204: Obstetric history

Introduction
Name, age, occupation
Current gestation
Gravidity/parity

Family history
Twins
Complications during pregnancy
Inherited conditions
History of diabetes, hypertension, thyroid
  problems

Drug and alcohol history
As per adult medicine

Past medical history
As per adult medicine, but specifically ask about
thromboembolic disease, hypertension, thyroid
disease and diabetes

Presenting complaint and history
Pain/bleeding/ruptured membranes/reduced
fetal movements/sickness

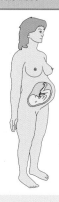

Systems review
Full inquiry as per adult medicine

Current pregnancy
LMP, current gestation
Pregnancy booking details
Screening test results/scan results
Complications previously and how managed
Fetal movements

Past obstetric history
Details of all pregnancies (weights, delivery,
ages, perinatal and neonatal problems)

Past gynaecological history
Menstrual history (menarche, menopause,
  cycle length duration and character, LMP,
  IMB or PMB)
Previous gynaecological investigations,
  operations and treatment
Contraception and sexual history
Last cervical smear, any previous abnormal ones

Station 205: Obstetric examination

COMPLETION
Perform urinalysis
Consider other examinations depending on
  individual cases, e.g. fundoscopy, CVS and
  neuro if pre-eclampsia

ABDOMEN – AUSCULTATION
Listen for a fetal heart with a Pinard
  stethoscope or doppler

ABDOMEN – PALPATION
A – Determine and measure the fundal height
B – Palpate with hands facing up the abdomen
  to determine the fetal lie by palpating the
  fetal parts and estimate liquor volume
C – Palpate with hands facing down the
  abdomen to determine presentation

ABDOMEN – INSPECTION
Shape and size   Striae/linea nigra
Scars   Fetal movements
Symmetry   Everted umbilicus

INTRODUCTION
REMEMBER THE ESSENTIALS CHECKLIST
Essential to have a chaperone and remember
  the importance of respecting dignity and
  maintaining good communication
Ask about any pain

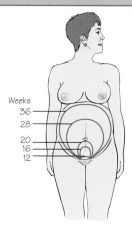

Weeks
36
28
20
16
12

EXPOSURE
Below breasts to symphysis pubis

POSITION
As flat as possible for examination of the
abdomen (will need to be semiprone in later
pregnancy)

GENERAL INSPECTION
Well/unwell   Febrile   Oedema
Height and weight   Pale

CVS
Pulse
BP: this should be measured semirecumbent at
  45°, using a correctly sized BP cuff and
  Korotkoff sound (V)

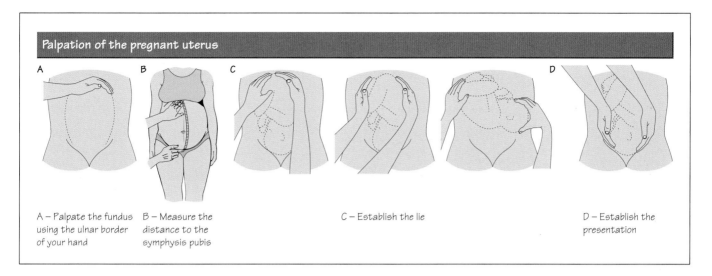

Palpation of the pregnant uterus

A – Palpate the fundus using the ulnar border of your hand

B – Measure the distance to the symphysis pubis

C – Establish the lie

D – Establish the presentation

Station 204: Obstetric history

• *A 26-year-old woman who is 25 weeks' pregnant presents to A&E with abdominal pain. Please take an obstetric history*

Hints and tips

• Follow the format described opposite
• Gravidity = total number of pregnancies including the current one
• Parity = number of births beyond 24 weeks' gestation
• The patient's general health is important; ask also about any problems of pregnancy and fetal movements
• Always ask about results of laboratory tests and ultrasound scans
• The validity of the expected delivery date (EDD) should be checked, asking about the LMP and usual cycle length
• For each preceding pregnancy, include all significant events – such as complications, modes of delivery, birth weights and the life and health of babies – as they may be relevant
• Take past gynaecological history including contraceptive history, surgical procedures and smear history
• Many medical conditions may have an important bearing on the pregnancy or, indeed, may be affected by the pregnancy, for example heart disease, epilepsy, asthma, thyroid disease or diabetes

• Drug history: history of allergies should be highlighted and any use/abuse of drugs during pregnancy should be noted. Arrangements may have to be made to wean the mother off the drug
• Family/social: it is vital to elicit hereditary illnesses or congenital defects

Station 205: Obstetric examination

• *Please demonstrate an examination of the pregnant uterus using the mannequin provided*
• *Please examine this 35-year-old pregnant patient*

Hints and tips

• Follow the routine described opposite

Discussion points

• At what date does the fundus become palpable?
• When might you perform a vaginal examination on a pregnant patient?
• Define engagement and how can you assess when the head is engaged?
• If the head is not engaged at term, what are the possible causes?

Station 206: Gynaecological history – pelvic pain

Introduction
Name, age, occupation
Planned or emergency appointment

Social history
As per adult medicine
Impact of the symptoms on the patient's life

Family history
As per adult medicine, but check about breast and gynaecological malignancy

Drug and alcohol history
As per adult medicine

Past medical history
As per adult medicine, but specifically ask about thromboembolic disease, hypertension, thyroid disease and diabetes

Presenting complaint and history
Pain/discharge/post-coital bleeding/intermenstrual bleeding (IMB)/dyspareunia/post-menopausal bleeding (PMB)/urinary symptoms/prolapse
Associated symptoms and relation to cycle
Previous treatments and response

Past gynaecological history
Menstrual history (menarche, menopause, cycle length duration and character, LMP, IMB or PMB)
Previous gynaecological investigations, operations and treatment
Contraception and sexual history
Last cervical smear, any previous abnormal ones
Previous termination of pregnancy

Past obstetric history
Details of all pregnancies (weights, delivery, ages, perinatal and neonatal problems)

Systems review
Full inquiry as per adult medicine
In particular remember the importance of endocrine-type questions, asking about mood and systemic questions, e.g. weight loss (?malignancy)

Station 207: Gynaecological examination

COMPLETION
Consider Sim's speculum
Consider DRE (see Station 117)
Consider further examination of CVS/respiratory/GI/endocrine depending on diagnosis and possibility of operation

↑

PERINEUM – CUSCO'S SPECULUM EXAMINATION
See Station 207

↑

PERINEUM – BIMANUAL EXAMINATION
See Station 206

↑

PERINEUM – INSPECTION
Skin changes, pubic hair, lumps, lesions, prolapse

↑

ABDOMEN – AUSCULTATION
Bowel sounds

↑

ABDOMEN – PERCUSSION
Dullness of masses
Shifting dullness

INTRODUCTION
REMEMBER THE ESSENTIALS CHECKLIST
Essential to have a chaperone and remember the importance of respecting dignity and maintaining good communication
Ask about any pain
Warm speculums

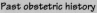

Inspect Percuss
Palpate Auscultate

Expose

Palpation towards the pelvis
Laparoscopy
Vertical   } Scars
Pfannensteil
Gynaecological masses arise from the pelvis

ABDOMEN – PALPATION
Tenderness
Peritonism
Masses – if a mass, could the patient be pregnant, where does it arise?

EXPOSURE
As per diagram initially

↓

POSITION
Supine initially
Supine with legs apart for examination of perineum

↓

GENERAL INSPECTION
Well/unwell   Pale
Height and weight   Signs of systemic disease
Febrile   Signs of endocrine disease

↓

CVS
Pulse/BP

↓

BREASTS
Screening test for breast cancer (see Chapter 49)

↓

ABDOMEN – INSPECTION
Scars   Linea nigra
Symmetry
Abdominal distension
Hair distribution
Striae
Herniae

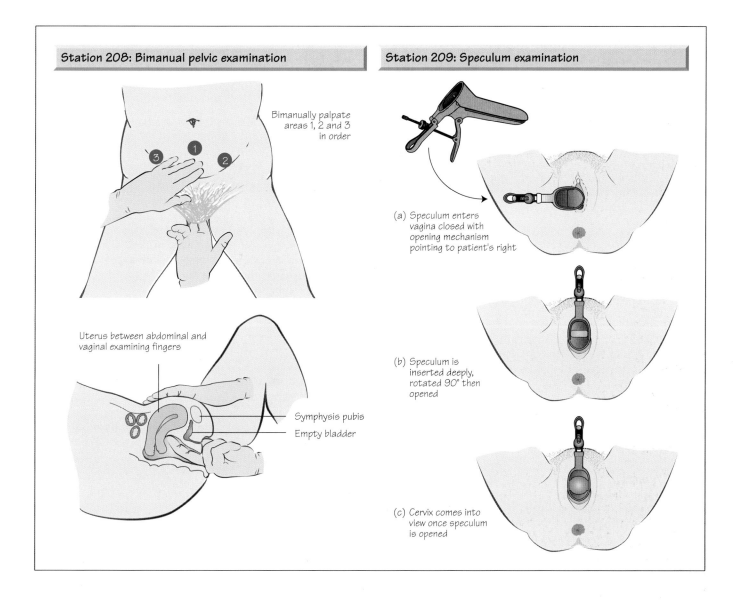

Station 208: Bimanual pelvic examination

Bimanually palpate areas 1, 2 and 3 in order

③ ① ②

Uterus between abdominal and vaginal examining fingers

Symphysis pubis

Empty bladder

Station 209: Speculum examination

(a) Speculum enters vagina closed with opening mechanism pointing to patient's right

(b) Speculum is inserted deeply, rotated 90° then opened

(c) Cervix comes into view once speculum is opened

Station 206: Gynaecological history – pelvic pain

• *You are a FY1 doctor working in general practice. Mrs HK is a 52-year-old female who has come to see you complaining of pelvic pain. Please take a gynaecological history*

Hints and tips

• Follow the format described opposite
• Pain is the presenting complaint, so enquire fully about this symptom first
• Nature of the pain? Uterine pain is colicky and felt in the sacrum and groins. Ovarian pain is often felt in the iliac fossae, radiating down the front of the thigh to the knee
• Dyspareunia – is it superficial or deep?
• The menstrual history is absolutely vital in the gynaecological history
• History: this should include the age at menarche, as well as the date of the last menstrual period (LMP) or menopause. Was the last period normal?
• Details of LMP are normally written as, for example, K5/28 (number of days bleeding/length of cycle, day 1 to day 1)

• Are periods regular? Are they heavy or light? Are there clots or flooding? How many pads/tampons are needed? Are they painful? Is there any bleeding between periods, post-coitally or since the menopause?
• Vaginal discharge: amount, colour, smell, itch and when it occurs. Is there any prolapse and incontinence? When? How bad?
• Sex and contraception: sexually active? Mode of contraception, and is patient happy with it? Problems of conception? Previous treatments for infertility? Sexually transmitted diseases (STDs)? When was the last smear – including result?
• Ask briefly about previous obstetric history
• Complete the history if permitted by the examiner and be prepared to offer a differential and management plan

Station 207: Gynaecological examination
See opposite.

Station 208: Bimanual pelvic examination

• *Please perform a bimanual digital examination on this 28-year-old patient, explaining the procedure to the patient but using the mannequin for the actual examination*

Hints and tips

- Communication is essential for this procedure
- It is not often painful but can be uncomfortable
- Explain the procedure first
- Request a chaperone
- Position the patient correctly (supine with knees flexed and hips abducted) and maintain dignity
- Wear gloves and use lubrication
- Explain to the examiner that you would perform the inspection first (see opposite)
- Gently insert two fingers into the vagina
- Place your left hand above the symphysis pubis and push down (see opposite)
- Palpate the uterus, cervix and adnexae
- Note any tenderness or masses
- Once complete, wipe off any excess lubricant, offering a towel to the patient

Station 209: Speculum examination

- *This 32-year-old lady needs a speculum examination performing. She has not had this procedure before. Please explain the procedure and then carry out the examination using the mannequin provided*

Hints and tips

- Communication is essential for this procedure
- It is not often painful but can be uncomfortable
- Explain the procedure first
- Request a chaperone
- Position the patient correctly (supine with knees flexed and hips abducted) and maintain dignity
- Wear gloves
- Choose appropriate size of speculum and check that it works and has been warmed
- Inspect the perineum first
- Explain to the examiner that you would like perform a bimanual examination initially
- Apply lubricating gel to the speculum and with your left hand gently part the labia
- Gently insert the closed speculum with the blades in the vertical plane (see opposite)
- Rotate 90° while gently advancing
- Once fully inserted, open the blades slowly under direct vision to visualise the cervix, looking for any obvious abnormalities
- The ratchet can be tightened at this point if desired
- State that a swab/smear could be taken
- Withdraw the speculum and close slightly
- Continue to slowly withdraw while inspecting the vagina and close fully to remove
- Clean off excess lubricant and hand the patient a towel

Sims' speculum

- This is used to visualise a prolapse
- The patient needs to be in the left lateral position with knees bent

Contraindications to a digital vaginal examination

- Suspected placenta praevia
- Premature rupture of the membranes

Station 210: Contraception

Method	Types	Failure rate (per 1000 woman years)	Mechanism of action	Advantages	Disadvantages	Contraindications
Combined OCP	e.g. Microgynon	0.2	Inhibit ovulation	Effective ↓ Period pain and bleeding ↓ Risk of ovarian neoplasia Protect against ovarian cysts and benign breast disease	S/Es – Nausea, weight gain, ↓ libido, headache, bloating, acne, spotting Risks – rare but important: thromboembolic disease, cardiovascular disease, ↑ BP, CVA, cervical and breast neoplasia	PMH of thromboembolism, IHD, CVA, liver disease, breast or endometrial neoplasia Pregnancy, breastfeeding Smoking Undiagnosed vaginal bleeding
Progestogen only (mini pill)	e.g. Micronor	1	Alters cervical mucus	Fewer risks than the combined OCP i.e. no increased risk of thromboembolic disease Safer if patient has CVS risk factors	Less effective than combined pill Timing window is smaller i.e needs to be taken at the same time each day S/Es – weight gain, acne, spotting, ↓ libido	Previous ectopic
Progestogen only depot	e.g. Depo-provera (3 monthly injection) Implanon (3 yearly implant)	<1	As above	Convenient	As above Some irregular bleeding initially followed by amenorrhoea	
Barrier	Male condom Female condom 4-8/100 Diaphragm Cap	Approximately 5-15	Barrier	↓ Risk of STDs particularly with the male condom Non hormonal	Less effective Inconvenient	
Intrauterine devices	Copper device Hormone device	<0.5	Inhibition of sperm migration, ovum transport, implantation and fertilisation	Safe No need to remember pills	Complications – perforation or migration, infection, risk of ectopic pregnancy	Endometrial or cervical neoplasia Past or current PID Pregnancy Undiagnosed vaginal bleeding Previous ectopic
Sterilisation	See Station 211	See below	Prevent delivery of sperm	Permanent Convenient	Complications of surgery Difficult to change mind!	

Station 211: Sterilisation

Female
Laparoscopic:
- Clips/rings
- Bipolar cautery
Minilaparotomy
- e.g. Pomeroy method

- Effective and permanent method
- Not reversible on NHS
- High initial cost
- Increased risk of ectopic pregnancy if fails
- Can be performed under local or general anaesthetic

Failure:
Can occur due to pregnancy at the time of sterilization, tube re-anastomosis, fistula formation, equipment failure or surgical error
Failure rate: 1 in 200

Fallopian tubes are cut or blocked to stop the egg travelling from the ovary to the uterus
- Fallopian tube
- Ovary
- Uterus
- Vagina

Male
Failure rate 1 in 2000
Sterility needs to be confirmed by two negative semen analyses

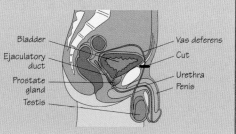

- Bladder
- Ejaculatory duct
- Prostate gland
- Testis
- Vas deferens
- Cut
- Urethra
- Penis

Station 212: Subfertility

Causes

Maternal

Ovulatory disorders	Hypothalamic-pituitary failure Hypothalamic-pituitary dysfunction (e.g. PCOS) Premature ovarian failure Hyperprolactinaemia
Tubal/uterine or cervical	Fallopian tube damage or blockage Endometriosis, fibroids, pelvic adhesions, cervical infections/stenosis
Other	Drugs Endocrine (thyroid/Cushing's) Neoplasia and its treatment

Paternal

Impaired production or function of sperm	Shape, motility, reduced sperm count Varicocele, undescended testis Infections
Impaired delivery	Impotence, blocked ducts, ↓ semen, retrograde ejaculation, hypospadias, absent vas deferens (e.g. cystic fibrosis)
Unexplained	Up to 25%

Station 210: Contraception

• *A 22-year-old female student has recently changed GP practice and has come to discuss contraception options with you*

Hints and tips

• Determine the patient's reason for attending
• Discuss previous contraception
• Ascertain relevant obstetric and gynaecological history
• Ascertain patient's current knowledge of contraception options
• Discuss advantages and disadvantages of different contraception including failure rates
• Summarise and agree a management plan

Station 210A: Missed pill

• *A 19-year-old female presents, having forgotten to take her oral contraceptive. What advice should be given?*

Hints and tips

• If a pill is missed, it should be taken as soon as possible and the next dose should be taken as usual
• If there are < 7 pills left, run two packs together
• Alternative contraception may be necessary depending on number of pills missed and where in cycle

Station 210B: Antibiotics and the pill

• *A 23-year-old female needs antibiotic treatment for a urinary tract infection. She is also taking the pill – what advice should be given?*

Hints and tips

• If taking antibiotics (or other interacting medication) for a short time, use another form of birth control for the duration of the treatment and for 7 days afterwards
• If these 7 days extend into the next month, run two packs back to back

Station 210C: Emergency contraception

• *A 16-year-old female presents to you, her GP. She had intercourse the previous evening, during which the condom split. What are her options?*

Hints and tips

• Prescribe levonorgestrel 1.5 mg stat dose, taken as soon as possible after the unprotected intercourse
• She should avoid unprotected intercourse and if there is no menses within 3 weeks, return for a pregnancy test
• Take this opportunity to discuss contraceptive issues and offer screening for STDs

Discussion points

• Discuss the different types of contraception

• What are the different types of oral contraception and can you tell me the side effects and contraindications for these?
• What are the risks associated with using an intrauterine contraceptive device (IUCD)?

Station 211: Sterilisation

Student info: *A 28-year-old female has come to see you (GP FY1) to request sterilisation*

Patient info: *You are a 28-year-old who has had two children who are now 5 and 2 years. You are not sure you would like to have more children. Your husband is adamant that you should have no further children and feels sterilisation is the best option. He refuses to wear condoms and you admit yourself that taking the pill was always a little haphazard. There has been no mention of him having a sterilisation. You have not discussed this with any of your family or friends and are not completely sure that you want the procedure. You are otherwise fit and well, taking no medication*

Hints and tips

• Determine the patient's reason for attending
• Establish previous obstetric history
• Establish reasons for wanting sterilisation
• Ascertain patient's knowledge of the options available and complications of sterilisation and also her knowledge of alternative forms of contraception
• Establish the fact that this patient is unsure
• Offer information in the form of leaflets
• Offer advice regarding the types of procedure available and the possible complications
• Stress the point that this is a permanent procedure and reversal, although not impossible, is not easy
• Discuss the fact that patients sometimes regret their decision (especially when younger, i.e. < 30 years old)
• Explain the one in 200 risk of failure *Lifetime*
• Offer thinking time and arrange a further appointment
• Suggest that you meet with both the patient and her husband to discuss matters further

Station 212: Subfertility

• *Please consult this couple who are concerned that they may have fertility problems. They have been trying for a baby for just over 12 months with no success*

Hints and tips

• Investigation of subfertility is indicated following 12 months without conception
• Earlier evaluation is indicated in women who have a history of oligomenorrheoa/amenorrhoea, are older than 35 or have suspected pelvic pathology *1° or 2°*
• This can be a very emotive subject so be extremely sensitive

RF ↑ age (male and female)
Smoking/alcohol/illicit drugs
↑ BMI or ↓ BMI
Excessive exercise

Mx Full history from both patients (in particular sexual and gynaecological histories)
Examination of both male and female (observe carefully for signs of endocrine disease/polycystic ovarian syndrome (PCOS); examine external genitalia and perform gynaecological examination)

Ix *General* FBC, U&E, TFT, Glc
Urinalysis
Male Semen analysis (3-monthly intervals if necessary)
Female Check LH/follicle-stimulating hormone (FSH)
Consider prolactin level
Hysterosalpingography (HSG) if no previous gynaecological co-morbidities, otherwise consider laparoscopy and dye

PCOS ⊃ ↑↑LH

Menopausal ⊃↑↑FSH

Rx
General Normalise weight
Smoking/alcohol cessation
Folic acid supplements
Ovulation disorder Clomiphene (used if adequate levels of oestrogen and gonadotrophins, e.g. hypothalamic pituitary dysfunction)
Gonadotrophins (used if low levels of gonadotrophins, e.g. hypothalamic pituitary failure *or* second line if clomiphene fails)
Metformin (PCOS)
Bromocriptine (if hyperprolactinaemic)
In vitro fertilisation (IVF)
Tubal/uterine/peritoneal disease Surgery
IVF
Unexplained infertility Clomid and intrauterine insemination (IUI)
Gonadotrophins and IUI
IVF

Station 213: Spontaneous miscarriage

History hints

- Vaginal bleeding most common ± abdominal pain
- Last menstrual period: work out gestation
- Pregnancy test - when and which test?
- What have they passed?
- Fresh blood/altered/products/fetus
- How much pain? Contractions? Post-coital bleeding? Shoulder tip?
- Planned pregnancy?
- Anaesthetic suitability?
- PHM/surgical history/maternal illness
- PID/IUCD/fertility

Examination hints

- Signs of shock
- Pyrexial
- Abdominal tenderness/peritonism/masses
- Genital tract: polyps/ectropion/cervicitis/vaginitis
- Pelvic exam: fundus size – does it correspond to dates?
- Cervix:
  Dilated = inevitable abortion/incomplete abortion Closed = threatened abortion/complete
- Speculum exam: local cause of bleeding, expulsion of products

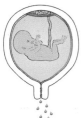
(a) Threatened miscarriage

(b) Incomplete miscarriage

(c) Missed miscarriage

Station 214: Recurrent miscarriage

Aetiologies of recurrent pregnancy loss

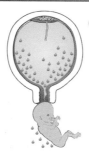

Idiopathic >50%

Infection 5%

Immunological factors 5–10%
- Antiphospholipid antibody syndrome
- Allommunity

Genetic factors 5–10%
- Parental chromosomal abnormalities

10–15%

10–15%

Reciprocal translocation

Robertsonian fusion

Anatomic factors

(a) Congenital malformations
- Müllerian fusion abnormalities

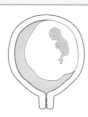

Arcuate

Septate

Didelphic

Bicornuate (complete)

- Abnormalities due to in utero DES exposure

(b) Acquired lesions

Uterine fibroids

Uterine synechiae (Asherman syndrome)

Endocrine factors
- Luteal phase deficiency
- Metabolic disorders (thyroid, diabetes)

Station 213: Spontaneous miscarriage

- *A 32-year-old woman presents with lower abdominal pain and vaginal bleeding. Her pregnancy test is positive. Please take a history and discuss her differential diagnosis, investigation and management*

Hints and tips

This station could involve taking a gynaecological history or include discussing miscarriage as a possible diagnosis with a patient.

- History and examination hints as opposite
- Miscarriage is defined as loss of pregnancy before 24 weeks
- Most occur in the second or third month
- 15–20% of miscarriages are clinically diagnosed pregnancies
NB. Over 50% of all conceptions abort spontaneously but most go unrecognised.

Discussion points

- What would be included in your differential diagnosis?
- How would you investigate this woman?
- Please tell me about the different types of miscarriage and the treatment of each
- What risk factors are you aware of for spontaneous miscarriage?

ΔΔ   Threatened abortion
     Ectopic pregnancy
     Haemorrhagic cyst
     Molar pregnancy

Classification of miscarriage

1 *Threatened*:
- Vaginal bleeding in early pregnancy
- Closed os ± lower abdominal pain
- Management: expectant management, Rhesus –ve women should receive anti-D prophylaxis if > 12 weeks' pregnant

2 *Inevitable*:
- Heavy bleeding and os open, with imminent miscarriage

3 *Incomplete*:
- Continuation of threatened abortion
- Bleeding ++ and abdominal pain
- Dilated cervix
- Cervix opens → conceptus into vagina
- If some of conceptus remains = incomplete miscarriage
- Management: evacuation of retained products of conception

4 *Complete*:
- Progression of incomplete miscarriage
- Pain ceases and vaginal bleeding slows
- Uterus involutes
- More likely to complete if > 16 weeks' pregnant (incomplete miscarriage more common if > 8–12 weeks' pregnant)
- Management: usually conservative

5 *Missed*:
- Fetus has died in utero
- Uterus smaller than dates and os closed
- Complete retention of products of conception
- Management: evacuation of retained products
- Bloods: β-HCG, G&S, Rhesus status (if +ve, perform Kleihauer's test), FBC, clotting, U&E
- Imaging: transvaginal US

General Mx   ABCDE (see Ch. 11)
           Admit to gynaecology ward and inform appropriate specialists
           Keep the patient informed of events – a very distressing time
           Consider IM ergometrine to reduce bleeding by contracting uterus (only in non-viable pregnancy)
           Options: expectant management, evacuation of retained products

Station 214: Recurrent miscarriage

- *A couple has been referred to clinic following a third miscarriage. Please could you take a history from them and discuss a management plan*
- *Please write short notes on how you would approach the investigation of a couple who have had several miscarriages*

Hints and tips

- Recurrent miscarriage is defined as more than three consecutive pregnancy losses
- This is an emotive situation for the couple, which needs to be recognised
- Take a full medical history from the female partner including obstetric and gynaecological histories
- Establish the characteristics of previous miscarriages, e.g. trimester
- Ask about possibility of consanguinity
- Determine environmental or infective risk factors
- Systems review: undiagnosed diabetes or thyroid disease?
- Family history: history of immunological or chromosomal disorders?

Ix   *Examination*   Evidence of infection
                        Uterine abnormalities
     Bloods   FBC, U&E, LFT, TFT, Glu
                        Antiphospholipid antibodies (lupus anticoagulant, anticardiolipin antibody)
                        LH, prolactin
                        Peripheral blood karyotyping
     Imaging   Pelvic US
     Micro   Screen for bacterial vaginosis
                        (NB. there is no benefit in screening for other infections, e.g. TORCH)
     Other   Hysteroscopy

Station 215: Ectopic pregnancy

History hints

Abdominal pain (98%)
Amenorrhea (65%)
Vaginal bleeding/spotting (80%)
Also nausea, vomiting, dizziness, syncope, referred shoulder pain and tenesmus
Usually occurs 6-8 weeks after last menstrual period

Examination hints

Signs of shock
Pyrexial
Palpable adnexal mass
Abdominal tenderness with guarding and rebound suggests ruptured or bleeding ectopic

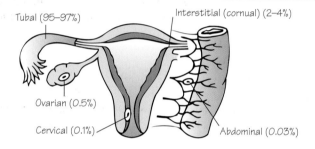

Tubal (95–97%)
Interstitial (cornual) (2–4%)
Ovarian (0.5%)
Cervical (0.1%)
Abdominal (0.03%)

Station 216: Termination of pregnancy

Ethical and legal aspects
- Opinion of two doctors needed
- > 1 criteria needs to be specified from the Regulations of the Abortion Act (1967) and Section 37 of the Human Fertilisation and Embryology Act (1990)

Criteria – termination allowed <24 weeks' gestation if:
- it reduces the risk to a woman's life
- it reduces the risk to her physical or mental health
- it reduces the risk to physical or mental health of her existing children
- the baby is at substantial risk of being seriously mentally or physically handicapped

There is no upper limit on gestational time if there is:
- Risk to the mother's life
- Risk of injury to the mother's physical/mental health
- Substantial risk that, if the child were born, it would suffer severe physical or mental abnormalities
- <1% of terminations are performed after 20 weeks
- If a doctor is of the opinion, formed in good faith, that a woman has grounds for an abortion, they are required to complete a certificate
- Any practitioner who terminates a pregnancy is required to notify the Chief Medical Officer

Station 217: Antepartum haemorrhage

Placental abruption hints
- Vaginal bleeding
- Abdominal pain
- Uterine contractions
- Fetal distress

Placenta praevia hints
- Painless vaginal bleeding
- Bright red blood (maternal origin)
- Fetal malpresentation

Causes of APH
Placental abruption (30%)
Placenta praevia (20%)
Vasa praevia (rare)
Other: cervicitis
     genital infection
     vaginal trauma
     polyps
     early labour

Classification of placental abruption

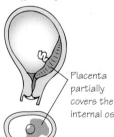

Revealed bleeding (80%)
Premature separation of placenta with retroplacental clot and vaginal bleeding

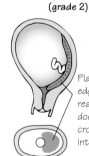

Concealed bleeding (20%)
The degree of separation is variable and ranges from partial to total with fetal demise

Definition: Premature separation of the placenta from the uterine side wall

Classification of placenta praevia

MAJOR

Complete placenta praevia (European classification grade 4)
Internal cervical os
Pelvic inlet
Placenta completely covers the internal cervical os

Partial placenta praevia (grade 3)
Placenta partially covers the internal os

MINOR

Marginal placenta praevia (grade 2)
Placental edge reaches but does not cross the internal os

Low-lying placenta (grade 1)
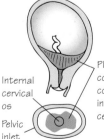
2 cm range from internal cervical os
Lower edge of placenta reaches into the lower uterine segment and within 2 cm of internal os, but does not cover it

Definition: Implantation of the placenta over the cervical os in advance of the fetal presenting part

Station 215: Ectopic pregnancy

• *A 21-year-old female presents to A&E with a positive urinary pregnancy test, lower abdominal pain and some vaginal spotting. Please assess this simulated patient and discuss your actions with the examiner*

Hints and tips

• Approach a patient with a possible ectopic pregnancy as a medical emergency; use the ABCDE approach (see Ch. 11)

Discussion points

• What are the risk factors for an ectopic pregnancy?
• What investigations would you request as the gynaecological FY1?
• Discuss the management of a patient with an ectopic pregnancy
• What are the indications and contraindications for medical management of an ectopic pregnancy?

RF   Previous ectopic or tubal surgery
        Pelvic inflammatory disease
        Infertility, endometriosis, anatomical anomalies
        Current IUCD

∆∆   Ectopic pregnancy; early intrauterine gestation; threatened miscarriage; functional ovarian cyst; pelvic inflammatory disease; non-gynaecological cause, e.g. appendicitis

Ix   *Urine*   β-HCG
         Bloods   Serum β-HCG (serial measurements); FBC, G&S
         Imaging Transvaginal US
         Other   Laparoscopy

General Mx   Oxygen, IV fluid resuscitation (blood if necessary)
                 Analgesia

Specific Mx

β-HCG < 1500 mIU/ml
US may not show a gestational sac. If stable and US is negative, manage at home

β-HCG > 1500 mIU/ml
An intrauterine pregnancy should be detectable on US by an experienced ultrasonographer in 95% of cases. If an intrauterine sac is not visible with a serum β-HCG of > 1500, suspicion of ectopic pregnancy is markedly increased

β-HCG > 6000 mIU/ml
If no intrauterine gestational sac is seen, assume it is an ectopic pregnancy

Rx   *Medical*   Expectant – observation if declining β-HCG
                     IM methotrexate for selected patients with serial β-HCG measurements
         Surgery   Salpingectomy or salpingostomy

Station 216: Termination of pregnancy

• *A 19-year-old girl presents approximately 8 weeks pregnant; she states that she does not wish to keep the baby. In your role as the obstetric FY1, please discuss this situation with her*

Hints and tips

• Confirm pregnancy
• Counsel her and make her aware of alternatives (e.g. adoption)
• Screen for *Chlamydia*
• Discuss future contraceptive needs
• Check Rhesus status, if negative needs anti-D
• Discuss possible management options and complications
• Offer follow-up and support

Mx

Up to 9 weeks	Medical abortion: oral mifepristone + vaginal misoprostol
Up to 12 weeks	Suction curettage Consider cervical ripening with misoprostol
12–24 weeks	Surgery less safe Mifepristone + vaginal prostaglandins ± oxytocin

Complications

• Infection: occur in up to 10% of terminations
• Cervical trauma: occur in about 1% of terminations
• Other complications: haemorrhage (1.5/1000), perforation of uterus (1–4/1000) and failed termination (2.3/1000 surgical, 6.0/1000 medical)
• Anaesthetic complications
• Psychological effects
• Increased rate of complications if gestational age < 6 weeks or > 16 weeks

Station 217: Antepartum haemorrhage

• *A 29-year-old multiparous woman has been referred by her GP with vaginal bleeding. She is 38 weeks' gestation. You are concerned that she may have a placenta praevia or a placental abruption. Please discuss these diagnoses with the patient and explain how you will manage further*

Hints and tips

• ABCDE (see Ch. 11)
• History and relevant examination (see Ch. 76)
• Avoid pelvic examination in a woman with antepartum haemorrhage (APH) until placenta praevia has been excluded

RF

For placental abruption
Previous episode; maternal hypertension; multiparity; smoking/ cocaine; anatomical anomaly of the uterus/fibroids; age (higher risk with age); preterm premature rupture of membranes

For placenta praevia
Previous episode; previous uterine scar; multiparity; smoking; age

Ix   *Bloods*   FBC, clotting, U&E, G&S/cross-match
         Imaging US
         Other   Cardiotocography

Placenta praevia

• Anti-D for Rhesus-negative patients
• Steroids if < 34 weeks
• Elective Caesarean section at 39 weeks
• Emergency section if bleeding is severe, despite transfusion, regardless of gestation
• If preterm gestation, expectant management is indicated in patients with no observed bleeding, reactive non-stress test and stable haematocrit
• Vaginal examinations should be avoided

Placental abruption

• < 34 weeks: if minor abruption and no fetal distress give steroids and observe
• > 37 weeks: if no fetal distress – induction of labour with continuous monitoring
• Fetal distress: urgent section

Station 218: Antenatal screening

Screening timeline in England

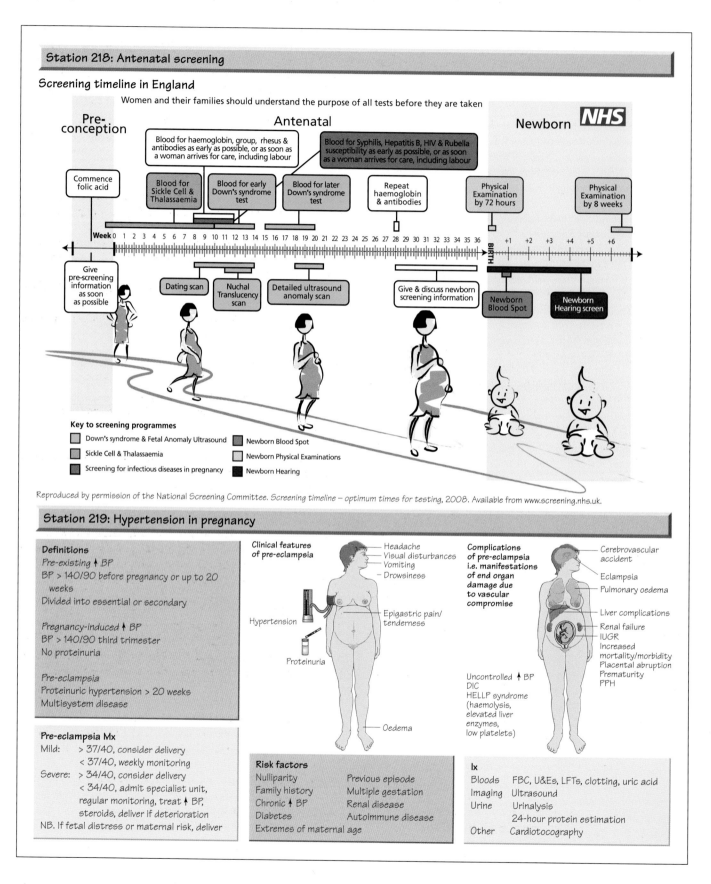

Women and their families should understand the purpose of all tests before they are taken

Pre-conception

Antenatal

Newborn NHS

Blood for haemoglobin, group, rhesus & antibodies as early as possible, or as soon as a woman arrives for care, including labour

Blood for Syphilis, Hepatitis B, HIV & Rubella susceptibility as early as possible, or as soon as a woman arrives for care, including labour

Commence folic acid

Blood for Sickle Cell & Thalassaemia

Blood for early Down's syndrome test

Blood for later Down's syndrome test

Repeat haemoglobin & antibodies

Physical Examination by 72 hours

Physical Examination by 8 weeks

Week 0 1 2 3 4 5 6 7 8 9 10 11 12 13 14 15 16 17 18 19 20 21 22 23 24 25 26 27 28 29 30 31 32 33 34 35 36 +1 +2 +3 +4 +5 +6

BIRTH

Give pre-screening information as soon as possible

Dating scan

Nuchal Translucency scan

Detailed ultrasound anomaly scan

Give & discuss newborn screening information

Newborn Blood Spot

Newborn Hearing screen

Key to screening programmes

Down's syndrome & Fetal Anomaly Ultrasound

Sickle Cell & Thalassaemia

Screening for infectious diseases in pregnancy

Newborn Blood Spot

Newborn Physical Examinations

Newborn Hearing

Reproduced by permission of the National Screening Committee. Screening timeline – optimum times for testing, 2008. Available from www.screening.nhs.uk.

Station 219: Hypertension in pregnancy

Definitions

Pre-existing ↑ BP
BP > 140/90 before pregnancy or up to 20 weeks
Divided into essential or secondary

Pregnancy-induced ↑ BP
BP > 140/90 third trimester
No proteinuria

Pre-eclampsia
Proteinuric hypertension > 20 weeks
Multisystem disease

Pre-eclampsia Mx
Mild: > 37/40, consider delivery
< 37/40, weekly monitoring
Severe: > 34/40, consider delivery
< 34/40, admit specialist unit, regular monitoring, treat ↑ BP, steroids, deliver if deterioration
NB. If fetal distress or maternal risk, deliver

Clinical features of pre-eclampsia
- Headache
- Visual disturbances
- Vomiting
- Drowsiness
- Epigastric pain/tenderness
- Hypertension
- Proteinuria
- Oedema

Complications of pre-eclampsia i.e. manifestations of end organ damage due to vascular compromise
- Cerebrovascular accident
- Eclampsia
- Pulmonary oedema
- Liver complications
- Renal failure
- IUGR
- Increased mortality/morbidity
- Placental abruption
- Prematurity
- PPH

Uncontrolled ↑ BP
DIC
HELLP syndrome (haemolysis, elevated liver enzymes, low platelets)

Risk factors
Nulliparity	Previous episode
Family history	Multiple gestation
Chronic ↑ BP	Renal disease
Diabetes	Autoimmune disease
Extremes of maternal age	

Ix
Bloods	FBC, U&Es, LFTs, clotting, uric acid
Imaging	Ultrasound
Urine	Urinalysis
	24-hour protein estimation
Other	Cardiotocography

Station 218A: Preconception care

• *A 29-year-old female has come to see her GP as she is planning on starting a family. Please discuss this situation with her and advise her accordingly*

Preconception advice

• Aim to prevent congenital anomalies and maximise maternal health
• Should be offered to all women of childbearing age as > 50% of pregnancies are unplanned
• Give advice on proper nutrition, exercise, smoking cessation, abstinence from alcohol and drugs, protection from radiation (X-rays) and workplace exposures, information on prescribed and over-the-counter (OTC) drugs to avoid teratogenicity, infection control (STD protection and treatment, rubella and hepatitis immunity status) and psychosocial counselling for planning a pregnancy

Dietary advice

• Calories: 30–35 kcal/kg/day plus 300 kcal
• Calcium: 300 mg extra calcium per day, which is a ≈ 250 ml of milk or one generic $CaCO_3$ tablet
• Iron requirements: 30 mg of elemental iron per day; more in multiple pregnancies. One dose of 324 mg ferrous sulphate provides 65 mg
• Folic acid requirements: 0.4 mg to 1 mg/day

Other general advice

• *Occupation*: abstinence from physical work may be recommended if there have been two previous premature deliveries, an incompetent cervix or fetal loss secondary to uterine anomalies, but general bed rest has no proven benefit
• *Exercise*: avoid in supine position after first trimester. Avoid exercise with potential for abdominal trauma
• *Alcohol*: ↑ risk of mid-trimester abortion, mental retardation and behaviour and learning disorders
• *Tobacco*: increases the risk of low-birth-weight infants, premature labour, spontaneous abortions, stillbirth and birth defects

Discussion points

• What are the aims of preconception care and who should be offered this?

Station 218B: Booking visit

• *A 24-year-old female has attended the antenatal clinic for the first time. She states she is 11 weeks' pregnant. You are the FY1 in the clinic. Please discuss with the examiner how you would approach this situation and explain to the patient what investigations you will perform*

Hints and tips

This station could be introduced in several ways and could test individual items involved in a booking visit.

• History and examination: see Chapter 75 for general advice
• General advice as for Station 218A + counsel patient about prenatal screening tests (see timeline opposite)

Booking Ix	*Bloods*	FBC (anaemia) and G&S
		Glucose
		Consider Hb electrophoresis
		Syphilis and rubella screening
		Offer hepatitis B and HIV testing
	Imaging	US
	Micro	Urine MC&S + urinalysis

Station 218C: Prenatal diagnostic tests

Student info: *You are the obstetric FY1 doctor. Please counsel this 35-year-old woman whose triple test result has shown a risk of her baby having Down syndrome as 1 : 200*

Patient info: *You are a senior lawyer who has been trying to conceive for 4 years. You have had no previous pregnancies and no medical history to note. You have a friend who had a similar consultation with her doctor 2 years ago and went on to have an amniocentesis. Unfortunately your friend lost her baby and the karyotype turned out to be normal. You and your husband, a cardiac surgeon, feel that you would not want to have a baby with Down syndrome. You are not sure of the exact meaning of the test results and need some further clarification about the risks to the baby*

Hints and tips

• Ascertain patient's reason for attending and prior knowledge
• Ascertain patient's thoughts on the possibility of having a baby with Down syndrome
• Explain that the tests so far have been for screening, i.e. to determine the risk, but it is now possible to perform a diagnostic test to know for sure, e.g. amniocentesis
• Explain the procedure of amniocentesis, discussing the benefits vs the risks (miscarriage 0.5–1%)
• Offer further advice (leaflets, arrange to see the consultant) and offer time to think about the situation

Diagnostic tests

• *Amniocentesis*:
  • performed in patients > 15 weeks pregnant
  • prenatal diagnosis of chromosomal and inherited problems
  • miscarriage risk of 0.5–1%
• *Chorionic villus sampling*:
  • performed earlier in pregnancy so if there is an abnormality, patient can consider abortion sooner
  • higher risk of miscarriage (1–2%)

Station 219: Hypertension in pregnancy

• *You are the FY1 doctor in the antenatal clinic and have been asked to review a patient who is 36 weeks pregnant with a BP of 155/100. Please discuss the management of this patient with the examiner, including possible causes, further investigations and management*

Hints and tips

This instruction suggests an examiner-led viva station, although the scenario could easily be played by an actor. Rather than discuss the management, you could be asked to take a relevant history or even communicate the diagnosis of pregnancy-induced hypertension.

Mx

Rx	*Medical*	Control BP if > 160/110; consider labetolol
		Prevent eclampsia – consider IV magnesium
		Promote fetal maturity – steroids if < 34 weeks
	Interventional	Delivery is the only effective treatment
	Location	Obstetric ward, consider high dependency unit
	Monitoring	See Ix opposite
		Maternal and fetal monitoring
		Strict fluid balance

Station 220: Dysmenorrhoea/pelvic pain

Acute pelvic pain

Gynaecological causes
- Ectopic pregnancy
- Pelvic inflammatory disease (PID)
- Ruptured ovarian cyst
- Adnexal torsion
- Miscarriage

Other causes
- Appendicitis
- Mesenteric adenitis
- Urinary tract infections
- Diverticulitis

Chronic pelvic pain

Gynaecological causes
- Dysmenorrhoea
- Endometriosis
- Adenomyosis
- Fibroids
- Chronic PID

Other causes
- Chronic gastrointestinal disease
- Chronic urinary tract disease
- Musculoskeletal problems

Dysmenorrhoea
- Primary – pain with no organic pathology, often starts at menarche
- Secondary – usually associated with pathology, often starts later in life

Station 221: Abnormal vaginal bleeding

Abnormal uterine bleeding

Organic causes

Pelvic causes
- Pregnancy-related conditions, e.g. miscarriage
- Neoplasia, e.g. cervical or uterine cancer
- Bengin tumours, e.g. fibroids
- Inflammatory, e.g. PID
- Trauma
- Iatrogenic, e.g. IUCD

Systemic causes
- Endocrine, e.g. hyper- or hypothyroidism, diabetes, adrenal disease
- Haematological, e.g. coagulation and platelet deficiencies
- Hepatic, e.g. chronic liver disease
- Drugs, e.g. steroids, anticoagulants

Unexplained/dysfunctional uterine bleeding (DUB)

Anovulatory
- Usually around menarche and menopause
- Irregular cycle and bleeding

Ovulatory
- Usually 35–40 years old
- Regular heavy periods
- Often physiological, e.g. related to LH surge

Management

Excessive bleeding

Exclude anaemia — Exclude malignancy — Exclude systemic cause

Symptom relief

To reduce volume – tranexamic acid or IUS

To regulate loss – progesterones or combined contraceptive

If fails

Surgery

Hysteroscopy ⟷ Hysterectomy

Causes of abnormal vaginal bleeding

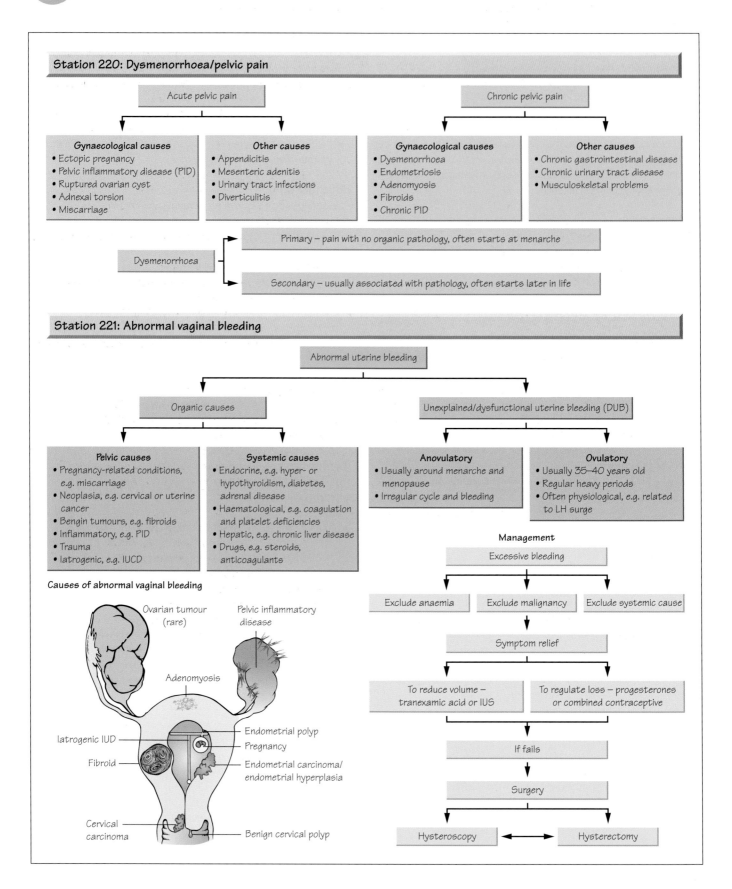

- Ovarian tumour (rare)
- Pelvic inflammatory disease
- Adenomyosis
- Iatrogenic IUD
- Fibroid
- Cervical carcinoma
- Endometrial polyp
- Pregnancy
- Endometrial carcinoma/endometrial hyperplasia
- Benign cervical polyp

Station 220: Dysmenorrhoea/pelvic pain

• *You are a FY1 doctor on your GP placement. A 19-year-old female has come to see you complaining of painful periods. Please take a structured gynaecological history and discuss your management plan*

Hints and tips

• The chances of pathology increases if the pain disturbs sleep
• 50% have a 'clear' laparoscopy, so always consider psychological problems
• Always consider other pathologies: non-gynaecological causes can coincide with menses
• Painful periods are depressing, but true clinical depression lowers pain threshold
• Determine patient's reason for attending
• Brief obstetric and gynaecological history
• Confirm age of menarche and character of periods since
• Establish detail about the pain, noting if it bothers her at night
• Confirm LMP and ask about presence or absence of symptoms of abdominal pain, breast soreness and mood change
• Take a sexual and contraceptive history
• Determine general health and systemic symptoms
• Structure a diagnosis and discuss some relevant investigations

Discussion points

• What are the causes of dysmenorrhoea?
• How would you approach the investigation of this patient?
• A 24-year-old woman presents to the A&E department with right iliac fossa pain. What would you include in your differential diagnosis and what features of the history would support each of these? How would you investigate this patient?

Ix	*Bloods*	FBC for menorrhagia, WCC for PID
		FSH, LH, prolactin, testosterone
	Imaging	Ultrasound
	Micro	Swabs – high vaginal and endocervical (*Chlamydia* and gonorrhoea)
		Urinalysis
	Other	Consider laparoscopy

Station 221: Abnormal vaginal bleeding

• *You are the FY1 in the gynae clinic. A 45-year-old patient has been referred by her GP with heavy periods. Please take a focused history and discuss a possible diagnosis and investigations*

• *A 38-year-old female has been referred to the gynae clinic with a history of intermenstrual bleeding. Please take a history from this patient and discuss possible causes*

Definitions

Menorrhagia	Heavy periods, i.e. ↑ volume
Intermenstrual bleeding (IMB)	↑ frequency
Postcoital bleeding (PCB)	Non-menstrual bleeding post intercourse
Postmenopausal bleeding (PMB)	Vaginal bleeding > 12 months after cessation of periods

Hints and tips

• Determine the patient's reason for attending
• Complete obstetric and gynaecology history
• Concentrate on characteristics and pattern of menstruation, e.g. cycle length, days bleeding, flooding
• Determine if there has been an alteration in the cycle and when this occurred
• Try and determine amount of blood loss
• Confirm sexual and contraceptive histories if appropriate age
• Check for symptoms of anaemia
• Check systems review, e.g. symptoms of thyroid disease
• Establish drug history
• Offer possible diagnoses and agree on a management plan including initial investigations

Ix	Check pregnancy test if appropriate	
	Bloods	FBC, iron studies, clotting
		Consider endocrine tests, e.g. TFT
	Imaging	Ultrasound
	Other	Cervical smear
		Consider hysteroscopy ± endometrial biopsy
		Consider use of menstrual diary
Rx	*Medical*	
	First line	Mirena intrauterine system
	Second line	NSAIDs (e.g. mefanamic acid)
		Tranexamic acid (antifibrinolytic)
		Stop if no improvement after three cycles
		Combined OCP
	Third line	Oral progestogen
	Surgical	Endometrial ablation
		Myomectomy (surgical removal of fibroids)
		Hysterectomy

Station 222: Cervical dysplasia

The NHS Cervical Smear Screening Programme

All women aged 25-64 are eligible

Age 25	- first invitation
25-49	- 3 yearly
50-64	- 5 yearly
>65	- if no smear since age 50 or previously abnormal

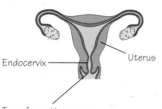

Endocervix

Uterus

Transformation zone – the area where most abnormal cell change occur

Aetiology/risk factors

Human papillomavirus (HPV)	Sexually active women
Smoking	Low social groups
Multiple sexual partners	Chlamydia
Young age at first coitus	Multiparity
+ve family history	Long-term OCP use
Rare in Jews/Muslims	

Result	Action
Negative	Manage incidental findings (e.g. infections) Recall according to screening programme guidelines
Inadequate	Manage incidental findings Repeat sample as soon as convenient if technically inadequate Refer for colposcopy after three consecutive inadequate samples
Borderline	Squamous cell change – refer for colposcopy after three tests in a series reported as borderline nuclear change Endocervical cell change – refer for colposcopy after one test reported as borderline nuclear change in endocervical cells
Abnormal result	Refer for colposcopy if > 3 tests reported as abnormal at any grade in a 10-year period. NB. three consecutive negative results are required >6 months apart before returning to routine screening programme
Mild dyskaryosis	Ideally, refer for colposcopy after one mild dyskaryosis result However, it is acceptable to recommend a repeat test < 6 months as many will have returned to normal by then Refer for colposcopy after two abnormal tests
Moderate dyskaryosis	Refer for colposcopy
Severe dyskaryosis	Refer for colposcopy

Station 224: Endometrial hyperplasia/neoplasia

Stages of endometrial carcinoma

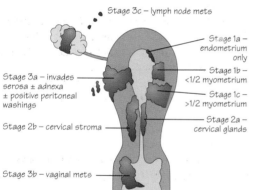

Stage 3c – lymph node mets

Stage 1a – endometrium only

Stage 3a – invades serosa ± adnexa ± positive peritoneal washings

Stage 1b – <1/2 myometrium

Stage 1c – >1/2 myometrium

Stage 2b – cervical stroma

Stage 2a – cervical glands

Stage 3b – vaginal mets

NB. Prognosis is also dependent on tumour grade

Stage 4b – distant mets

Brain

Lung

Liver

Bone

Stage 4a – Bowel or bladder

History hints

Post-menopausal bleeding
Inter-menstrual bleeding
Menorrhagia

Aetiology/risk factors

Early menarche	Late menopause
Nulliparity	Infertility
Tamoxifen (Nolvadex) use	Ovarian dysfunction
Obesity	Diabetes
HRT (oestrogen replacement)	
Chronic exposure to unopposed oestrogens	
Hereditary chronic anovulation	
Family history of breast, ovarian or colon cancer	

Protective factors
Smoking   Combined OCP   Multiparity

Management

Hyperplasia – depends on:
• Severity of symptoms
• Presence of atypical cells
• Surgical risk
• Future childbearing wish

Options
Without atypia: progestins
With atypia: hysterectomy or high-dose progestins if high surgical risk or fertility desired (regular endometrial surveillance essential)

Management

Neoplasia
TAH and BSO
± lymph node dissection
Radiotherapy
Brachytherapy
Palliation

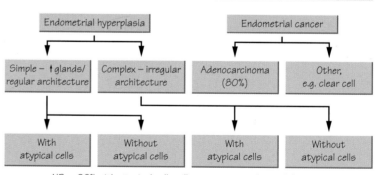

Endometrial hyperplasia → Simple – ↑ glands/regular architecture → With atypical cells / Without atypical cells

Complex – irregular architecture

Endometrial cancer → Adenocarcinoma (80%) → With atypical cells / Without atypical cells

Other, e.g. clear cell

NB. > 20% with atypical cells will progress to endometrial cancer

Station 222: Cervical dysplasia

• You are an FY1 doctor in GP. A 29-year-old female has come for the results of her smear test. She saw one of the other GPs on her last visit. The result has been reported as showing severe dyskaryosis. This is the first smear she has had

Hints and tips

The station could be examined in a variety of ways: purely discussing the result and agreeing a course of action or taking a full history, explaining the result and also discussing the risk factors.

• Determine the patient's reason for attending

• Take a brief obstetric and gynaecological history (if required); otherwise move to the explanation part of the consultation

• Explain the result in non-jargon terms, clarifying that this result does not equate to a diagnosis of cancer but that there is evidence of slightly abnormal cells which need to be further investigated

• Explain that the danger of having no further investigation is that over time these cells could lead to invasive cancer

• Explain that the further investigation will require referral to a specialist gynaecologist who will need to perform a colposcopy

• A pregnancy test will need to be performed before this test

• Colposcopy is performed to visualise and obtain diagnostic information of any abnormal areas

• Explain that the procedure is carried out in the out-patient clinic and no anaesthetic is required; a speculum will be passed and the doctor will then visualise the cervix with a set of powerful binoculars (the colposcope)

• Various substances can be placed on the cervix (e.g. saline, acetic acid) in order to visualise any abnormal areas. Biopsies may then be taken from these areas and sent to be examined under a microscope for further evaluation and a further appointment will be made to discuss the result of the biopsy

• End the consultation by confirming the plan and checking if the patient has any questions

Discussion points

• What are the risk factors for developing cervical cancer?

• Can you tell me about the NHS cervical screening plan?

• Discuss the pros and cons of screening programmes

• What is the management of a patient with cervical intraepithelial neoplasia (CIN) 2?

Management of CIN

Treatment should be offered for biopsy-proven CIN 2 and 3 and CIN that is persistent over 12 months. Options are:

• Ablation
• Cryotherapy
• Loop excision
• Cone excision

Management of invasive neoplasia

This depends on the staging. Management often use a combination of therapies, primary and adjuvant:

• Cone biopsy/simple hysterectomy
• Radical hysterectomy
• Chemotherapy
• Radiotherapy
• Brachytherapy (local radiation implants)
• Palliation

Station 223: Cervical smear

• A 25-year-old patient has attended for her first cervical smear. Please explain this procedure and gain consent

Hints and tips

This station could test several domains depending on the actual instruction: you could be asked to carry out the procedure using a model, explain the procedure or gain consent for the procedure. Please review the communication skills section and Chapter 76 (performing a speculum examination).

• Check the patient's prior knowledge and understanding of the procedure

• Explain the procedure, including reasons for performing it and any possible side effects

• Perform a speculum examination (see Ch. 76) to view the squamo-columnar junction of the cervix

• Liquid-based cytology (LBC) is now the method of choice: a brush is used rather than a spatula, which is rotated against the squamocolumnar junction (usually in the cervical canal)

• The end of the brush is then broken off into a container of preservative fluid, and sent to the laboratory

• The advantages of LBC over previous methods are that reporting time is reduced and there are less inadequate smears. The inadequate rate is 9.1% with Pap smears compared to 1.6% with LBC. LBC is also 12% more sensitive than older methods

• Complete the request form with the clinical information

• Make a clear plan as to how to inform the patient of the result

Station 224: Endometrial hyperplasia/neoplasia

• A 58-year-old patient comes to see you complaining of post-menopausal bleeding. Please take an appropriate history and inquire about risk factors for endometrial hyperplasia/carcinoma

Hints and tips

• Follow a similar routine to Station 221 (Ch. 81)

Ix Cervical smear
    Pelvic US
    Dilation and curettage (D&C)
    Hysteroscopy + endometrial biopsy

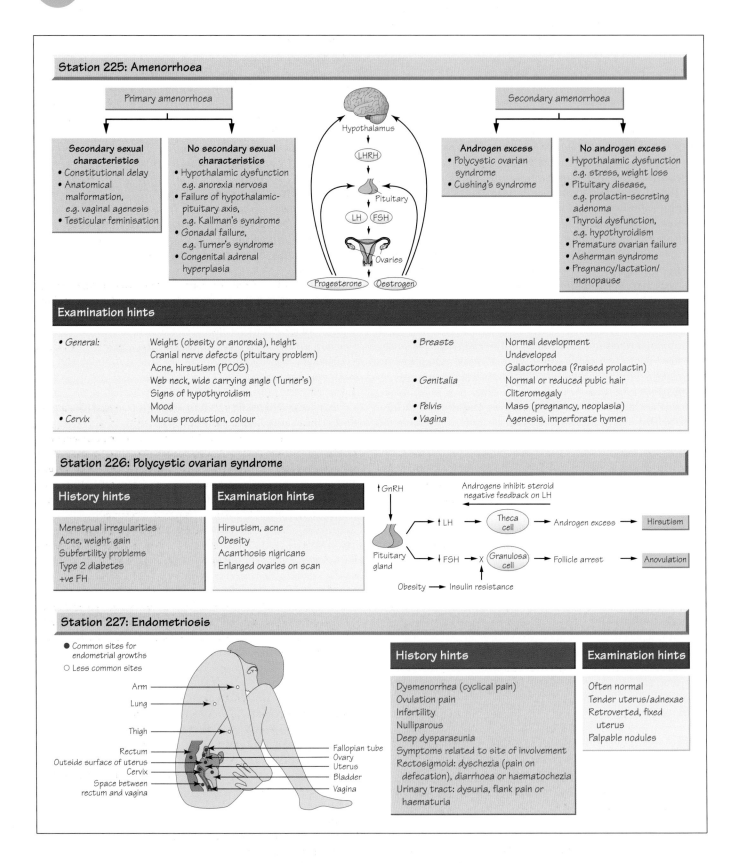

Station 225: Amenorrhoea

Primary amenorrhoea

Secondary amenorrhoea

Hypothalamus
LHRH
Pituitary
LH FSH
Ovaries
Progesterone Oestrogen

Secondary sexual characteristics
• Constitutional delay
• Anatomical malformation, e.g. vaginal agenesis
• Testicular feminisation

No secondary sexual characteristics
• Hypothalamic dysfunction e.g. anorexia nervosa
• Failure of hypothalamic-pituitary axis, e.g. Kallman's syndrome
• Gonadal failure, e.g. Turner's syndrome
• Congenital adrenal hyperplasia

Androgen excess
• Polycystic ovarian syndrome
• Cushing's syndrome

No androgen excess
• Hypothalamic dysfunction e.g. stress, weight loss
• Pituitary disease, e.g. prolactin-secreting adenoma
• Thyroid dysfunction, e.g. hypothyroidism
• Premature ovarian failure
• Asherman syndrome
• Pregnancy/lactation/ menopause

Examination hints

• *General:* Weight (obesity or anorexia), height
Cranial nerve defects (pituitary problem)
Acne, hirsutism (PCOS)
Web neck, wide carrying angle (Turner's)
Signs of hypothyroidism
Mood
• *Cervix* Mucus production, colour

• *Breasts* Normal development
Undeveloped
Galactorrhoea (?raised prolactin)
• *Genitalia* Normal or reduced pubic hair
Cliteromegaly
• *Pelvis* Mass (pregnancy, neoplasia)
• *Vagina* Agenesis, imperforate hymen

Station 226: Polycystic ovarian syndrome

History hints

Menstrual irregularities
Acne, weight gain
Subfertility problems
Type 2 diabetes
+ve FH

Examination hints

Hirsutism, acne
Obesity
Acanthosis nigricans
Enlarged ovaries on scan

↑GnRH

Androgens inhibit steroid negative feedback on LH

Pituitary gland

→ ↑LH → Theca cell → Androgen excess → Hirsutism

→ ↓FSH → X Granulosa cell → Follicle arrest → Anovulation

Obesity → Insulin resistance

Station 227: Endometriosis

● Common sites for endometrial growths
○ Less common sites

Arm
Lung
Thigh
Rectum
Outside surface of uterus
Cervix
Space between rectum and vagina

Fallopian tube
Ovary
Uterus
Bladder
Vagina

History hints

Dysmenorrhea (cyclical pain)
Ovulation pain
Infertility
Nulliparous
Deep dysparaeunia
Symptoms related to site of involvement
Rectosigmoid: dyschezia (pain on defecation), diarrhoea or haematochezia
Urinary tract: dysuria, flank pain or haematuria

Examination hints

Often normal
Tender uterus/adnexae
Retroverted, fixed uterus
Palpable nodules

Station 225: Amenorrhoea

• *You are a FY1 doctor in your GP placement. A 25-year-old female has come to see you concerned that she has not had a period for 4 months. Please take a relevant history and discuss your further management including investigations*

Hints and tips

• Determine the patient's reason for attending
• Take a brief obstetric and gynaecological history
• Ask about possibility of pregnancy and ask about contraception
• Confirm age of menarche and character of periods since
• Confirm LMP and ask about presence or absence of symptoms of abdominal pain, breast soreness and mood change
• Determine history of chronic illness, trauma or surgery
• Full DH
• Obtain a sexual history
• SH: substance misuse, exercise, diet and home situation
• Elicit any psychosocial issues
• Comprehensive review of symptoms including vasomotor symptoms, hot flushes, virilising changes, galactorrhoea, headache, fatigue, palpitations, nervousness, hearing loss and visual changes
• Associated symptoms (looking for an endocrine disorder such as hypothyroidism)

Discussion points

• What are the causes of amenorrhoea?
• How would you approach the investigation of this patient?
• Tell me what you know about Turner's syndrome
• For each of the causes of amenorrhoea you have discussed, tell me about the treatment

Definitions

Primary amenorrhoea	Absence of menses by age 16 years
Secondary amenorrhoea	Cessation of menstruation for at least 6 months or for at least three cycles
Oligomenorrhoea	Menstruation less than every 35 days

NB. Unless there is a suspected organic problem or investigation for subfertility is needed, it is usual to wait 6 months before commencing investigations.

Ix	*Pregnancy test*	
	Bloods	FBC, U&E, TFT, Glc, ESR, LFT
		FSH, LH, prolactin, testosterone
	Other	Progestin challenge (?withdrawal bleed)
	Imaging	MRI brain (pituitary tumour, empty sella)
		US (PCOS, anatomical anomaly)
General Rx		Patient education
		Treat underlying causes, e.g. hypothyroidism, depression, anorexia
Specific Rx		Gonadal failure: OCP
		Hypothalamic dysfunction: OCP
		Anatomical anomaly: surgery
		Pituitary adenoma: surgery
		Ovarian failure: oestrogen replacement

Station 226: Polycystic ovarian syndrome

• *A 21-year-old attends her GP for a review. Her friend has recently been diagnosed as having PCOS and she is concerned that she also has the condition because she has noticed some fine hair on her face. Take a relevant history and discuss features that would suggest PCOS was the cause*

Hints and tips

• Follow the hints and tips from Station 227

Ix	*Bloods*	↑ LH : FSH ratio
		↑ testosterone and dehydroepiandrosterone sulphate levels
		Glc
	Imaging	Ultrasound
	Other	Consider endometrial biopsy at any age if there is prolonged amenorrheoa or oligomenorrhoea
ΔΔ		Late-onset adrenal hyperplasia
		Androgen-producing ovarian or adrenal neoplasia
		Cushing's syndrome
		Idiopathic hirsutism

Future sequelae

• Gynaecological: subfertility, amenorrhoea, dysfunctional uterine bleeding, increased risk of endometrial cancer, possible increased risk of breast cancer
• Dermatological: hirsutism, alopecia, acne
• Cardiovascular: lipid changes, increased risk of cardiovascular disease
• Endocrine: insulin resistance

Management

• Weight loss may reduce hirsutism and reverse the menstrual disturbance
• *Hormonal therapy*: treat menstrual irregularity with medroxyprogesterone or oral contraceptives. Can induce fertility with clomiphene
• *Hirsutism*: weight loss, depilation and electrolysis. Oral contraceptives may improve hirsutism (especially those with norgestimate). An alternative is Depo-Provera. Spironolactone is an anti-aldosterone diuretic and an anti-androgen, which can be used alone or with hormones. Second-line agents (flutamide, finasteride) have more adverse effects
• *Insulin resistance*: consider screening with a 75 g glucose tolerance test. If positive, metformin is useful to reduce insulin resistance, promote weight loss and prevent long-term complications

Station 227: Endometriosis

• *A 29-year-old lady has been referred to the gynaecological clinic with symptoms of dysmenorrhoea and dyspareunia. You are the FY1 doctor in clinic. Please take a relevant history and discuss possible investigations*

Hints and tips

• Establish patient's reason for attending
• Take a full obstetric and gynaecological history
• Check for specific points as opposite
• Clarify FH of obstetric and gynaecological problems
• Establish management plan
• Answer any questions and offer further information (leaflets, help groups, senior review)

Causes

There are several theories, which include:
• Retrograde menstruation
• Metaplastic conversion of coelomic epithelium

- Haematogenous or lymphatic spread
- Altered immune response

Ix *Bloods* CA-125 (may be raised, but not specific or sensitive)
   Imaging US/CT pelvis (may pick up large deposits)
   Other Laparoscopy (direct visualisation is necessary to confirm the diagnosis as clinical diagnosis is wrong 30–40% of the time)
   Laparoscopy will help assess the extent and stage of the disease as well as tubal patency. Patient-assisted laparoscopy can improve the diagnostic yield

Classification

The American Fertility Society system divides endometriosis into stages I–IV (minimal, mild, moderate or severe).

Management

This depends on disease severity.

Mild

Diagnosis is suspected but not confirmed as laparoscopy is usually not indicated. Treatment consists of:
- Observation ± NSAIDs
- Combined OCP (> 6 months, response rate 75%)
- Depo-Provera 150 mg IM, 3-monthly

Moderate

Confirm diagnosis with laparoscopy before treatment.
- 'Pseudomenopause': danazol is a synthetic androgen that suppresses gonadotropins and causes amenorrhoea. Response rate is ≈ 90%. Begin on the first day of menstruation. Side effects: vasomotor symptoms such as atrophic vaginitis, weight gain, fluid retention, migraines, dizziness, fatigue, depression and acne
- 'Pseudopregnancy': continuous OCP (i.e. without break). Increase dose if breakthrough bleeding occurs, up to 3–4 pills daily, although nausea may limit therapy. Maintain amenorrhoea for 6–9 months: 80% response rate.
- Progesterone treatment: useful if pseudopregnancy is not tolerated or is contraindicated. Initiate therapy during menses. As effective as other treatments
- Conservative surgery to laparoscopically remove extrauterine endometrial tissue is often performed at the time of laparoscopic diagnosis. Recurrence rate: 19% over 5 years

Severe

- Definitive surgery: hysterectomy and bilateral oophorectomy. Recurrence: 10% over 10 years
- Gonadotrophin-releasing hormone (GnRH) agonists such as leuprolide acetate (IM), goserelin (subcutaneous implant) or nafarelin (nasal spray) induce an artificial menopausal state. Side effects are similar to menopause, including decreased bone mineral density. Response rate: 90%

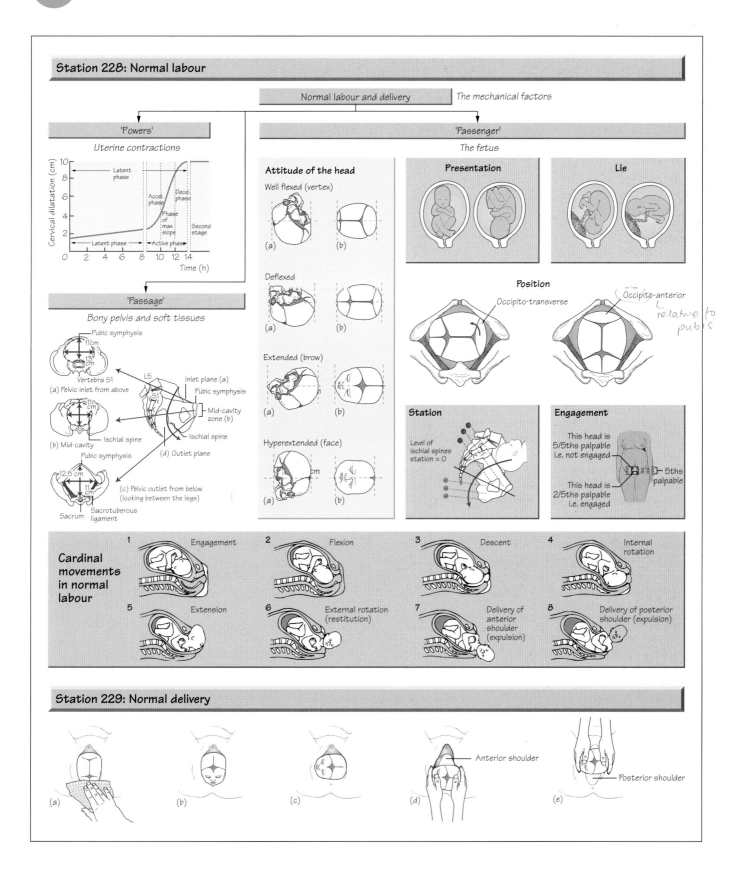

Station 228: Normal labour

Normal labour and delivery — *The mechanical factors*

'Powers'

Uterine contractions

'Passage'

Bony pelvis and soft tissues

- Pubic symphysis
- 11cm
- 13 cm
- Vertebra S1
- (a) Pelvic inlet from above
- 11 cm
- Ischial spine
- (b) Mid-cavity
- Pubic symphysis
- 12.5 cm
- 11 cm
- Sacrum
- Sacrotuberous ligament
- (c) Pelvic outlet from below (looking between the legs)
- L5
- Inlet plane (a)
- Pubic symphysis
- Mid-cavity zone (b)
- Ischial spine
- (d) Outlet plane

Attitude of the head

Well flexed (vertex)
(a)   (b)

Deflexed
(a)   (b)

Extended (brow)
(a)   (b)

Hyperextended (face)
(a)   (b)

'Passenger'

The fetus

Presentation

Lie

Position

Occipito-transverse

Occipito-anterior
relative to pubis

Station

Level of ischial spines station = 0

Engagement

This head is 5/5ths palpable i.e. not engaged

This head is 2/5ths palpable i.e. engaged

5ths palpable

Cardinal movements in normal labour

1 Engagement
2 Flexion
3 Descent
4 Internal rotation
5 Extension
6 External rotation (restitution)
7 Delivery of anterior shoulder (expulsion)
8 Delivery of posterior shoulder (expulsion)

Station 229: Normal delivery

(a)   (b)   (c)   (d) Anterior shoulder   (e) Posterior shoulder

Station 228: Normal labour

• *Please describe the stages of labour and the mechanics behind it, and then demonstrate the anatomy of the pelvis using the models provided*

Stages of labour

Stage 1 Onset of labour until full cervical dilation; subdivided into phases (see partogram opposite):
  • *Latent phase*:
    • can be prolonged
    • cervix up to 3 cm dilated
  • *Active phase*:
    • dilation of cervix 0.5–1 cm/h

Stage 2 Full cervical dilation until delivery of the fetus:
  • *Passive stage*: full dilation until head reaches pelvic floor
  • *Active phase*: maternal pushing

Stage 3 Delivery of the fetus until delivery of placenta

Definitions

Presentation	Leading body part occupying the lower pelvis (e.g. cephalic or breech)
Lie	Long axis of the fetus relative to the long axis of the uterus (longitudinal, transverse or oblique)
Attitude	Degree of flexion or extension of the head
Position	Relationship of a selected part of the fetus to a fixed part of the maternal pelvis (e.g. in cephalic presentation the selected part is the occiput)
Station	Level of descent of the presenting part – assessed on vaginal examination and described in relation to the ischial spines
Engagement	The widest diameter of the presenting part has passed the pelvic brim – assessed by abdominal examination (expressed as fifths palpable)

Station 229: Normal delivery

• *Please guide the examiner through the delivery of a baby using the mannequin provided*

Hints and tips

This station could involve a delivery simulator, a discussion with the examiner or a demonstration of a delivery using an anatomical model.
• Once crowning occurs, delivery is imminent (the baby's head no longer recedes between contractions)
• Wash hands and wear gloves
• Place your hand over the head using a swab to control the delivery (rapid expulsion can lead to perineal tears)
• Ask the patient to stop pushing and to pant
• Once the head is out, check for the cord and reduce if necessary
• Once external rotation of the head has occurred, the anterior shoulder can be delivered by holding the head on each side and applying gentle downward traction
• Lift the head gently until the posterior shoulder appears and then the torso and legs will follow
• Double clamp the cord and then cut
• Monitor the baby and mother, keeping the baby warm
• Assess 1 minute apgar score for baby
• Await third stage of labour

Discussion points

• Please describe the stages of normal labour and discuss the reasons for dystocia
• Discuss the management of the third stage of labour
• Discuss the immediate management of the newborn
• What are the indications for a term induction of labour?
• What is the Bishop score and how is it used?
• What are the contraindications for induction of labour?
• What methods of augmentation of labour are you aware of and when would these be used?

Station 230: Preterm labour

• *A 24-year-old primip starts to have regular, sustained contractions at 34 weeks of pregnancy. How would you assess her and what can be done to try to prevent premature labour?*

Hints and tips

• For obstetric history and examination hints, see Chapter 75
• Estimate fetal weight and age – use US if necessary
• Assess fetal heart rate and presence of uterine activity with monitoring
• Pelvic examination to check the cervix (ideally by speculum)
• Check membranes/presence of amniotic fluid/swabs
• Obtain urinalysis and culture

Discussion points

• What are the risk factors for premature labour and what are the management principles?
• Can you mention some tocolytic agents and their mechanism of action?

RF	Previous episode
	Genital tract infection/UTI
	Intra-amniotic infections
	Uterine anomalies
	Congenital abnormalities
	Multiple gestations
	Smoking/cocaine
	Low socioeconomic status
Specific Mx	Steroids < 34 weeks to promote pulmonary maturity
	Tocolysis to delay delivery
	Vaginal delivery if possible
	Close monitoring and support from neonatologist if necessary

Tocolysis

1 What are the contraindications to tocolysis?
  • Fetal distress, fetal anomalies, abruptio placentae and placenta previa with heavy bleeding
2 What are the risks and warnings involved?
  • If rupture of membranes, ↑ risk of cord prolapse and amnionitis
  • Mother may experience tachycardia, nervousness or pulmonary oedema secondary to medication
  • Prepare to deliver
3 What is the aim of tocolysis?
  • To arrest labour long enough for exogenous steroids to stimulate fetal surfactant production so as to prevent the pulmonary complications of preterm birth

4 What drugs (tocolytics) are available?

- Calcium channel antagonist, e.g. nifedipine
- Oxytocin receptor antagonist, e.g. atosiban

Station 231: Preterm, prelabour rupture of the membranes [1]

• A 19-year-old primip has a gush of fluid PV, but without contractions at 34 weeks of pregnancy. How is premature rupture of the membranes (PROM) defined and managed?

Hints and tips

- Preterm prelabour PROM is defined as rupture of the membranes occurring at 24–37 weeks' pregnancy without regular uterine activity
- For obstetric history and examination hints see Chapter 75
- Check for clinical signs of infection, i.e., chorioamnionitis ($\uparrow$ HR, pyrexia, uterine tenderness, vaginal discharge, fetal tachycardia)
- Check routine bloods including FBC and CRP
- Sterile speculum examination (fluid in the posterior fornix)
- High vaginal swab
- Avoid digital vaginal examination
- Consider US – ?oligohydramnios
- Monitor fetus (cardiotocography)
- Admit for continued monitoring

Complications   Preterm delivery
Infection
Prolapse of umbilical cord
Fetal immaturity

Mx   Risk of fetal immaturity must be weighed against the risk of infection
Administer steroids
Prophylactic erythromycin
Close monitoring
Tocolysis only if there are uterine contractions (see above)
Manage expectantly until the fetus is mature *unless* chorioamnionitis is present, fetal distress develops or labour cannot be inhibited with tocolysis
If expectant management, aim induction at c. 34 weeks
Deliver if amnionitis is present; signs include maternal or fetal tachycardia, maternal fever, uterine tenderness, foul cervical discharge, uterine contractions, leukocytosis and the presence of leukocytes or bacteria in amniotic fluid
IV antibiotics for chorioamnionitis

[1] Royal Society of Obstetricians and Gynaecologists. *Guideline No. 44.* Nov 2006. Available from www.rcog.org.uk.

Station 232: Instrumental vaginal delivery

Parts of forceps

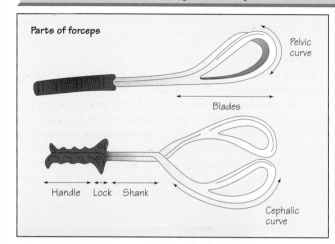

Pelvic curve

Blades

Handle Lock Shank

Cephalic curve

Types of forceps

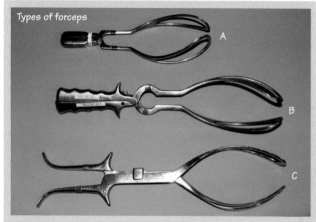

A

B

C

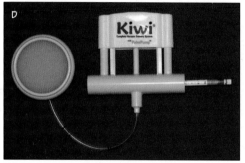

D

E

F

Station 233: Caesarean section

Emergency	Elective
Labour dystocia (problem with powers, passenger or passage)	Elective repeat
Failed induction of labour	Maternal disease
Large abruption	Previous uterine surgery
Fetal distress	Placenta praevia
Cord prolapse	Malpresentation
Severe pre-eclampsia	Macrosomia/anomaly
	Outlet obstruction e.g. fibroids
	Multiple gestation
	Patient request

Station 234: Postpartum haemorrhage

Labour stage 3

Signs of placental separation
- Sudden loss of blood
- Apparent lengthening of the umbilical cord
- Elevation and contraction of the uterus

Management of third stage
Delivery of the placenta

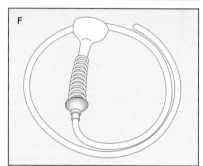

Suprapubic pressure

Uterus

Placenta

Gentle continuous traction

Causes and sites of postpartum haemorrhage (PPH)

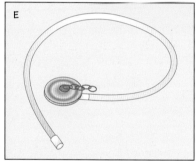

Rare

Common

Retained placental fragments

Uterine rupture

Atonic uterus

Cervical tear

High vaginal tear

Perineal trauma

Aetiology	Management
Uterine atony	Uterine massage Oxytocin infusion Other uterotonic therapies (e.g. prostaglandins)
Retained placenta	Manual removal (ERPC)
Trauma (haematoma, lacerations)	Repair
Coagulopathy	Correct abnormalities
Abnormal placentation	ERPC ± hysterectomy
Uterine rupture	Repair hysterectomy
Uterine inversion	Manual or hydrostatic (warm saline) replacement

Station 232: Instrumental vaginal delivery

• *Please name the different pieces of equipment and discuss the indications, contraindications and complications of instrumental vaginal delivery*

Hints and tips
• Used to shorten the second stage of labour in the best interest of the mother or the fetus
• A fully dilated cervix and experienced physician are required
• Advantages must be weighed against the increased risk of maternal lacerations

Types of instruments
• Wrigley forceps (outlet forceps): Fig. A
• Neville Barnes forceps (low/mid cavity forceps): Fig. B
• Kielland forceps (rotational forceps): Fig. C
• Hand-held ventouse ('Kiwi omnicup'): Fig. D
• Metal cup ventouse (for posterior application): Fig. E
• Siliastic cup ventouse: Fig. F

Indications
• Prolonged second stage (varies according to gravidity and regional anaesthesia)
• Fetal distress
• Maternal exhaustion
• Inadequate maternal efforts (e.g. neuromuscular disease)
• Prophylactic – if maternal contraindication to pushing (e.g. cardiac disease)
• Control of after-coming head in a breech delivery

Criteria	Adequate analgesia
	Informed consent
	Fetal head engaged and vertex presentation
	Position of head known exactly
	Membranes ruptured and bladder empty
	Cervix fully dilated
	No placenta praevia
	No evidence of cephalopelvic disproportion
	Experienced operator with capability of performing Caesarean section if required
Complications	Perineal injury
	Fetal injury – head injuries, bruising, lacerations

Classification [1]
• *Outlet forceps*:
  • fetal scalp visible without separating the labia
  • fetal skull has reached the pelvic floor
  • sagittal suture is in the AP diameter or right or left occiput anterior or posterior position (rotation does not exceed 45°)
  • fetal head is at or on the perineum
• *Low forceps*:
  • leading point of the skull (not caput) is at station plus 2 cm or more and not on the pelvic floor
  • two subdivisions: rotation of 45° or less; rotation more than 45°
• *Mid forceps*:
  • fetal head is one-fifth palpable per abdomen
  • leading point of the skull is above station plus 2 cm but not above the ischial spines
  • there are two subdivisions as per low forceps

Station 233: Caesarean section

• *A 24-year-old nulliparous woman is due to have an elective Caesarean section due to placenta praevia. Please consent the patient and answer any questions that she has*

Hints and tips
In practice this would be carried out by a more senior doctor but general communication skills and generic consent skills can be assessed at this type of station (see Chs 3, 8 and 9)

Indications

Labour problems	Failed induction or progression of labour
Anatomical problems	Cephalopelvic disproportion
	Obstruction to the birth canal (e.g. fibroids)
	Previous uterine surgery (classic Caesarean section, uterine rupture or myomectomy)
Placental	Placenta praevia (unless marginal)
	Abruption placentae
	Cord prolapse
Fetal	Malposition
	Distress
	Anomaly
Co-morbidities	Pre-eclampsia
	Diabetes
	Cardiac disease
Other	Elective repeat Caesarean section
Complications	Infection; bleeding (occasionally requiring puerperal hysterectomy); fetal injury; injury to other abdominal structures, e.g. urinary tract, bowel; anaesthetic risks; prolonged recovery; future risk of uterine dehiscence or rupture

Station 234: Postpartum haemorrhage

• *You have been asked to review a 19-year-old multiparous female who continues to have PV bleeding following delivery. This station makes use of a simulated patient*

Hints and tips
Use ABCDE approach (see Ch. 11).

RF	Previous postpartum haemorrhage (PPH); previous Caesarean section; multiparity; manual removal of placenta; placental abruption/praevia; polyhydramnios; multiple gestations; prolonged labour	
Classification	*Early PPH*	< 24 hours after delivery
	Late PPH	> 24 hours to < 6 weeks
General Mx	ABCDE (see Ch. 11)	
	Oxygen	
	IV access × 2	
	Bloods for FBC, cross-match and clotting	
	Bimanual examination to help try to determine cause	
	Call for expert help	
	Good communication to the patient to keep informed of events	
Specific Mx	See chart opposite	

[1] Royal College of Obstetricians and Gynaecologists. *Guideline No. 26.* Oct 2005. Available from www.rcog.org.uk.

Station 235: Fetal heart rate monitoring

Electronic fetal heart rate monitoring (non-stress test) may be performed by means of external Doppler, or direct scalp lead when membranes are ruptured

Indications

Induction of labour	Oligohydramnios	Diabetes	Antepartum or intrapartum haemorrhage
Augmented labour	Hypertension	Multiple gestation	Malpresentation
Reduced fetal movements	Previous caesarean	Prolonged rupture of membranes	

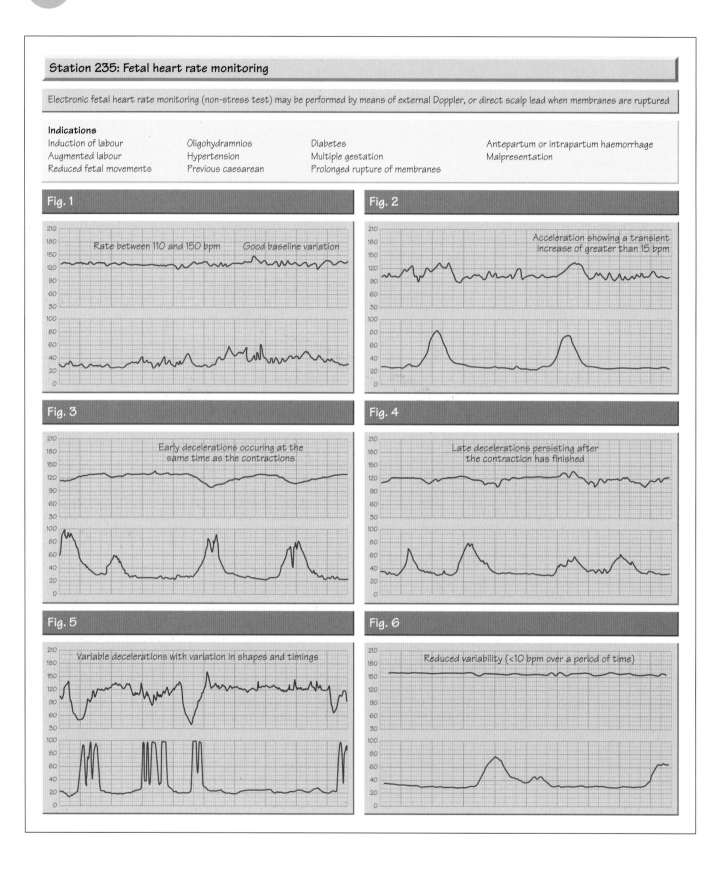

Fig. 1 — Rate between 110 and 150 bpm — Good baseline variation

Fig. 2 — Acceleration showing a transient increase of greater than 15 bpm

Fig. 3 — Early decelerations occuring at the same time as the contractions

Fig. 4 — Late decelerations persisting after the contraction has finished

Fig. 5 — Variable decelerations with variation in shapes and timings

Fig. 6 — Reduced variability (<10 bpm over a period of time)

• *Please study the following cardiotocograms (CTGs) and discuss the findings with the examiner*

Hints and tips

This station could be presented in several ways: a structured viva, a written station or a simulated patient with monitoring leads attached.
• Treat the patient, not just the CTG
• Remember the importance of an adequate history and examination, taking note of gestational age

Assess baseline fetal heart rate

• Assess the fetal heart rate between contractions
• Normal range = 110–160 bpm
• Bradycardia = < 110 bpm; tachycardia = > 160 bpm

Causes of bradycardia	Fetal hypoxia
	Epidural anaesthetics
	Drugs: β-blockers, oxytocin
Causes of tachycardia	Fetal hypoxia
	Maternal fever
	Drugs: β-agonists
	Maternal anxiety
	Fetal infection

Assess fetal heart rate variability

Normal fluctuations in the heart rate.
1 *Short-term variability*: beat-to-beat variation, normally 5–10 bpm
2 *Long-term variability*: a waviness of the fetal heart rate tracing, which normally has a frequency of 3–10 cycles/min and an amplitude of 10–25 bpm
  • Moderate variability: 6–25 bpm around the baseline (normal)
  • Decreased variability: < 5 bpm
  • Marked variability: > 25 bpm
3 *Decreasing variability*: this may indicate fetal distress. Causes of decreased variability are:
  • Fetal hypoxia
  • Fetal sleep
  • Prematurity

Periodic heart rate changes

These are changes in heart rate associated with contractions.
1 *Accelerations*:
  • Normally the fetal heart rate should increase or remain the same during contractions
  • Accelerations = transient increase in heart rate of greater than 15 bpm for at least 15 seconds
  • It is a reassuring sign if there are two or more accelerations in 20 minutes
2 *Decelerations*:
  • Transient decreases in fetal heart rate are normally associated with uterine contractions
  • Classified into early, variable, late and prolonged
3 *Early decelerations*:
  • Occur with uterine contractions

• Associated with head compression
• Vagally mediated
• They are not a sign of fetal distress
4 *Variable decelerations*:
  • Variable duration and timing in relation to contraction
  • Reflex pattern
  • Secondary to umbilical cord compression
  • Only of concern if prolonged or persistent
5 *Late decelerations*:
  • Transient but repetitive deceleration of the fetal heart rate
  • They occur late in the contraction phase
  • Due to fetal hypoxia
  • They indicate uteroplacental insufficiency
  • Ominous sign if persistent
6 *Prolonged decelerations*:
  • Last > 120 seconds
  • Seen with maternal hypotension, maternal hypoxia, tetanic contractions and prolapsed umbilical cord
  • Poor prognostic sign

Non-periodic heart rate changes

These are heart rate changes that are not associated with contractions and can be described as above.

Fetal heart rate patterns

1 *Reassuring patterns*:
  • Accelerations as described above
  • Moderate variabilty
  • Mild variable decelerations
  • Early decelerations
2 *Non-reassuring patterns*:
  • Bradycardia/tachycardia
  • Decrease in baseline variability
  • Decrease in baseline fetal heart rate
  • Late decelerations
3 *Ominous patterns*:
  • Persistent late decelerations with decreasing variability
  • Variable decelerations with loss of variability
  • Absence of variability
  • Severe bradycardia

Example cases (see opposite)

• Fig. 1: rate between 110 and 150 bpm, good baseline variation
• Fig. 2: accelerations with transient increases above 15 bpm
• Fig. 3: early decelerations occurring at the same time as contractions
• Fig. 4: late decelerations lasting longer than the duration of contraction
• Fig. 5: variable decelerations
• Fig. 6: reduced variability

Discussion points

• Name some methods of assessing fetal well being
• Describe the Apgar scoring system
• What fetal heart patterns are you aware of?
• Describe the reassuring/non-reassuring features of a CTG tracing

Station 236: Dermatology history

History of presenting complaint
Time since onset of the lesion/rash (hours, days, months or years)
Location of the lesion/symmetry
Duration of individual lesions
Do the lesions come and go, and do they occur in the same site or in differing sites?
Previous episodes of this lesion
Relationship to physical agents
Ask about irritants on the skin in hand eczema, e.g. detergents and about working practices and hobbies
Relationship to sun exposure
Associated pruritus (severe itching preventing sleep suggests scabies or dermatitis herpetiformis)
Associated pain
Size or colour change in pigmented lesions
Evidence of weeping or bleeding of the lesion
Increasing in diameter or depth

Family history
Family history of skin conditions
Current affected members
Genetically determined, e.g. atopic eczema
FH of skin cancer
Infective problems, e.g. scabies
Atopy

Systems enquiry
Systemic symptoms, e.g. headache, fever, loss of appetite and weight

Social history
Occupation/hobbies
Pets
Contact with irritants
Cosmetic use
Change in wash powder
Duration of sun exposure
Travel

Past history
Previous history of skin conditions or allergic reactions
History of eczema, asthma or hay fever
History of sun exposure
Previous history of systemic disease e.g. diabetes
Assessment of skin type may also help:
• Type I: always burns, never tans
• Type II: always burns, sometimes tans
• Type III: sometimes burns, always tans
• Type IV: never burns, always tans
• Type V: racially pigmented skin

Drug history
A drug history is vital to determine whether medications are responsible for the skin condition or have helped treat the condition so far
• Treatments tried so far and did they help?
• Ointments/creams/tablets
• Possibility of drug-induced rash
• Ask about over-the-counter and alternative remedies
• Current drug history
• Known allergies

Station 237: Dermatology examination

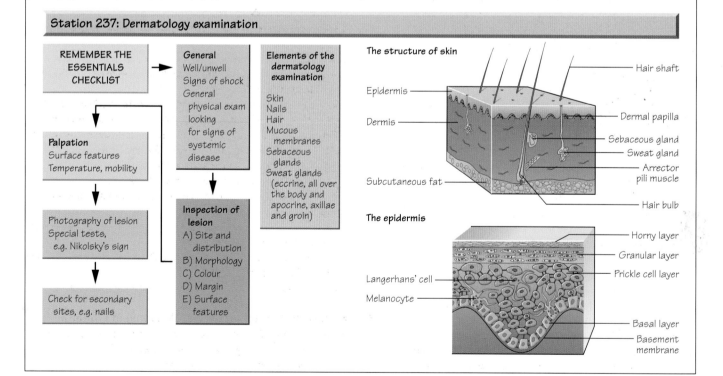

REMEMBER THE ESSENTIALS CHECKLIST

General
Well/unwell
Signs of shock
General physical exam looking for signs of systemic disease

Elements of the dermatology examination
Skin
Nails
Hair
Mucous membranes
Sebaceous glands
Sweat glands (eccrine, all over the body and apocrine, axillae and groin)

Palpation
Surface features
Temperature, mobility

Photography of lesion
Special tests, e.g. Nikolsky's sign

Check for secondary sites, e.g. nails

Inspection of lesion
A) Site and distribution
B) Morphology
C) Colour
D) Margin
E) Surface features

The structure of skin
Epidermis
Dermis
Subcutaneous fat
Hair shaft
Dermal papilla
Sebaceous gland
Sweat gland
Arrector pili muscle
Hair bulb

The epidermis
Langerhans' cell
Melanocyte
Horny layer
Granular layer
Prickle cell layer
Basal layer
Basement membrane

• *A 21-year-old male presents with a rash affecting his left arm. Please discuss the important elements when describing a dermatological lesion*
• *Please describe the lesions seen on these photographs and suggest possible diagnoses*

Hints and tips

• Do not forget the importance of taking a full history from patients with a dermatological condition, even if you feel the diagnosis is obvious
• Use the hints opposite for taking a focused dermatology history

Examination routine

• *Exposure*: essential for detailed inspection
• *General inspection*: do not forget a general inspection of the patient as described in previous chapters as many systemic illnesses are associated with skin conditions, e.g. malar flush – mitral stenosis, vitiligo – diabetes
• *Specific inspection*: describe each lesion carefully as summarised in this chapter and then check the rest of the skin for any other lesions
• *Palpation*
• *Special tests*: if appropriate
• Check for secondary sites
• Consider photographing and measuring the lesion
• *Completion*: general physical exam if necessary

Describing a lesion/rash

Site and distribution

• *Symmetrical*: involving both sides of the body to a similar extent; usually due to endogenous causes (e.g. eczema, psoriasis, acne)
• *Asymmetrical*: involving predominantly one side only; usually due to external causes (e.g. bacterial or fungal infections)
• *Sun exposed*: involving face, 'V' of neck and dorsum of hands
• *Discrete*: separated by normal skin from other similar lesions
• *Unilateral*: restricted to one side only (e.g. varicella zoster)
• *Generalised*: covering most of the body surface
• *Disseminated*: widespread discrete lesions
• *Grouped*: multiple lesions grouped in one area
• *Annular*: grouped in a ring
• *Linear*: arranged in a line due to:
  • Koebner's phenomenon, where lesions occur at a site of trauma (e.g. psoriasis, lichen planus, warts)
  • birthmark (e.g. epidermal naevus)
  • confined to a dermatome (e.g. varicella zoster)
• *Reticulate*: 'Net like' usually when a pattern of subcutaneous blood vessels becomes visible

Morphology

• Flat or raised
• Surface or deep (within the dermis or in the subcutaneous tissues)
1 *Primary lesions*:
  • *Macule* (size < 1 cm) and patch (size > 1 cm): circumscribed flat lesion due to localised colour change only
  • *Papule* (size < 1 cm): circumscribed elevated lesion
  • *Nodule* (size > 1 cm): palpable elevated lesion that has a rounded surface
  • *Plaque* (size > 1 cm): a raised lesion where the diameter is greater than the thickness. Usually due to epidermal pathology with scale, crust, keratin or maceration on the surface
  • *Vesicle* (size < 1 cm): circumscribed, elevated, fluid-filled lesion (blister)
  • *Bulla* (size > 1 cm): circumscribed, elevated, fluid-filled lesion (blister)
  • *Pustule* (size < 1 cm): a pus-filled lesion (if in doubt prick the lesion and pus comes out)
  • Larger lesions are either abscesses or pseudocysts
2 *Secondary lesions*: these have developed from primary lesions
  • *Erosion*: partial loss of the epidermis, heals without scarring
  • *Ulcer*: full-thickness loss of epidermis and some dermis, which will heal with scarring
  • *Atrophy*: depression of the surface due to thinning of the epidermis or dermis. Blood vessels easily seen under the skin, and there may be fine surface wrinkling
  • *Scar*: caused by dermal damage

Colour

• *Red*: due to blood; can be due to either inflammatory or non-inflammatory conditions
• *Red erythema*: redness that blanches on pressure (blood within the blood vessels)
• *Red purpura*: red, purple, orange or brown, which does not fade on pressure (blood outside the vessels)
• *Red telangiectasia*: small, dilated blood vessels, visible to naked eye
• *White*: due to loss of pigment
• *Brown*: due to melanin or haemosiderin.
• *Yellow*: usually due to lipids in the skin

Margin

• *Well defined or circumscribed*: able to draw a line around the lesion with confidence
• *Poorly defined*: have a border that merges into normal skin or outlying ill-defined papules
• *Active edge*: border of lesion is raised or shows increased scaling with relative clearing in the centre
• *Raised border*: centre of lesion is depressed compared to the edge

Surface features

• *Scaly*: dry/flaky surface due to abnormal stratum corneum, with accumulation or shedding of keratinocytes
• *Keratin/horn*: rough, uneven surface due to abnormal keratin, which is difficult to pick off. Seen in solar keratoses and chronic eczema
• *Exudate*: serum, blood or pus that has accumulated on the surface, either from an erosion or ruptured blister/pustule
• *Friable*: surface bleeds easily after minor trauma
• *Crust*: dried serum, pus or blood, looks like keratin
• *Warty/papillomatous*: surface consisting of minute finger-like or round projections
• *Excoriation*: localised skin damage due to scratching, consists of linear or pinpoint erosions or crusts
• *Lichenification*: thickening of the epidermis with increased skin markings due to persistent scratching
• *Umbilicated*: surface contains a round depression in the centre

Summary of common dermatology investigations

Bloods   To investigate possible underlying systemic problems, e.g. coeliac serology in dermatitis herpetiformis
Micro   Skin swab, scraping, nail clipping
Other   Woods light; skin biopsy/skin curette; patch testing

Station 238: Pruritus

Introduction
- Itching is a normal physiological process
- Pruritis is a mild itching sensation due to trivial stimuli
- It becomes pathological when the itching sensations interfere with well being and cause damage
- It is mediated by histamine, prostaglandins, acetylcholine, kinins and proteases
- Common 'itch spots' are located in warm areas where sweat is retained, especially the groin, foot and scalp
- It may occur spontaneously or be precipitated by the presence of chapped, dry skin, retained sweat or psychological factors such as anxiety or depression

Causes of pruritus

Skin disorders

Infections	Scabies, pediculosis, mites
Bites	Insects
Contact dermatitis	
Irritant dermatitis	Fibreglass, foreign bodies
Urticaria/eczema	
Other	Lichen planus, dermatitis

Miscellaneous

Psychogenic	Delusions of parasitosis
'Senile' pruritus	Elderly patients, no apparent cause

Systemic disorders

Endocrine	Hypo- and hyperthyroidism
Haematology	Iron deficiency anaemia, polycythaemia rubra vera
Hepatic	Cholestatic disease (e.g. primary bilary cirrhosis, drugs, extrahepatic obstruction)
Infections	Onchocerciasis, echinococcosis
Neoplastic	Lymphoma, leukaemia
Neurological	Multiple sclerosis
Renal	Uraemia
Drugs	Allergic reaction (e.g. penicillin)
	Vasoactive drugs (e.g. caffeine, alcohol)
	CNS drugs (e.g. opiates, amphetamines)
Other	Pregnancy

Station 239: Urticaria

Introduction
- Characterised by a transient, pruritic, patchy eruption
- Consists of lightly erythematous papules or wheals
- Superficial skin layers
- If the deeper layers are involved = angioedema
- Lesions vary in size (2–30 cm)
- Either circular or irregularly shaped
- Usually affects the trunk, but can occur anywhere

Urticaria can be:

Acute	Hives persisting < 6 weeks, occurs frequently in atopic individuals, with common causes being foods, drugs and infections, but frequently without an identifiable cause
Angioedema	As acute, but attacks manifest as large irregular areas of subcutaneous swelling, causes similar to urticaria but may also include hereditary angioedema or ACE inhibitors
Chronic	Attacks persist for > 6 weeks or more. Patients are not usually atopic

Types of urticaria

Idiopathic	30% of acute and 70% of chronic cases of urticaria	
Physical	Approx. 25% of cases	
	Several types:	
	1. Dermatographism	Reaction to firm stroking of the skin, last for around 5-10 minutes
	2. Cholinergic	Due to exercise or sweating, affects young people, 1-2 mm wheals
	3. Cold/heat	Uncommon reaction to cold and/or rewarming after cold exposure
	4. Solar (rare)	Rapid-onset pruritus and erythema, followed by urticaria, due to exposure to light
Immunological	Allergic reactions	Contact, e.g. plants or animals
		Ingestion of food, e.g. nuts, shellfish
		Ingestion of drugs, e.g. aspirin, penicillin
Hereditary angiodema	Autosomal dominant. May mimic a surgical abdomen. Low C1-esterase inhibitor levels are diagnostic. Give fresh frozen plasma pre-procedure or prevent attacks with danazol therapy	
Infections	Bacterial, protozoal, viral	

Station 238: Pruritus

Student info: *Mrs AD is a 46-year-old female who has come to see you complaining of a generalised itch. You are the FY1 doctor in a GP surgery and she is new to the practice. Please take a full history and discuss with your examiner a differential diagnosis*

Patient info: *You are Mrs AD, aged 46 years. PMH: gallstones were diagnosed 3 years ago. You have recent weight loss and decreased appetite over the last 2 months, and a 7-day history of generalised itch. You have been feeling generally unwell, and also complaining of night sweats. You have no respiratory system or CVS symptoms and no change in bowel habit or sickness. You have no current medications, although you have recently been taking an antihistamine. Your mother has hypothyroidism and father has type II diabetes. You initially thought it may have been due to a change in washing powder but you have stopped using this now. You really are at a loss to explain the symptoms*

Hints and tips
- Determine the patient's reason for visiting the GP
- Determine symptomatology
- Take a full dermatology history (see Ch. 87)
- Elicit the constitutional symptoms
- Establish correct FH
- Assess impact of the symptoms on the patient's life
- Address ideas, concerns and expectations of the patient

Discussion points
- What is your differential diagnosis?
- How would you investigate this patient?
- What treatments are available for pruritus?
- What features would you look for on examination of this patient?

Examination hints for this patient
Look for:
- Excoriations, lichenification and hydration
- Signs of systemic infection
- Gastrointestinal examination
- Haematological examination, i.e. lymph nodes and spleen
- Cachexia

Ix	*Bloods*	FBC, ESR, Glc, U&E, LFTs, TFTs, iron studies
	Other	Need to be directed to possible cause
Mx		
Conservative		Treat underlying systemic disorder
		Irritant avoidance, cool water compresses, nail trimming
Drugs		H_1-blockers, e.g. non-sedating histamines
		H_2-blockers, e.g. ranitidine
		Tricyclic antidepressants, e.g. amitriptyline
		Consider oral prednisolone (last resort)
Topical		Emollients, tar compounds, topical steroids, topical anaesthetics
Other		Localised ultraviolet B phototherapy or intralesional injections of corticosteroid

Station 239: Urticaria

Student info: *Mrs ES is a 60-year-old female who has been admitted with a chest infection. You are the on-call ward FY1 doctor and the nursing staff have asked you to see her as they have noticed a rash on her back. On examination she has a widespread raised erythematous rash on her trunk. Please ask Mrs ES some pertinent questions and be able to offer a differential diagnosis*

Patient info: *You are Mrs ES, a 60-year-old female who was admitted to hospital 24 hours ago with a chest infection. PMH: hysterectomy. DH: nil regular. You are allergic to an antibiotic but you cannot remember the name. You developed an itchy rash which you noticed earlier in the day over the trunk*

Hints and tips
- Determine the patient's understanding of why they are in hospital
- Ascertain the current problem and associated symptoms
- Dermatology history as per Chapter 87
- Elicit the allergy history
- Address the ideas, concerns and expectations of the patient

Discussion points
- What is the most likely diagnosis?
- What are the causes of urticaria?
- What treatments are available for a patient with urticaria?

Ix: acute urticaria	Laboratory tests are not generally needed
Ix: chronic urticaria	Exclude physical agents, then search for an occult systemic illness
Bloods	FBC, ESR, U&E, LFT, Ca, TFTs, ANA, autoimmune screen
	Consider cryoglobulin, hepatitis serology, rheumatoid factor, complement, immunoglobulins
Imaging	CXR
Micro	Urine culture
Other	Skin biopsy
Mx	
Conservative	Eliminate or limit exposure to the causative agent, treat any underlying disease
Drugs	Antihistamines
	H_1-blockers, e.g. cetirizine
	H_2-blockers, e.g. ranitidine
	Propanolol for stress-related urticaria
	Doxepin for cold urticaria
	Oral steroids
Topical	Application of capsaicin or local anaesthetic can suppress reactions in local heat urticaria

NB. Topical or systemic corticosteroids should be reserved for patients with refractory symptoms.

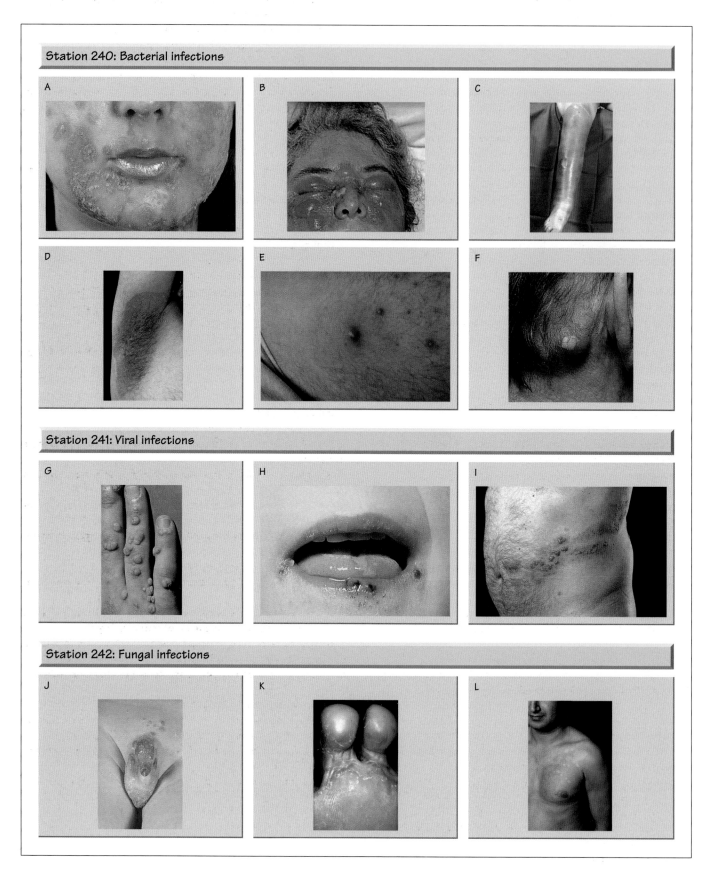

Station 240: Bacterial infections

A

B

C

D

E

F

Station 241: Viral infections

G

H

I

Station 242: Fungal infections

J

K

L

Station 240: Bacterial infections

• *What are the common bacterial infections of the skin, how and where do they present and how are they treated?*

• *Look at the following pictures, describe the skin problem and offer a diagnosis*

Hints and tips

Impetigo (Fig. A)

• Caused by group A *Streptococcus* or *Staphylococcus*

• Appears as small vesicles with yellowish crusts, with itching, pain and tenderness; moderately contagious

• Treat with anti-staphylococcals and good personal hygiene

Erysipelas (Fig. B)

• Caused by β-haemolytic streptococci

• Presents as a well-demarcated, painful tender, rapidly advancing erythematous plaque, sometimes with fever and leucocytosis

• Usually on face or extremities

• Treated in the same way as cellulitis

• Recurrence is common

Cellulitis (Fig. C)

• Caused by same organisms as impetigo

• Infection of the dermis and subcutaneous tissue, due to trauma or a break in the skin

• Presents with poorly defined erythema, tenderness and warmth, with possible lymphangitis, lymphadenopathy and systemic symptoms

• Treated with oral or IV antibiotics

• Observe for necrotising fasciitis and gangrene, which requires surgical excision

Erythrasma (Fig. D)

• Superficial intertriginous infections

• Caused by porphyrin-producing corynebacteria

• Treatment is with oral erythromycin or topical clindamycin

• Responds to miconazole and clotrimazole, but recurrence rate high

Furuncle (boil) (Fig. F)

• Caused by *Staphylococcus aureus*

• An acute, localised, perifollicular abscess of the skin and subcutaneous tissue

• Red, hot, tender inflammatory nodule that exudes pus

• Usually on the buttocks, axillae, breasts or nape of the neck

• Treat with systemic antibiotics ± incision and drainage

Station 241: Viral infections

• *What are the common viral infections of the skin, how and where do they present and how are they treated?*

Hints and tips

Warts (verruca vulgaris) (Fig. G)

• Focal lesions of epithelial hyperplasia

• Caused by human papilloma viruses (HPV)

• Commonly on the hands, feet, anogenital area (condylomata) and face

• Infectious and auto-inoculable

• Common in children, the elderly and the immunodeficient

• Treat with keratolytic agents (salicylic/lactic acid/podophyllin preparations) or cryotherapy

• Recurrence is common

Herpes simplex (types I and II) (Fig. H)

• Caused by DNA viruses

• Early lesions are multiple, 1–2 mm diameter, yellowish, clear vesicles on an erythematous base

• The vesicles can ulcerate and become painful

• Type I are usually peri-oral; Type II are genital

• Diagnosis is clinical or from viral titres, biopsy or culture

• Lesions may be preceded by a prodrome of pain and tingling

• Treatment is symptomatic. Antivirals (e.g. aciclovir) have limited effect unless taken early but can shorten lesion duration if used during the prodrome

Herpes zoster (shingles) (Fig. I)

• Reactivation of latent varicella zoster virus present in the sensory ganglia

• Classically described as grouped vesicles in one unilateral dermatome

• Thoracic and trigeminal nerve dermatomes are most common

• Symptoms are of pain, dysaesthesia and pruritus

• Healing takes 2–3 weeks

• Infectious until lesions are crusted over

• It is more common in the elderly

• Diagnosis is usually clinical or by biopsy, or by viral culture

• Oral aciclovir is effective if initiated within 2 days of onset of rash

Station 242: Fungal infections

• *What are the common fungal infections of the skin, how and where do they present and how are they treated?*

Hints and tips

Candidiasis (Fig. J)

• Caused by *Candida albicans*

• Seen as thrush, nappy dermatitis, perineal infections and intertriginous dermatitis

• Diagnosed by clinical examination and microscopic examination of skin scrapings

• Treat with topical imidazole creams, oral fluconazole or amphotericin B if severe

• Underlying disease, steroids and antibiotics are predisposing factors

Dermatophytoses (tinea) (Fig. K)

• Caused by fungi that infect the stratum corneum of the epidermis, hair and nails

• Labelled according to location: nails (unguium), foot (pedis), perineum (cruris), body (corporis), beard (barbae) and scalp (capitis)

• Presents as pruritic, grey, scaly patches that may lead to scalp alopecia

• Skin scrapings show fungal hyphae

• Treatment is with antifungals, as appropriate for the region affected

Tinea (pityriasis) versicolor (Fig. L)

• Lightly pigmented plaques on the neck, trunk and arms, which appear hypopigmented with sun exposure

• Diagnosis is made clinically and with potassium hydroxide preparations of skin scrapings

• Treated with topical imidazoles, oral antifungals or zinc/selenium shampoos

Station 243: Malignant melanoma

History hints

- Any other moles
- Previous sun exposure and sun burn
- Previous skin lesions and diagnoses
- Family history
- Recent changes in this and other moles

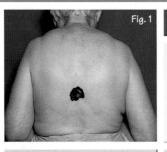
Fig. 1

Examination hints

Major signs	Minor signs
Change in size	Inflammation
Change in shape	Bleeding
Change in colour	Sensory changes
Diameter > 7 mm	Crusting

Four main types of melanoma (below)

Superficial spreading 65%
- Middle age
- Female : male ratio 2:1
- Sites: lower leg in women and trunk in man
- Usually slightly elevated lesion with variable colour

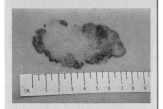

Nodular 27%
Aggressive tumour
Younger age group
Female : male ratio 1:2
Early vertical growth phase
Uniform colour, early ulceration and bleeding

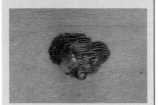

Lentigo maligna 7%
Least malignant
Usually found on face of elderly
Long radial growth phase
Presents as flat light brown macule

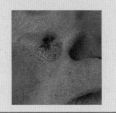

Acral lentiginous 1%
Aggressive tumour
Commonest type found in Blacks and Orientals
Soles of feet and palms
Subungual melanomas included in this group

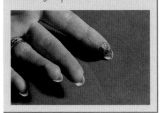

Station 244: Basal cell carcinoma

Hints
Commonest skin malignancy (a.k.a. rodent ulcer)
Mostly occur on sun-exposed skin
Commonest site: face above line from mouth to ear
BCC is locally invasive
Metastases extremely rare
Clinical types of BCC
Nodular or noduloulcerative/cystic/pigmented
Sclerosing/cicatricial/superficial
Predisposing factors
Xeroderma pigmentosa and radiotherapy
Sun exposure
Burns
Skin type
Immunosuppression

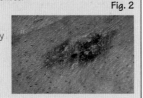
Fig. 2

Ulcerated basal cell carcinoma

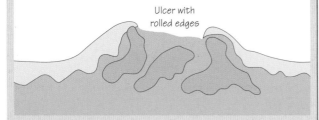
Ulcer with rolled edges

Station 245: Squamous cell carcinoma

Hints
Second commonest cutaneous malignancy
Commonest site: face and hands
Arises from keratinising cell layer
Differential diagnosis
Keratoacanthoma/BCC
Amelanotic melanomas /skin adnexal tumours
Predisposing factors
Solar keratoses/Bowen's disease /chronic ulceration
Family history
Sun exposure
Radiotherapy
Immunosuppressed

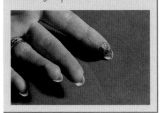
Fig. 3

Squamous neoplastic cells

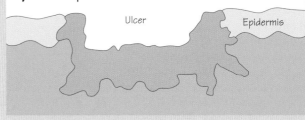
Ulcer
Epidermis

Station 243: Malignant melanoma

• *You are a FY1 doctor in your GP placement. Please assess this 50-year-female who has attended with concerns regarding a mole that her partner has noticed on her back. Please take a focused history and then describe the lesion shown in Fig. 1 (see opposite) to the examiner*

Hints and tips

For history and examination hints see opposite and Chapter 87.

Discussion points

• Discuss a differential diagnosis
• Discuss some of the treatment options available for a patient diagnosed with melanoma
• Please describe the epidemiology of melanoma
• Do you know any risk factors for developing melanoma?
• Do you know any prognostic indicators for melanoma?

Epidemiology	Incidence is doubling every 10 years
	Incidence of 40/100,000/year in Queensland
	Incidence of 4/100,000/year in Scotland
	1000 deaths/year in the UK
RF	History of sun exposure
	Giant melanocytic naevus
	Total number of naevi
	Dysplastic naevus syndrome
Pathology	60% arise in pre-existing naevi
	Initially radial, then vertical growth phase

Staging (American Joint Committee on Cancer)

T Thickness of tumour

Most important prognostic factor for local and distant recurrence and survival

Breslow's classification (thickness in mm + 10-year survival):

< 0.75	95–99%
0.76–1.49	80–90%
1.5–3.99	60–75%
> 4.0	< 50%

With regional lymphadenopathy 10-year survival is less than 10%

N Lymph **n**ode involvement

Intransit: < 2% of tumours, appear as 'satellites', usually associated with regional lymphadenopathy

Lymph node: commonest metastatic presentation, reduces survival by 50%

70–80% patients with regional lymphadenopathy have distant disease

M Distant **m**etastases

Rx

Surgery	Resection
	Resection margins:
	impalpable = 1 cm
	palpable = 2 cm
	nodular = 3 cm
	Regional lymphadenectomy – no improvement in survival and high risk of complications, e.g. lymphoedema
Adjuvant chemotherapy	Consider in 'high-risk' tumours (i.e. thick or +ve lymph nodes)
	No standard therapy
	Interferon α2b looks promising and provides an increase in disease-free and overall survival
Isolated limb perfusion	This is essentially intra-arterial chemotherapy
	Commonly used agents include melphalan ± TNFα

Station 244: Basal cell carcinoma

• *Please look at Fig. 2 (see opposite), describe the lesion and discuss your diagnosis*

Discussion points

• What are the predisposing factors for basal cell carcinoma (BCC)?
• How is BCC treated?

Rx	*Surgery*	Local excision with 0.4 cm margins
		Cure rate > 95%
		May require full-thickness graft
	Radiotherapy	
	Curettage/cryotherapy	For superficial lesions

Station 245: Squamous cell carcinoma

• *Please look at Fig. 3 (see opposite), describe the lesion and discuss your diagnosis*

Discussion points

• What is your differential diagnosis?
• What are the predisposing factors for squamous cell carcinoma (SCC)?
• What is the treatment for SCC?

Rx	*Surgery*	Wide local excision ± lymph node dissection
	Radiotherapy	

Station 246: Acne

Development of acne

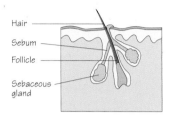
1. Normal hair follicle

Hair
Sebum
Follicle
Sebaceous gland

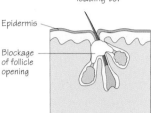
2. Blockage and infection leading to:

Epidermis
Blockage of follicle opening

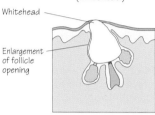
3. Closed comedo (whitehead)

Whitehead
Enlargement of follicle opening

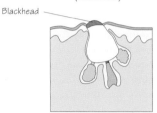
4. Open comedo (blackhead)

Blackhead

Acne classification by lesion

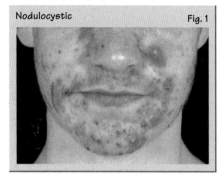
Nodulocystic   Fig. 1

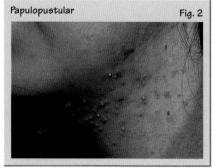
Papulopustular   Fig. 2

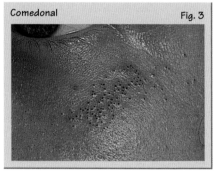
Comedonal   Fig. 3

Station 247: Psoriasis

History hints

Family history
Exacerbating and relieving factors:
  stress/emotion
  trauma
  preceding infection
  improvement with sunlight
  drug history – antimalarials, lithium, β-blocker
Non-itchy
Associated arthritis

Examination hints

Erythematous papules and plaques with grey/white silvery scale, especially extensor aspects of elbows and knees
Nails – pitting or oncholysis   Fig. 4   Fig. 5
Scalp – areas of scaling of the scalp
Flexural psoriasis
Palmoplanto pustulosis
Psoriatic arthropathy (DIP joints, single large joint)

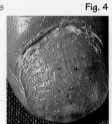
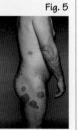

Station 248: Other papulosquamous disease

Lichen planus hints
- Pruritic eruption with violaceous, polygonal papules
- Occur in linear, annular or confluent groups
- Buccal mucosa also affected: whitish, reticulated, lacy plaques - Wickham's striae
- Exhibits the Koebner phenomenon
- If seen on vulva this has malignant potential and should be referred to gynaecology
- Rx: disease is chronic, but self-limiting; use of topical corticosteroids, antihistamines and intralesional corticosteroids are effective

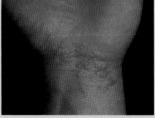
Fig. 6

Pityriasis rosea hints
- Characterised by the 'herald patch', which is larger than other lesions, usually bright red, round or oval, sharply demarcated plaque (2–5 cm) with scaly margins and central clearing
- 2–14 days later, a generalised reaction occurs, often in a 'fir tree' pattern
- ? Caused by human herpes virus 7 (HHV-7)
- Pruritus may be severe
- Rx: conservative, as the condition is self-limiting within 4–10 weeks

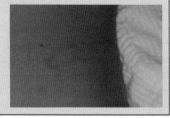
Fig. 7

Station 246: Acne

- *You are a FY1 doctor on your GP placement. Please assess this 22-year-old male who has attended with concerns regarding spots on his face. Please take a focused history and then describe the lesion shown in Fig. 1 (see opposite) to the examiner*
- *Please describe the different types of acne demonstrated in Figs 1–3 (see opposite) and discuss treatment options*

Hints and tips

For history and examination hints see opposite and Chapter 87.

Discussion points

- Describe the underlying pathology of acne
- Describe the different types of acne
- What conditions are associated with acne?
- How would you manage a patient with acne vulgaris?

A note on acne

- Common condition
- Significant morbidity for those affected
- Usually occurs during puberty
- *Contributing factors*:
  - increased sebum
  - hormones (raised androgens)
  - pore occlusion
  - bacteria (propionibacterium acnes)
  - genetic
- *Primary sites*: face, upper neck, chest and back
- *Aggravating factors*:
  - drugs (especially steroids)
  - irritants (e.g. cosmetics)
  - comedogenic agents
  - picking and squeezing
- *Associated conditions*:
  - infantile acne
  - chemical exposure (oils, paraffins)
  - acne medicamentosa (e.g. steroids)
  - polycystic ovarian disease
  - congenital adrenal hyperplasia
  - Cushing's syndrome

Classification and management

Comedones

- Appear as whiteheads and blackheads (closed and open comedones, respectively)
- Optimum treatment is with topical agents, taking a minimum of 2 weeks to show any improvement
- Benzoyl peroxide should be applied frequently to produce drying and even scaling
- Tretinoin (retin A), applied as a cream or gel nightly, usually requires 3–5 months of treament
- Azelaic acid, which is useful in hyperpigmentation, it is antibacterial and antikeratinising, but can lead to erythema and skin irritation
- Adapalene (Differin), which is a retinoid like tretinoin, used daily is effective

Papulopustular acne

- Significant inflammatory component with inflamed papules and pustules

- Treatment is similar to that for comedonic acne, but with the addition of antibiotics (e.g. topical erythromycin, clindamycin, tetracycline)
- In moderate to severe cases, systemic antibiotics can be used

Nodulocystic acne

- Typified by comedones, inflammatory papules and pustules, and deep, inflamed nodules and cysts
- Can result in scarring
- Hypertrophic scars often form on the chest and back
- Treatment can be similar to the treatments listed above or with oral isotretinoin (Roaccutane) but take caution with possible pregnancies. Liver function tests and serum lipid levels need to be monitored
- Other therapies include:
  - combined oral contraceptives
  - spironolactone for a patient with evidence of androgen excess
  - comedo extraction

Station 247: Psoriasis

- *Please examine this patient's elbows and discuss your findings, including any further examinations you would like to perform*
- *Please describe the lesions seen in Figs 4 and 5 (see opposite)*

Hints and tips

- Lesions are erythematous papules and plaques with grey/white, silvery scales
- A full examination of the patient's skin is necessary, looking for the different patterns of disease:
  - extensor surfaces of elbows and knees
  - scalp
  - nails
  - flexures
  - palms and soles
  - guttate psoriasis – small, diffuse plaques, may occur after an antecedent upper respiratory tract infection
- May present as Koebner's phenomenon, with lesions appearing at sites of trauma, e.g. an excoriation
- Nails manifest as pitting and stippling or onycholysis
- Psoriatic arthritis can affect the distal interphalangeals (DIPs) and metacarpophalangeals (MCPs), with rheumatoid factor usually negative, so state you would perform a full musculoskeletal examination

Discussion points

- What are the precipitating factors for psoriasis?
- What different patterns of psoriasis do you know?
- What would your differential include?
- What treatments are you aware of?

ΔΔ Psoriasis, pityriasis rosea, discoid eczema, secondary syphilis
Rx *Local*
 Moisturisers; vitamin D analogues, e.g. calcipotriene (as effective as corticosteroids; but no skin atrophy or tachyphylaxis); coal tar formulations; dithranol; topical corticosteroids
 UV light Psoralen + ultraviolet A
 Systemic Methotrexate; hydroxyurea

Station 248: Other papulosquamous disease See opposite.

Station 249: Dermatitis

Dermatitis overview

- The terms eczema and dermatitis are interchangeable
- Dermatitis means inflammation of the skin
- Presents with pruritus and erythema ± distinct margins
- The specific look of the rash depends on the chronicity:
  - Acute dermatitis – blisters
  - Subacute dermatitis – scaling and crusting
  - Chronic dermatitis – lichenification

Diagnosis	Primarily clinical, based on history and dermatological appearance
Investigations	Limited to skin patch tests or a KOH test to identify fungal infection
Treatment	Depends on type of dermatitis but general principles are:

- Keep skin well hydrated with emollients
- Reduce itching and scratching with topical medications (e.g. steroids) or antihistamines
- Avoid irritants and drying agents
- Treat other rashes, especially fungal infections

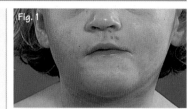

Fig. 1

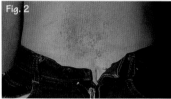

Fig. 2

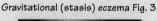

Gravitational (stasis) eczema Fig. 3

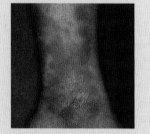

Seborrheic eczema Fig. 4

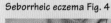

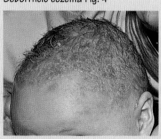

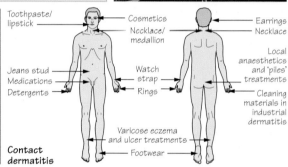

Contact dermatitis

Toothpaste/lipstick — Cosmetics
Necklace/medallion
Jeans stud — Watch strap
Medications — Rings
Detergents
Earrings
Necklace
Local anaesthetics and 'piles' treatments
Cleaning materials in industrial dermatitis
Varicose eczema and ulcer treatments — Footwear

Station 250: Erythemas

Erythema nodosum
Causes
Bacterial: TB, leprosy, streptococcus
Viral
Fungal
Drugs, e.g. OCP
Systemic disease:
  sarcoidosis, IBD

Fig. 5

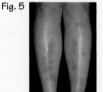

Erythema multiforme
Causes
Idiopathic
Infections, e.g. herpes, mycoplasma
Collagen disease, e.g. SLE
Neoplastic, e.g. Hodgkin's
Autoimmune, e.g. Wegener's
Drugs, e.g. sulphonamide
Pregnancy

Fig. 6

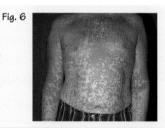

Station 251: Bullous disease

Fig. 7

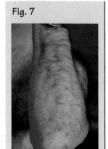

Fig. 8

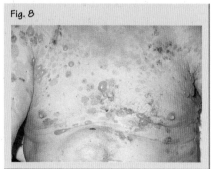

Fig. 9

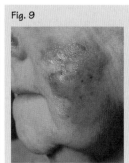

Bullous disease presents with eruptions of blisters. The causes are varied:
- infections (e.g. impetigo)
- physical injury (e.g. heat)
- drugs (e.g. barbiturates)
- acquired skin disorders (e.g. pemphigoid)
- metabolic disease (e.g. diabetes)

Station 249A: Atopic eczema

• *You are a FY1 doctor on your GP placement when a 6-month-old child attends with erythema, vesiculation and crusting affecting the face, scalp, arms and legs – particularly the popliteal and antecubital fossae. Please examine this young patient's face and describe the problem (Fig. 1)*

Discussion points

• What associations of atopic eczema are you aware of?
• What treatment would you consider?

Association Hay fever, asthma and urticaria

Mx Promote healing (emollient creams and topical corticosteroids); control infection (topical or systemic antibiotics); relieve pruritus (consider antihistamines); short course of systemic corticosteroids can be used in severe cases; avoidance of environmental triggers

Station 249B: Contact eczema

• *A 19-year-old male has attended your GP surgery complaining of a rash on his abdomen (Fig. 2). Please assess and discuss your thoughts with the examiner*

Discussion points

• Name some common precipitants implicated in contact eczema
• What is the immunological mechanism?
• How can the diagnosis be confirmed and what is the treatment?

Immunology Type IV (delayed cellular) hypersensitivity mechanism
The reaction requires a prior exposure

Ix Patch testing (dilute solution of suspected culprits allowed to react with normal skin)

Mx Symptomatic care (e.g. emollients); wet to dry soaks of astringent solutions (Burow's solution) and antipruritics (e.g. diphenhydramine, hydroxyzine); NSAIDs will help with pruritus; oral corticosteroids are effective and indicated for the treatment of severe cases with involvement of large areas of the skin, swelling of the face or genitalia, or large areas of bullae; steroids should be tapered over several weeks; avoid allergen

Station 250: Erythemas

• *A 42-year-old female has been admitted to hospital. Please inspect the patient's legs and describe your findings (Fig. 5)*

Discussion points

• What are the causes of erythema nodosum?
• What investigations should be performed?
• What are the causes of erythema multiforme?

Erythema nodosum

• Inflammation of subcutaneous fat
• Immunological reaction
• Typical presentation: painful, red nodules on the legs or forearms
• A careful history is needed

Ix Will depend on clinical suspicion of the cause; mantoux test antistreptolysin titre; CXR

Rx Depends on the cause; antibiotics for bacterial infection; NSAIDs for the pain; consider oral steroids

Erythema multiforme

• Typical presentation: pink, oedematous papules that evolve into flat, dull red macules with central clearing mainly around the palms, soles and extensor extremities (Fig. 6)
• A careful history is needed: recent infection, recent drug use and other symptoms (e.g. fever, malaise, myalgias and upper respiratory tract infection symptoms)

Ix Will depend on clinical suspicion of the cause; CXR; if not resolving or recurrent, may need to investigate for underlying malignancy

Rx Depends on cause; usually self-limiting within a week; consider antibiotics/antivirals depending on cause; consider prednisolone

Station 251A: Dermatitis herpetiformis

• *A 38-year-old male presents with an itchy rash on his elbows. He also complains of weight loss and intermittent diarrhoea. Please examine the rash (Fig. 7); describe your findings and offer a diagnosis*

Discussion points

• What is dermatitis herpetiformis associated with?
• What is the treatment for dermatitis herpetiformis?

Sx Itchy vesicular rash; found on elbows, knees and buttocks (extensor surfaces); associated symptoms of coeliac disease

Ix *Bloods* Antigliaden antibodies; anti-endomysial antibodies; iron studies

  Other Skin biopsy; consider jejunal biopsy

Associations Coeliac disease and its associated symptoms; small bowel lymphoma

Mx Gluten-free diet; dapsone (need to check FBC and LFTs to monitor for agranulocytosis and dapsone-induced hepatitis)

Station 251B: Pemphigoid

• *A 74-year-old male presents to his GP with the rash shown in Fig. 8. Please describe the lesions and discuss your diagnosis*

Hints and tips

• Autoimmune, chronic, itchy, blistering disease
• 70% patients have IgG antibodies to basement membrane
• More common in elderly patients
• Disease often remits in 1–2 years; relapse in 10%?

Discussion points

• What bullous skin disorders are you aware of?
• What causes pemphigoid? What treatment is available?

Ix *Bloods* IgG antibodies
  Skin biopsy

Rx Steroids
  Steroid-sparing immunosuppressive agents, e.g. azathioprine

Station 251C: Pemphigus

• *A 62-year-old female presents to hospital with the rash shown in Fig. 9. Please describe the lesions and discuss your diagnosis*

Hints and tips

• Potentially life-threatening autoimmune disease
• IgG antibodies to antigens within the epidermis
• Flaccid blisters and erosions
• Positive Nikolsky sign – superficial layer of skin 'slides' off the deeper layers when a light pressure is applied
• > 50% patients have lesions involving the mouth

Discussion points

• What causes pemphigus?
• How would you manage a patient with pemphigus?

Ix *Bloods* IgG antibodies
  Skin biopsy

Mx involve dermatology early; high-dose steroids; steroid-sparing immunosuppressive agents, e.g. azathioprine; consider plasmapharesis; mouth care; careful monitoring of nutrition and hydration; monitoring for secondary infection

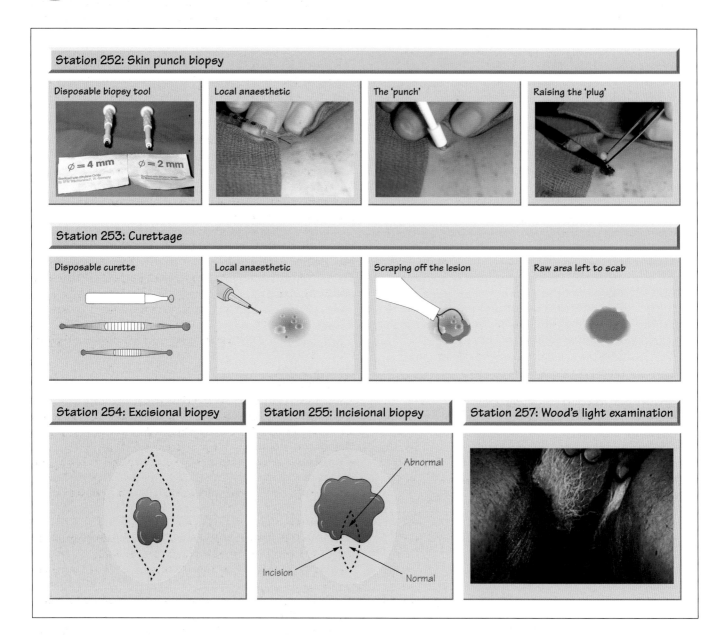

Station 252: Skin punch biopsy
Disposable biopsy tool | Local anaesthetic | The 'punch' | Raising the 'plug'
Ø = 4 mm Ø = 2 mm

Station 253: Curettage
Disposable curette | Local anaesthetic | Scraping off the lesion | Raw area left to scab

Station 254: Excisional biopsy | Station 255: Incisional biopsy | Station 257: Wood's light examination
Abnormal
Incision
Normal

In dermatology, a good history and examination can allow a large proportion of diagnoses to be made. However, as there are many conditions that present in a similar way, there are several investigations which are important to be able to describe and interpret and could easily be employed in the OSCE situation.

Station 252: Skin punch biopsy

• *Mr HI has developed a lesion on his arm that requires a skin biopsy. Please name three methods and describe one technique in detail. Discuss the types of lesions that a biopsy helps distinguish*

Hints and tips
• Introduction

• Check he is the correct patient
• Explanation of reason for carrying out procedure
• State that you would check the platelet and clotting results
• Check equipment (sterile gloves, aseptic tray, local anaesthetic, punch biopsy needle, suture and dressing)
• Using an aseptic technique, clean the required area
• Administer local anaesthetic
• Make a tubular punch (diameter ≈ 2 mm) through to the subcutis using a circular motion
• Raise the plug of tissue and snip off at its base avoiding compressing the tissues too hard with the forceps
• Apply steristrip dressings or insert a suture
• Place sample in specimen jar and correctly label

Station 253: Curettage

Hints and tips

- To remove epidermal lesions
- Local anaesthetic
- Scoop the lesion from the edge while stretching the skin
- Specimen to histology

Indications   Solar keratoses
                    Small basal cell carcinoma

Station 254: Excisional biopsy

Hints and tips

- Used for most small tumours
- Diagnosis and cure are achieved with complete excision
- Includes small borders of normal skin
- If the lesion is pigmented, it should be excised deeply
- Incision should follow tension or wrinkle line
- Administer local anaesthetic
- Make an elliptical incision around the lesion
- This incision should be vertical rather than slanting
- Specimen to histology
- Suture the wound

Station 255: Incisional biopsy

Hints and tips

- Can be used for larger lesions to get histological information
- Need to include adequate amount of normal tissue to compare with the abnormal
- Incision should follow tension or wrinkle line
- Same technique as for excisional biopsy

Station 256: Viral cultures

Discussion points

- When might you use viral cultures to assist with a diagnosis in dermatology?
- What other tests are available to assist with a diagnosis in dermatology?
- When might you use the Tzanck test to assist with a diagnosis in dermatology?

Hints and tips

- Viral cultures are more sensitive and easier to interpret than the Tzanck test
- Identifications can usually be made within 2 or 3 days
- If a viral infection is suspected, vesicle fluid can be put into special transport media for culture at most medical centres
- Other dermatology tests include: patch tests for allergic contact dermatitis, darkfield examination for syphilis, skin scrapings for scabies, hair counts for alopecia
- Tzanck test can be quick and reliable for diagnosing herpes simplex, herpes zoster and pemphigus
- A smear of cellular material is scraped from the base and sides of a vesicle and stained with Wright's or Giemsa stain

- Multinucleated giant cells are seen in herpes simplex, herpes zoster and varicella but not in vaccinia
- Pemphigus can be diagnosed by finding typical acantholytic cells that have very large nuclei and scant cytoplasm that are no longer attached to each other

Station 257: Wood's light examination

- *When might you use Wood's light examination to assist with a diagnosis in dermatology?*

Hints and tips

- This involves viewing the skin in a dark room under UV light filtered through a Wood's glass ('black light')
- Tinea versicolor fluoresces two subtle gold colours
- Erythrasma fluoresces a bright pink-red
- The earliest clue to a *Pseudomonas* infection, especially in burns, may be green fluorescence

Station 258: Microscopic examination

Discussion points

- When might you use microscopic examination to assist with a diagnosis in dermatology?
- When might you use microbial culture and sensitivity to assist with a diagnosis in dermatology?
- When might you use fluorescence microscopy to assist with a diagnosis in dermatology?

Hints and tips

- Take a scraping if fungal infection is suspected
- Ideally, scales are taken from the active, advancing border of the lesion, covered with 20% potassium hydroxide
- In dermatophyte infections, hyphae are primarily seen
- In tinea versicolor and candidal infections, budding yeast and hyphae are seen
- Microbial culture is useful for acute bacterial skin infections
- Microbial culture should not delay treatment
- For a pustular lesion a swab sample is sufficient
- In chronic infections (e.g. TB, deep fungi), specimens such as deep biopsy must be cultured and special media may be needed
- *Indirect immunofluorescence tests* (evaluation of serum for circulating antibodies):
    - in pemphigus or bullous pemphigoid the serum may contain specific antibodies that bind to different areas of the epithelium
    - in pemphigus, the antibody titre may correlate with the severity of the disease
- *Direct immunofluorescence tests* (evaluation of a patient's skin for in vivo antibody deposition):
    - biopsy specimens of patients with pemphigus, pemphigoid, dermatitis herpetiformis, herpes gestationis, systemic lupus erythematosus and discoid lupus erythematosus show diagnostic patterns of antibody deposition
- The direct immunofluorescence test is more definitive than ordinary histology for diagnosing most of these diseases

History hints

Presenting symptoms
Trauma
Pain
Irritation
Loss of vision
Blurred vision
Double vision
Headache
Previous trauma
For each symptom determine the pattern and speed of onset and relationship to other symptoms

Past ophthalmic history
Past ophthalmic history is vital
Are glasses or contact lenses worn?
Date of last eye examination and testing

Drug history
Medicines prescribed for non-ocular conditions can also lead to eye problems in susceptible individuals, e.g. anticholinergic drugs may precipitate acute closed-angle glaucoma or topical β-blockers may produce bradycardia
Previous eye drops
History of OCP or HRT
OTC meds, e.g. aspirin

Past medical history
Past ocular history
Cardiovascular or cerebrovascular disease due to risk of emboli
Diabetes and hypertension due to ocular complications
Systemic disease, e.g. sarcoid and inflammatory bowel disease, due to their ocular manifestations

Social/family/occupational history
History of irritants or possible foreign bodies
Use of protective glasses, e.g. welder
Smoking
FH of eye conditions including in childhood
FH of systemic disease

Station 259: Vision and driving

DVLA rules	Domain	Group 1: Ordinary driving licence	Group 2: Vocational driving licence
	Acuity	Requisite: 'Read in good light (with the aid of glasses or contact lenses if worn) a registration mark fixed to a motor vehicle and containing figures 79 mm high and 50 mm wide at a distance of 20 m'	Uncorrected acuity in both eyes must be 3/60. Corrected acuity (using lenses if necessary) has to be 6/9 in the better eye and 6/12 in the worse eye
	Visual fields	Requisite: 'A field of at least 120° on the horizontal measured using a target equivalent to the white Goldman III4e settings with no defect in the binocular field within 20 degree of fixation above or below'	Normal binocular field of vision is required, i.e. any area of defect in a single eye is totally compensated for by the field of the other eye
	Double vision	Cease driving on diagnosis Resume when controlled by glasses or patch	Patching not acceptable

Station 260: Eye examination

The eye and systemic disease

System	Diagnosis	Eye problem
Cardiology	Hypertension	Retinopathy
	Endocarditis	Roth spots
	↑ Lipids	Corneal arcus, lipaemia retinalis
	Hypertension	Central retinal artery or vein occlusion
	Marfan's	Dislocation of the lens
Endocrinology	Diabetes	Retinopathy, cataract
	Thyroid	Graves' ophthalmopathy
	Pituitary	Visual field defect
Gastroenterology	Wilson's	Kayser–Fleischer rings
	IBD	Uveitis
Haematology	Sickle cell	Retinopathy
	Leukaemia	Hypopyon
Infection	HIV	Retinopathy
	CMV	Retinitis
	Syphilis	Iritis, vasculitis, Argyll Robertson pupils
	Toxoplasmosis	Uveitis
Neurology	Amaurosis fugax	Transient loss of vision
	Migraine	Transient loss of vision
	Papilloedema	See Chapter 97
	Multiple sclerosis	Optic neuritis
	Myotonic dystrophy	Cataract
	Myasthenia gravis	Ptosis
Respiratory	Sarcoidosis	Uveitis
	Pancoast's tumour	Horner's syndrome
Rheumatology	Giant cell arteritis	Optic neuropathy
	Rheumatoid arthritis	Scleritis
	Seronegative arthropathies	Iritis (anterior uveitis)
	Sjogren's syndrome	Dry eyes
	Bechet's disease	Uveitis

- Know basic eye anatomy:
Externally: eyelids, lacrimal gland, nasolacrimal duct, conjunctiva (covers eye and loops around, so cannot get foreign body behind an eye), cornea (transparent)
Anterior segment: sclera (outer coating), aqueous humour (nutrients), iris (colourful part), pupil, lens (focuses light), ciliary body (produces aqueous and focuses lens)
Posterior segment: vitreous humour (space), retina and optic nerve head (generate visual impulses), choroid (blood/nutrient supply), sclera
- Measure visual acuity
- Visual field testing and blind spot
- Examine pupils: include light reflex
- Examine accommodation reflex: ability of lens to change focus to see something up close. Ciliary muscle contracts; causes zonules (hold lens in place) to relax
- Examine eye movements: innervation of extraocular muscles – aide memoire $LR_6 (SO)_4$ + III nerve
- Perform fundoscopy and detect red reflex (be able to detect diabetic and hypertensive eye problems)
- Recognise common conditions
- Recognise ophthalmic emergencies, e.g. red eye

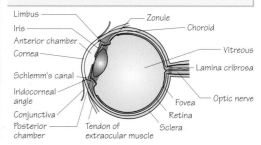

Limbus, Iris, Anterior chamber, Cornea, Schlemm's canal, Iridocorneal angle, Conjunctiva, Posterior chamber, Tendon of extraocular muscle, Zonule, Choroid, Vitreous, Lamina cribrosa, Optic nerve, Fovea, Retina, Sclera

Ophthalmology example stations

- A 38-year-old male presents with a history of red, itchy, painful eyes and intermittent swelling of several joints. Please take a full history
- A 25-year-old female presents with a discharge from both her eyes. Please take a history and formulate a differential diagnosis and management plan
- Please look at the photographs provided and suggest a differential diagnosis and three management points for each one

Station 259: Vision and driving

Student info: *You are the FY1 doctor in the ophthalmology clinic. A 48-year-old male has been referred after seeing his GP and optician with deterioration in his vision. Please take a focused history. You do not need to perform an examination. The optician has documented visual acuity to be 6/12 in both eyes after correction of his vision*

Patient info: *You are a 48-year-old male. You have not been to see either your GP or optician previously despite the fact your eye sight has been deteriorating over several years. You are a taxi driver and have been scared that you would lose your licence. You first noticed the problem as a difficulty with driving at night but it has now got to the stage where you have had a couple of near misses while driving. PMH: hypertension for which you take ramipril 5 mg OD. FH: your father died in his forties from heart problems and you believe he suffered from some form of inherited eye problem, but you are unsure of the exact name. Otherwise you are in good health and currently feel well. You live with your wife who is a housewife and looks after your four children. If you lose your job, the financial consequences would be hard. You feel there is something seriously wrong but have been unwilling to accept this until now. If the doctor suggests you will have to stop driving, then initially state you cannot. If they explain the reasons why you must, then agree at least in principle*

Hints and tips

- Ascertain the patient's prior knowledge of the situation including the reason for referral
- Determine symptomatology
- Determine timing of symptoms
- Elicit PMH, DH and SH
- Establish the FH of an unknown eye problem
- Establish the fact that the patient is a taxi driver
- Address any concerns the patient has, in particular the fact that driving is essential for his occupation

Discussion points

- What advice would you give this patient with regard to his driving?
- Can you discuss the DVLA rules regarding vision and application for an ordinary licence?
- Are the rules different for a passenger-carrying vehicle licence?

Station 260: Eye examination

Hints and tips

- Many aspects of the examination of the eye are summarised in the cranial nerve examination station (see Ch. 33)
- It is important to remember the importance of the eye as part of systemic disease – a brief revision list is documented opposite
- Actual 'hot' cases will be rare in the OSCE but the differential diagnosis, particularly of the red eye, is essential for all medical practitioners
- Always examine the right eye first

- Below is a generic examination routine, although it would be usual in an OSCE for the examination to be broken down and tested in steps

Examination routine

- Introduction/consent/ask about pain
- *General inspection*: remember the importance of generalised inspection of the patient (e.g. signs of myotonic dystrophy – consider cataracts; signs of a stroke – consider a visual field defect; signs of thyroid disease – consider Graves' ophthalmology)
- *System-specific inspection*: look at the eyes
- *Visual acuity* (see Chs 33 and 97): consider pinhole visual acuity
- *Visual fields* (see Ch. 33)
- *Pupils and papillary reflexes* (see Ch. 33)
- *Eye movements* (see Ch. 33)
- Examine the eye from the front to the back (periocular region, lids, conjunctiva, cornea, anterior segment, lens, vitreous, macula, retina and optic nerve): use of a slit lamp will not be examined, but you would be expected to examine the eye with a torch and ophthalmoscope
- Consider intraocular pressure measurement (you would not be expected to perform this)
- Finally, once happy with the above, consider dilation of the pupils to aid with examining the posterior structures
- *Fundoscopy* (see Ch. 34)
- *Completion*:
  - consider colour vision assessment
  - consider systemic examination depending on findings so far

Important notes on the red eye

- Know conditions that require urgent referral: corneal infections, chemical injuries, scleritis, iritis, orbital cellulitis, hyphema and acute glaucoma
- Acute alkali injury is worse than acid. Needs immediate irrigation until pH is 6
- In acid injuries irrigate until pH is 8. No neutralising
- Herpes simplex virus keratitis: the blue eye picture. There is inflammation of the cornea, which looks like snowflakes. Treat with topical/oral antivirals; *avoid* steroids (can blind the patient)
- Iritis (otherwise known as anterior uveitis): painful red eye with small pupil. Check rest of the body for inflammation, and treat with steroids. Associated with autoimmune diseases. Cornea is clear
- Orbital cellulitis: pain with motility; big infected eye (orbit is swollen). Treatment is an emergency; requires hospitalisation. Infection can spread from the sinuses to the orbit and then the brain

Summary of ophthalmology investigations

The investigations will depend on the underlying diagnosis, e.g. autoimmune screen, vasculitic screen.

Bloods	As per underlying diagnosis (e.g. glucose)
ECG	Consider if there is a vascular problem
Imaging	Ultrasound
	CT and MRI (or orbital X-ray)
Micro	Eye swab
Other	Slit lamp examination including measurement of intraocular pressure
	Retinoscopy
	Exophthalmometer
	Electrophysiological tests
	Fluorescein angiography
	System-specific investigations

Station 261: Glaucoma

	Acute angle closure glaucoma	Primary open angle glaucoma (POAG) + chronic angle closure glaucoma (CACG)
Symptoms	Painful red eye Blurring of vision, haloes Severe headache, nausea and vomiting History of similar episodes in the past	Usually asymptomatic until advanced stages of the diseases
Visual acuity	Decreased	Normal/decreased in advanced stages
Conjunctiva	Injected	Normal
Cornea	Hazy in symptomatic eye	Clear
Anterior chamber	Shallow in both eyes Positive 'eclipse sign'	Deep in both eyes
Gonioscopy	Closed angles	POAG - open angles CACG - closed angles
IOP	Much higher than 21 mmHg and the eye may feel harder than fellow eye on digital palpation	Usually higher than 21 mmHg
Pupil	Mid-dilated in symptomatic eye	Relative afferent pupillary defect (RAPD) if asymmetrical involvement
Optic disc	May be difficult to examine due to hazy cornea Can be normal, hyperaemic or cupped if there have been previous neglected attacks	Vertical cup disc ratio ± 0.7 in a normal-sized disc Increase in cup disc ratio over time Asymmetry in cup disc ratio ± 0.2 between the two eyes Splinter haemorrhages

Anatomy: Normal and cupped optic nerve heads in chronic primary open angle glaucoma

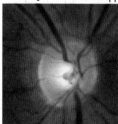
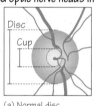

Disc
Cup

(a) Normal disc
Cup disc ratio approx 0.3

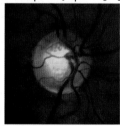
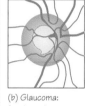

(b) Glaucoma: focal notch

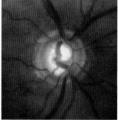
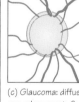

(c) Glaucoma: diffuse cup enlargement. Cup disc ratio approx 0.8

Station 262: Uveitis

History hints

Painful red eye
Blurred vision
Photophobia
Symptoms due to associated diseases

Associations

Idiopathic
Infectious Toxoplasmosis
               Herpes zoster
               CMV
Systemic   Ankylosing
               spondylitis
               Reiter's
               disease
               IBD
               Sarcoidosis

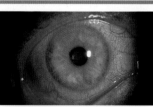

External ocular appearance in a patient with uveitis. Note inflammatory response at the limbus

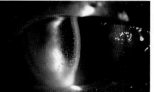

Keratic precipitates on the corneal endothelium

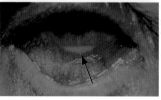

A hypopyon, white cells collected to form a fluid level in the inferior anterior chamber

Classification

Anterior uveitis	Usually limited to the iris (iritis) Associated with autoimmune diseases, e.g. rheumatoid arthritis or ankylosing spondylitis Most common in young and middle aged
Pars planitis	Area between the iris and the choroid. Usually young men and is generally not associated with any other disease, although may be related to Crohn's or multiple sclerosis
Posterior uveitis	Usually choroiditis If the adjacent retina is also involved it is called chorioretinitis. Posterior uveitis may follow a systemic infection or occur in association with an autoimmune disease. Also CMV retinitis in AIDS

Station 261: Glaucoma

Hints and tips

• Eye disorder characterised by progressive eye damage, partly due to intraocular pressure.
• Normal intraocular pressure (IOP) is 11–21 mmHg; this level may not necessarily be healthy for all people
• Some people with normal pressure develop optic nerve injury (normal- or low-pressure glaucoma)
• In contrast, many patients have pressure > 21 mmHg without any optic nerve injury
• 1–2% prevalence in white Causasians over 40 years old
• Can occur at any age
• Classification:
  • primary or secondary
  • open or closed angle
  • acute or chronic
  • congenital, juvenile or adult
  • normal or high pressure

Primary open-angle glaucoma

• Glaucoma with an open anterior chamber angle
• Most common form (65%) of glaucoma
• Usually both eyes are affected
• Vision lost by glaucoma cannot be recovered

Mx   Aim is to lower the IOP, to prevent optic nerve and visual field damage
'Goal' = 33% drop from presenting IOP
Baseline tests, visual fields and optic disc photography serve as a baseline for future comparison

Rx
Medical   Lantanoprost – increases uveoscleral drainage, generally considered first line once a day and has fewer side effects
Topical β-blockers, e.g. timolol, given in increasing concentration until control is satisfactory
Systemic carbonic anhydrase inhibitors, e.g. acetazolamide, reduce aqueous formation
Surgery   Argon laser burns to the trabecular meshwork
Or if a more extensive approach is required, a conventional trabeculectomy
Introduction of adjunctive antimetabolite treatment at the time of glaucoma surgery has helped to improve surgical success rates – this is particularly true in those patients where the natural healing processes tend to obliterate the drainage channel created

Closed-angle glaucoma

• Glaucoma associated with a closed anterior chamber angle
• Accounts for about 10% of all glaucomas
• Can be primary due to pupillary block, or secondary due to something pulling or pushing the iris up into the angle

Rx
Medical   Initial treatment for an acute closed-angle glaucoma attack is medical
Topical β-blockers, IV or oral carbonic anhydrase inhibitor, and topical α2-selective adrenergic agonists should be given immediately + 2% pilocarpine (1 drop every 15 minutes for 1 hour) to 'open up' the angle by rotating the ciliary body
An osmotic drug is used if response to the other treatment is inadequate
Surgery   Laser peripheral iridotomy is the definitive treatment for acute-angle glaucoma. When the cornea is not clear or the eye is extremely inflamed the iridotomy is deferred; otherwise it is performed as soon as the condition of the eye permits
Because the contralateral eye has an 80% chance of developing an acute attack, a prophylactic peripheral iridotomy must be performed on that eye

Station 262: Uveitis

• *This 28-year-old male patient has a recent history of bloody diarrhoea and is now complaining of a painful right eye. Please examine his eyes, discussing your findings with the examiner as you progress*

Hints and tips

• Examine the eyes as for the routine in Chapter 94
• This sort of case would be rare in an OSCE but a simulated patient could be used and photographic materials referenced
• The general observation of the patient will be even more essential for this case due to the association with other systemic conditions

Examination   Ciliary injection (engorgement of vessels around the limbus)
Keratic precipitates
Mx   Analgesia
Steroids, topical if mild; systemic for more severe case
Dark glasses
Short-acting dilators (e.g. cyclopentolate) may be given to keep the pupil dilated and to prevent ciliary spasm and the formation of posterior synechiae
It is important to treat the complications
Intraocular pressure may be reduced by a carbonic anhydrase inhibitor
Treat associated diseases
Complications   Glaucoma
Cataracts
Fluid within the retina
Retinal detachment
Vision loss

Discussion points

• What are the causes of uveitis?
• How can uveitis be classified?
• What is the treatment?
• What disease associations are there?
• What are the treatment priorities?

Station 263: Diabetic retinopathy

National Screening Committee
- UK National Guidelines on Screening for Diabetic Retinopathy

Background – level 1
• Microaneurysms
• Retinal haemorrhage ± exudates

Preproliferative – level 2
• Venous beading
• Venous loop
• Intraretinal microvascular abnormality (IRMA)
• Multiple deep, round or blot haemorrhages
• Cotton wool spots

Proliferative – level 3
• New vessels on disc (NVD)
• New vessels elsewhere (NVE)
• Pre-retinal or vitreous haemorrhage
• Pre-retinal fibrosis ± tractional retinal detachment

Maculopathy
• Exudate within 1 disc diameter (DD) of the fovea
• Circinate or group of exudates within the macula
• Retinal thickening within 1DD of the centre of the fovea
• Any microaneurysms or haemorrhage within 1DD
  of the fovea

Examination hints

Dots and blots	= capillary microaneurysms and retinal haemorrhages
Hard exudates	= small areas of white plaque which indicate leakage of lipid deposits from the vessels
Cotton wool spots	= areas of retinal infarction
Neoproliferation	= development of new vessels
Chorioretinal atrophy	= areas caused by laser photocoagulation

Station 264: Hypertensive retinopathy

Examination hints – grading

Grade 1	Increased tortuosity of retinal vessels with increased reflectiveness (silver wiring)	
Grade 2	As above plus AV nipping of some vessels	
Grade 3	As above plus retinal haemorrhages and cotton wool exudates	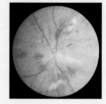
Grade 4 (photo)	Papilloedema, retinal oedema and hard exudates often in the shape of a macular star	

Station 265: Cataract

History hints

Gradual reduction in visual acuity	No pain or redness
Increased glare from sunshine or car lights	Monocular diplopia
Altered colour perception	

Examination hints

Loss of red reflex
Well-developed cataracts appear as grey or yellow-brown opacities in the lens
Examination of the dilated pupil with the ophthalmoscope held about
  30 cm away usually discloses subtle opacities
Small cataracts stand out as dark defects in the red reflex
A dense cataract may obliterate the red reflex
Slit-lamp examination provides more details about the character,
  location and extent of the opacity

Station 266: Age-related macular degeneration

History hints

Gradual onset reduction in vision
Shadowy areas in central vision
Distortion of vision centrally esp. colour, fine detail
NB. Commonest cause of blindness in the elderly

Age-related maculopathy (ARM)
Initial change, characterised by Drusen (yellow deposits)
± changes in the retinal pigment epithelium (RPE)

↓ Progression leads to...

Age-related macular degeneration (AMD)

Geographic atrophy (dry AMD) 90% of cases	**Choroidal neovascularisation** (wet AMD) 10% of cases but 90% of cases are of severe visual loss

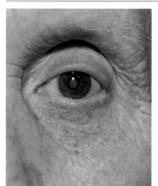

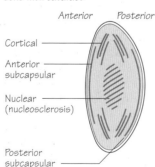
Lens with cataract

Anterior   Posterior

Cortical

Anterior
subcapsular

Nuclear
(nucleosclerosis)

Posterior
subcapsular

Choroidal neovascularisation (CNV)

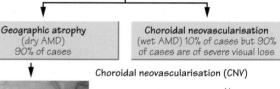
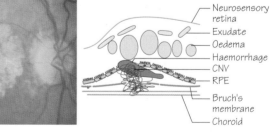

Neurosensory
retina
Exudate
Oedema
Haemorrhage
CNV
RPE
Bruch's
membrane
Choroid

These fundoscopy stations could involve real patients with actual retinal changes or simulated patients on whom the student performs the technique of fundoscopy, with the examiner then having photos of specific abnormalities for the student to discuss

Station 263: Diabetic retinopathy

• *This patient has type 1 diabetes, please perform a fundoscopy. Please comment on the abnormalities shown on the picture provided*

Hints and tips
• Perform fundoscopy as described in Chapter 98
• Look for any other clues around the patient – diabetic diet sign, evidence of other vascular disease, evidence of dialysis fistula, amputation
• Look for the abnormalities listed in the examination hints section (see Ch. 94)

Discussion points
• What eye complications occur in diabetics?
• What are the different types of diabetic retinopathy?
• What causes cotton wool spots and exudates?
• When is laser photocoagulation considered?
• What eye symptoms might a diabetic patient complain of and why?
• What are the treatment priorities in a patient with background diabetic retinopathy?

Mx	
Rx	Optimise glycaemic control and vascular risk factors
	Laser therapy
Monitoring	Annual screening, monitoring of diabetic control
Specialists	Ophthalmologist (refer patient with maculopathy, preproliferative or proliferative retinopathy or decreased visual acuity)
	Diabetologist

Station 264: Hypertensive retinopathy

• *This patient is on bendrofluazide 2.5 mg daily. Please perform fundoscopy and comment on your findings. Now point out some abnormalities shown on the picture*

Hints and tips
• Perform fundoscopy as described in Chapter 98
• Look for any other clues around the patient – evidence of other vascular disease
• Ask a question if allowed
• Look for the abnormalities listed opposite
• NB. Many diabetic patients also have hypertensive retinal changes.

Discussion points
• What are the different grades of hypertensive retinopathy and how do they differ?
• As an FY1, what urgent tests would you carry out if you noted grade 4 retinopathy on a patient who presented to hospital?
• What are the causes of hypertension?

Station 265: Cataract

• *Please take a brief history and perform fundoscopy on this 74-year-old patient who has noticed some deterioration in vision in his right eye*

Hints and tips
• Perform fundoscopy as described in Chapter 98

• Look for any other clues around the patient as in previous cases
• Look for the abnormalities listed opposite
• State to the examiner that you would like to take a full history and complete your examination of the eye including performing a formal test of visual acuity

Discussion points
• What are the causes of cataract?
• What treatment options are available for a patient with a cataract?
• What symptoms might this patient complain of?
• Describe a classification of cataracts
• What are the complications of cataract surgery?

Causes	Ageing
	Congenital
	Systemic disease (e.g. diabetes)
	Drugs (e.g. steroids)
	Inherited (e.g. Marfan's, myotonic dystrophy)
	Trauma
	Radiation
Rx	
Conservative	Frequent eye examinations and prescription changes initially to maintain vision
Surgery	Indicated if cataract impairs everyday life or if lens threatens to cause glaucoma or uveitis
	Lens extraction is the mainstay of modern cataract surgery, usually under local anaesthesia

Station 266: Age-related macular degeneration (ARMD)

• Please take a history from this 76-year-old female who has noticed poor eye sight and measure her visual acuity

Hints and tips
Use the hints in Chapters 94 and 98 for ophthalmology history and visual acuity measurement.

Discussion points
• What are the risk factors for ARMD?
• What treatment options are available for a patient with ARMD?
• Describe a classification of ARMD

Ix	Fundoscopy – may show pigmentary or haemorrhagic disturbance in the macular region
	Fluorescein angiography – may demonstrate a neovascular membrane beneath the retina
RF	Smoking
	Genetic predisposition
	Association with hypertension
Mx	
Rx of wet ARMD	Photodynamic therapy with 'cold' laser
	Intravitreal injections of triamcinolone (steroid) or an anti-VEGF (vascular endothelial growth factor) agent (avastin)
	Laser photocoagulation of lesion
Monitoring	Vision, blind register
MDT	Talking books, clocks, home visit, optical aids
Specialists	Ophthalmologist
Education	Seek medical advice early if 'other' eye deteriorates

Station 267: Refractive errors

Emmetropia (normal) – entering light rays are focused on the retina by the cornea and the lens, which is elastic. During accommodation, the ciliary muscles adjust the lens shape to properly focus images. Refractive errors cause blurred vision due to a failure of focusing

Myopia (nearsightedness) – the point of focus is in front of the retina as the cornea is too steeply curved or the axial length of the eye is too long. Distant objects are blurred, but near objects can be seen clearly. To correct this, a concave (minus) lens is used. Myopic refractive errors frequently increase until growth stops

Hypermetropia (or farsightedness) – the point of focus is behind the retina because the cornea is too flatly curved or the axial length is too short. Near objects are blurred. To correct this, a convex (plus) lens is used

Astigmatism – non-spherical curvature of the cornea or lens causes light rays to focus at different points. To correct astigmatism, a cylindric lens (a segment cut from a cylinder) is used. Cylindric lenses have no refractive power along one axis and are concave or convex along the other axis

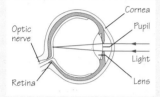 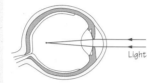 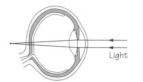 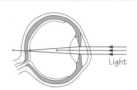

Presbyopia is loss of the lens' ability to change shape to focus on near objects due to ageing. Typically, presbyopia becomes noticeable by the time a person reaches his/her 40s. A convex (plus) lens is used for correction when viewing near objects, which can be a separate pair of glasses, or combined into bifocals or variable focus lenses

Station 268: The red eye

Causes of a red eye

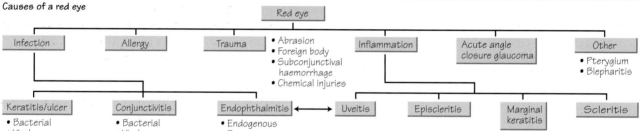

Loss of vision

Loss of vision associated with headache or painful eye movements (non-inflamed eye)	Sudden painless loss of vision	Gradual loss of vision
Optic neuritis/retrobulbar neuritis	Retinal detachment	Refractive errors
Giant cell arteritis/temporal arteritis	Vitreous haemorrhage	Cataracts
Migraine	Central retinal vein occlusion	Age-related macular degeneration
Benign intracranial hypertension	Central retinal artery occlusion	Primary open angle glaucoma
Pituitary haemorrhage	CVA/TIA	Retinal disease, e.g. diabetes
		Tumour

Station 269: Optic nerve disease

Pale optic disc

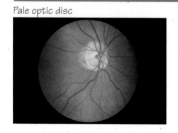

Normal optic disc

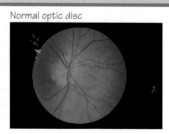

Papilloedema

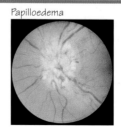

Acute right papillitis

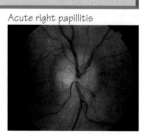

Station 267: Refractive errors

- *This 24-year-old patient has been referred by the GP complaining of headaches and blurred vision. Please perform a pinhole test of vision*
- *Please examine the diagrams shown opposite and discuss with the examiner the refractive error each patient would have and the management*

Hints and tips: pinhole test

- This test is used to determine small to moderate refractive errors
- Introduce yourself and explain the purpose of the test
- Perform a visual acuity test using the Snellen chart
- Reassess using a pinhole to see if the vision improves
- If the vision improves, then the patient may have a refractive error or early lens opacity. Vision does not improve with a retinal or optic nerve abnormality

Station 268: The red eye

A candidate is unlikely to encounter a patient with an acute loss of vision or red eye in an OSCE but the causes, especially of the red eye, are essential knowledge for a FY1. This could be examined in the form of a structured viva or written question using photographic material.

Hints and tips: conjunctivitis

Classification
- *Viral*:
  - take swabs; self-limiting, lasting about 1 week
  - consider antibiotics to prevent bacterial infection
  - if severe, consider steroids, but they can worsen herpes infections
- *Bacterial*:
  - take swabs; often self-limiting
  - antibiotics usually prescribed
- *Gonococcal*:
  - take swabs; usually self-limiting
  - prescribe antibiotics if severe, e.g. ciprofloxacin
  - treat actual and presumed bacterial infections
  - rare complications include corneal ulceration, abscess, perforation and blindness
- *Allergic*:
  - avoidance
  - topical OTC antihistamine
  - topical corticosteroids if severe

Discussion points
- What are the management principles for acute conjunctivitis?
- What choice of antibiotic eye drop would you use?

Hints and tips: episcleritis

Examination	Watery discharge
	Corneal findings uncommon
	Anterior uveitis in up to 10%
Causes	Idiopathic (most common)
	Connective tissue disease, e.g. RA, SLE, IBD
	Miscellaneous, e.g. foreign body
Mx	No treatment – usually self-limiting
	Artificial tears
	Topical steroids for more severe attacks
	Systemic NSAIDs can be considered
	Sunglasses

Hints and tips: scleritis

- May cause inflammation of anterior ± posterior segments of the eye
- Often causes severe pain; often described as a deep, boring ache which interferes with sleep
- Bilateral in c. 50% patients
- Ask about previous episodes and underlying systemic illnesses

Causes	Coexists with systemic disease in c. 50% cases
	RA, SLE, ankylosing spondylitis, sarcoidosis
Mx	Timely ophthalmology referral
	Analgesia
	Systemic steroids or other immunosuppressive agents
	Important to make diagnosis due to potential loss of sight

Station 269: Optic nerve disease
Hints and tips: papilloedema

Examination	Swelling of the optic nerve head due to increased intracranial pressure
	Usually bilateral
	Visual acuity may be normal or reduced
	Patient may have transient episodes of visual loss
	Reduced colour vision
	Enlarged blind spot in more severe cases
Causes	Raised intracranial pressure, e.g. space-occupying lesion (SOL), hydrocephalus, benign intracranial hypertension, saggital sinus thrombosis
	Malignant hypertension
	Infection. e.g. meningitis
	Infiltrative, e.g. lymphoma
	Toxic, e.g. chloramphenicol
Ix *Bloods*	FBC, WCC, U&E, ESR
Imaging	CT head, MRI or magnetic resonance angiogram to exclude saggital sinus thrombosis if no SOL on CT
Micro	Lumbar puncture if CT is normal

Unilateral disc swelling
- Papilloedema by definition is caused by raised intracranial pressure which usually causes bilateral disc swelling
- Unilateral disc swelling can occur due to:
  - demyelination, e.g. multiple sclerosis
  - inflammatory causes, e.g. uveitis
  - vascular causes
  - infective causes, e.g. toxoplasmosis

Hints and tips: optic neuritis

Examination Inflammation of optic nerve; optic disc may appear swollen (papillitis); sudden onset loss of vision, often painful; reduced colour vision; mild retinal phlebitis; young adults; females > males

Causes Idiopathic; demyelination; infectious; autoimmune

Hints and tips: optic atrophy

Examination Atrophy of the optic nerve; produces a pale disc; visual acuity is normally reduced, but can affect colour vision in early stages; it is *not* a diagnosis but a sign of chronic optic nerve disease

Causes Vascular, e.g. central retinal artery occlusion; hereditary, e.g. autosomal dominant and recessive forms, Leber's optic atrophy; inflammatory, e.g. sarcoidosis, polyarteritis nodosa; nutritional, e.g. vitamin B_{12} deficiency; demyelination, e.g. multiple sclerosis

Station 270: Direct ophthalmoscopy

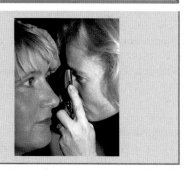

Station 271: Instilling eye drops

Mydriatic drops: cautions
Contraindicated in closed angle glaucoma
May precipitate glaucoma in patients
  with hypermetropia and a shallow
  anterior chamber
Warn patients that the drops will cause
  stinging and occasionally local irritation
Warn patients that their vision will blur
Patients should not drive until the effects
  have worn off

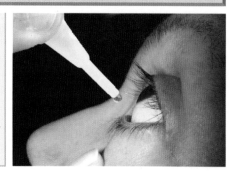

Ocular pharmacology at a glance

Mydriatics (cause pupil dilation)
- Antimuscarinics   e.g. tropicamide 0.5–1% – reduces parasympathetic innervation causing relaxation of the sphincter pupillae and cycloplegia (loss of accommodation)
- Alpha-adrenergics   e.g. phenylephrine 2.5% – stimulates iris dilators but not as good an effect as anticholinergic because the dilator pupillae is a weaker muscle. Higher doses of phenylephrine should be avoided due to risk of systemic side effects

Steroids
- Do not use on fungus or herpes simplex or rheumatoid corneal melt!
- Treatment of inflammatory problems (must have justifiable reason for use). Long term can develop glaucoma and cataracts

Glaucoma – two mechanisms to lower pressure in eye:
- ↓ Production of aqueous humour
  - β-blockers   e.g. timolol – can induce bronchospasm, hypotension, depression
  - Alpha-2 agonist   e.g. brimonidine – can cause arrhythmias/hypertension (note mydriatic cautions above)
  - Carbonic anhydrase inhibitors e.g. acetazolamide
- ↑ Outflow
  - Parasympathomimetic   e.g. pilocarpine (cause miosis)
  - Prostaglandin analogues   e.g. latanoprost (need to monitor eyes as can get discoloration)

Station 272: Visual acuity assessment

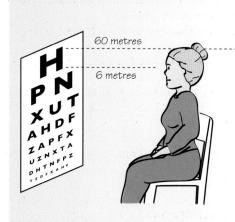

60 metres

6 metres

At 6 metres I can only read what the
girl behind me can read at 60 metres

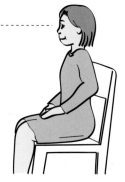

Poor lady. Her vision is only
6/60 as good as mine

Standard
Snellen chart

H	6/60
P N	6/36
X U T	6/24
A H D F	6/18
Z A P F X	6/12
U Z N X T A	6/9
D H T N F P Z	6/6
T Z D F X A H V	6/5

Station 270: Direct ophthalmoscopy

Take time while on the wards to familiarise yourself with several examples of ophthalmoscopes, in particular how to put them together and turn them on. Some students state they find it impossible to close their opposite eye when using the ophthalmoscope. This is actually encouraged by some specialists because it reduces accommodation spasm. The best advice is just to practise a lot to get used to the technique.

If you wear glasses for distance, keep them on. Ask the patient to remove their glasses. Contact lenses can be kept in.

Hints and tips

- Introduction/consent
- Explanation of reason for carrying out procedure
- Ask about any pain or change in vision if allowed
- Perform a brief external examination of the eyes (do not forget to perform a brief general examination of the patient)
- Ask the patient to sit in a chair and look straight forward
- Assemble the ophthalmoscope if necessary and check it works
- Darken the room
- Adjust the ophthalmoscope so that the light is no brighter than necessary
- Adjust the aperture to a plain white circle
- Set the dioptre dial to zero unless you have determined a better setting for your eyes
- Use your right hand and right eye to examine the patient's right eye
- Ask the patient to look straight ahead
- Sit at arm's length, looking through the aperture and pointing the light source at the pupil
- You should see the retina as a 'red reflex'
- Follow the red colour to move within a few inches of the patient's eye (warn the patient you will be moving very close to them!)
- Adjust the dioptre dial to bring the retina into focus
- Find a blood vessel and follow it to the optic disc
- Inspect outward from the optic disc in at least four quadrants and note any abnormalities
- Move laterally from the disc to observe the macula
- Ask the patient to look at the light to observe the fovea
- Ask the patient to look at extremes of gaze
- Now repeat the procedure using your left hand and left eye to examine the patient's left eye

A note on dioptres

Dioptres are used to measure the power of a lens. The ophthalmoscope actually has a series of small lens of different strengths on a wheel (positive dioptres are labelled in green/black, negative in red). When you focus on the retina you 'dial in' the correct number of dioptres to compensate for both the patient's and your own vision. For example, if both you and your patient wear glasses with −2 dioptre correction you should expect to set the dial to −2 with your glasses on or −4 with your glasses off. It is easier to view anterior structures with a positive dioptre (e.g. +5), but as you draw nearer to the patient dial negative.

- Hypermetropic eye – dial more plus
- Myopic eye – dial minus

Station 271: Instilling eye drops

It is unlikely that there would be enough patients available for an OSCE station to have their pupils dilated, so in general a placebo drop is substituted. It is worth knowing a few examples of ophthalmology drugs and their mechanisms of action (see opposite).

• *It is necessary to perform fundoscopy on this patient, but in order to do this it is first necessary to dilate the eye using a mydriatic drop. Please instill 2 drops of the correct drug into the patient's right eye*

Hints and tips

- Introduction/consent
- Give a brief explanation of the reason for carrying out the procedure
- Check the patient has not driven to the clinic
- Choose carefully from the preparations a suitable dilating drop e.g. tropicamide 1%
- Explain to the patient the immediate effects, e.g. stinging, watering eye, blurring of vision
- Gently pull the lower eyelid down
- Hold the bottle with the nozzle about 0.5 cm vertically above the eye
- Administer 1 drop without the bottle touching the eye
- The patient can dab their cheek if the eye waters but should not wipe the eye

Discussion points

- What dilating drops are you aware of and what is their mechanism of action?
- What are the contraindications and cautions to administering a mydriatic?
- What is the mechanism of action of tropicamide?

Station 272: Visual acuity assessment

This is a basic test of vision, but again is another discriminator in an OSCE as students have often not performed the test alone. Remember to test each eye in turn and test acuity before other elements of an eye exam and definitely before administering drops.

• *Please assess this 74-year-old man's visual acuity using the Snellen chart provided*

Snellen chart

- The chart has rows of different-sized letters on it (other charts are available for patients who cannot read)
- It should be placed at a distance of 6 m from the patient (this is usually done using a mirror at 3 m)

The acuity is recorded as the reading distance (i.e. 6 metres) over the row number of the smallest letter seen

- A normal-sighted person should be able to see the largest letter at 60 m
- If a patient can only see the top letter at 6 m, their vision is 6/60
- A normal-sighted person should see the letters on the 6m row at 6 m = 6/6 vision
- If a patient's vision is better than this, then the acuity measurement could be 6/5 or 6/4
- The patient should wear their glasses
- Test *each* eye separately (ask the patient to cover their other eye)
- Ask the patient to read as far down the rows as possible
- If the vision is less than 6/9, use a pinhole to see if it improves (a refraction problem that can be corrected with glasses)
- If vision is worse than 6/60, move the patient closer to the chart
- If the patient still cannot see, proceed to test acuity as discussed in Chapter 33

Station 273: Ear history

Symptoms of ear disease:

Deafness   Tinnitus   Discharge (otorrhoea)
Pain (otalgia) Vertigo   Balance problems

Other relevant features in the history:
• Previous ear surgery or history of head injury
• Systemic disease (e.g. stroke or multiple sclerosis)
• Ototoxic drugs (antibiotics, diuretics, cytotoxics)
• Exposure to noise at work or recreation (e.g. shooting)
• FH of deafness
• History of atopy and allergy in children
• Pain may be referred, so enquire about any other head and neck symptoms
• Associated systemic symptoms (e.g. fever)
• Recent upper respiratory tract illness
• PMH of diabetes and multiple sclerosis

Causes of ear pain
External
• Trauma
• Otitis externa
• Furunculosis
Middle ear
• Acute otitis media
• Acute mastoiditis
Referred
• Teeth, larynx, pharynx, neck

Causes of ear discharge
Serous
• Otitis externa
Mucoid/purulent
• Otitis media
Clear/blood stained
• Consider CSF if head injury
Foul smelling
• Cholesteatoma

Ear history stations
Hearing loss   Tinnitus   Vertigo   Earache   Ear discharge

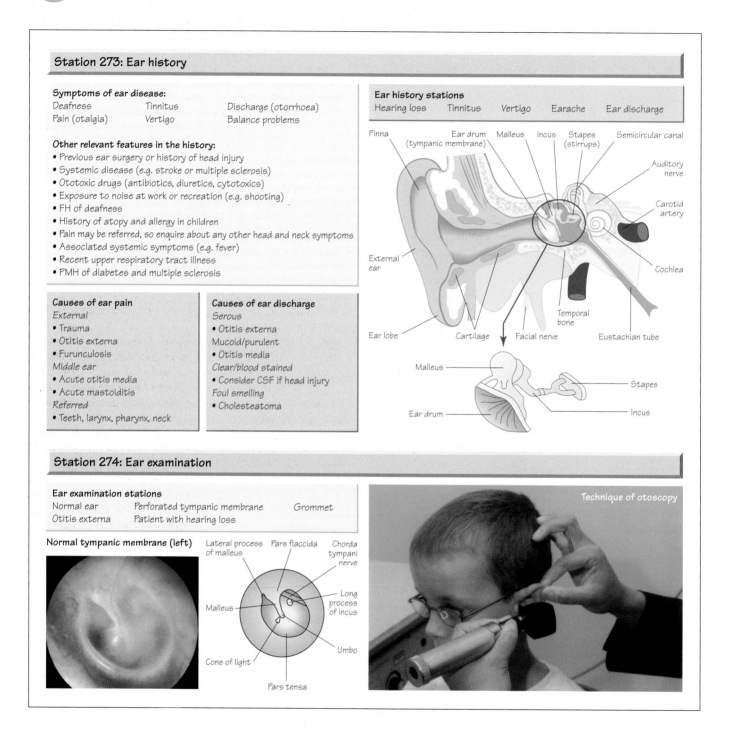

Station 274: Ear examination

Ear examination stations
Normal ear   Perforated tympanic membrane   Grommet
Otitis externa   Patient with hearing loss

Normal tympanic membrane (left)

Station 273: Ear history
• *A 43-year-old woman has been referred to the ENT clinic with unilateral hearing loss. You are the FY1, please take a history and formulate a differential diagnosis*
• *A 62-year-old female has come to see you (her GP) with dizziness. Please take a structured history*

Hints and tips
Ear history stations may involve a real or simulated patient or indeed, as many ear problems affect children, it may be necessary to take the history from a parent.
• Ascertain the patient's reason for attending
• Establish the main and associated symptoms

- Be clear about the time course, nature and progression of any symptoms. Are they bilateral or unilateral?
- With symptoms of pain, try to establish whether this is local or referred
- Five nerves can refer pain to the ear:
  - auricular branch of trigeminal = sinus or teeth
  - greater auricular nerve = neck
  - sensory branch of facial nerve = geniculate herpes
  - vagus nerve = throat
  - tympanic branch of glossopharyngeal = throat
- If there is discharge, is it accompanied by pain in the affected ear? What is the nature of the discharge? When does it occur? Chronic ear discharge is not normally associated with pain
- There are five important causes of discharge:
  - furunculosis
  - otitis externa
  - *acute suppurative otitis media*
  - *chronic suppurative otitis media with cholesteatoma*
  - *chronic suppurative otitis media without cholesteatoma*
- Deafness – what does the patient mean? The term can be used to describe anything from partial to complete loss of hearing
- The deafness must be classified as conductive or sensorineural (can be mixed)
- This must be confirmed on examination, but clues may be given from symptoms of exposure to loud noise, foreign body, ototoxic drugs, trauma or infection
- Tinnitus is described by patients as a ringing or buzzing in the ears. Whilst a cause may not be found, treatable causes (e.g. drug related or acoustic neuroma) need excluding
- Vertigo is the inappropriate sensation of movement. Subjective vertigo – sensation of imbalance; objective vertigo – demonstrable nystagmus
- How long does the symptom last? Is it associated with other symptoms such as nausea and vomiting, tinnitus or hearing loss? Is it affected by head movement?
- Most ear causes of vertigo can be divided into diagnoses depending on the length of history, i.e. labyrinthitis (days to weeks), menieres (minutes to hours) or benign paroxysmal positional vertigo (seconds to minutes)
- Establish the presence of other important or worrying symptoms or points in the history (see opposite)
- Ask general questions regarding the patient's health
- Assess the impact of the symptoms on the patient's life
- Address any concerns the patient has

Station 274: Ear examination

- *This patient presents with a history of ear ache; please examine her ears*
- *Please demonstrate the technique of otoscopy on this man's right ear*
- *Please use this auroscope to examine the mannequin's ears and then using the example picture, point out some anatomical features*

Hints and tips

The station could involve a real patient, a simulated patient or a mannequin. Photographs could be used for descriptions. Before performing the examination, the external ear should be inspected for any obvious abnormality including the following:
- Size and shape of the pinna
- Extra cartilage tags/pre-auricular sinuses or pits
- Evidence of trauma to the pinna
- Suspicious skin lesions on the pinna including skin cancers
- Skin conditions of the pinna and external canal
- Obvious infection of the external ear and canal with frank discharge
- Evidence of previous surgery (scars) (look behind pinna)
- Assessment of facial nerve function

Hints and tips: auroscope/otoscope examination

- Introduction/check correct patient
- Explanation of procedure and clinical indication
- Obtain verbal consent
- Determine which is the better hearing ear
- Ask about any pain in or around the ears
- Perform a brief external examination of the ear
- Assemble the auroscope and check equipment
- Select an appropriately sized speculum (use the largest one that will fit)
- Start with the better hearing ear
- Before examining, palpate the pinna for tenderness (especially the tragus)
- Grasp the pinna between the forefinger and thumb and pull outwards, upwards and backwards during examination (this straightens the canal and allows better inspection of the tympanic membrane or eardrum)
- Examine the canal, noting the condition of the canal skin, the presence of any wax and any foreign body or discharge
- Examine the tympanic membrane, noting any bulging or perforation
- Remember to examine both ears or tell the examiner that you would normally do this using a model
- Thank the patient and clear away your equipment

NB. Hold the otoscope like a pencil (not like a hammer) and near the eyepiece – you will have more control and are therefore less likely to cause the patient discomfort by making sudden or exaggerated movements.

Tympanic membrane

You will have to carefully and gently move the otoscope about to see the whole drum in several different views. You may be asked to identify the following:
- Otitis externa
- Perforations
- Tympanosclerosis
- Glue ear/middle ear effusion
- Retractions of the drum
- Grommet (tympanostomy tube)
- Foreign body

State to the examiners that you would complete your examination by performing an assessment of hearing and by performing a cranial nerve examination (see Ch. 33).

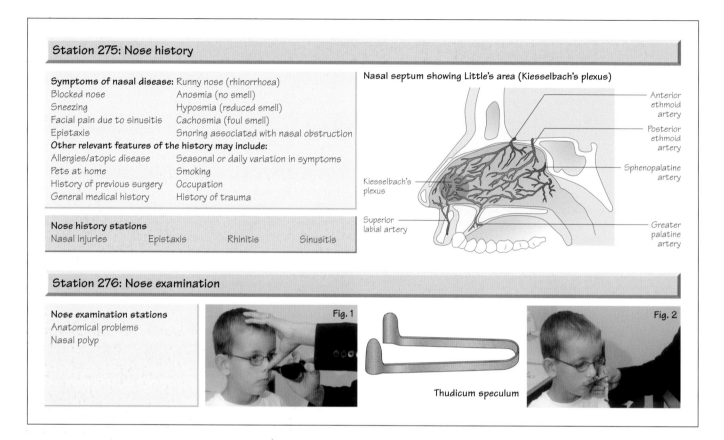

Station 275: Nose history

Symptoms of nasal disease: Runny nose (rhinorrhoea)
Blocked nose   Anosmia (no smell)
Sneezing   Hyposmia (reduced smell)
Facial pain due to sinusitis   Cachosmia (foul smell)
Epistaxis   Snoring associated with nasal obstruction
Other relevant features of the history may include:
Allergies/atopic disease   Seasonal or daily variation in symptoms
Pets at home   Smoking
History of previous surgery   Occupation
General medical history   History of trauma

Nose history stations
Nasal injuries   Epistaxis   Rhinitis   Sinusitis

Nasal septum showing Little's area (Kiesselbach's plexus)

Anterior ethmoid artery
Posterior ethmoid artery
Sphenopalatine artery
Kiesselbach's plexus
Superior labial artery
Greater palatine artery

Station 276: Nose examination

Nose examination stations
Anatomical problems
Nasal polyp

Fig. 1

Thudicum speculum

Fig. 2

Station 275: Nose history

- *This patient has a 2-month history of difficulty breathing through his nose. Please take a relevant history*

Hints and tips
- The key points to cover in the history are summarised above
- Ascertain the patient's reason for attending and determine the main and associated symptoms
- Remember to assess impact of the symptoms on the patient's life and work. Anosmia may be very important to a wine taster!
- Address any concerns the patient has

Station 276: Nose examination
Hints and tips
- *Inspection*:
  - look at the external nose from all angles
  - often deformities are best seen from above
  - look specifically for the following:
    - obvious bend, deformity or swelling
    - scars or abnormal creases across the nose
    - redness or evidence of skin disease
    - discharge, crusting or offensive smell
  - to inspect the nose, first look into the very front of the nose (anterior nares) by tipping the tip of the nose up with a finger and looking inside without a speculum

- After this you will need a Thudicum speculum to open up the nose and a light source (head light/mirror) to examine the inside of the nose
- Alternatively you can use an otoscope with a large end piece (especially in children – Fig. 2)
- You should be able to identify: nasal septum, inferior turbinate, middle turbinate, evidence of inflammation (rhinitis), deviation of the septum, nasal polyp (grey/yellow colour and insensitive)
- In children, a foreign body may occasionally be seen inside the nose, this is usually accompanied by an offensive, unilateral nasal discharge if it has been there for some time
- To assess the nasal airway there are a variety of bedside techniques:
  - hold a cold metal tongue depressor under the nose while the patient exhales. If there is reasonable airflow, there should be some condensation under both nostrils (Fig. 2)
  - occlude one nostril with a thumb and ask the patient to sniff. This gives a reasonable idea of the patency of the airway
- Smell is not routinely assessed in nasal examination as this can be very subjective. On occasions where there is a need to assess smell, this is done using a series of bottles containing specific odours. Usually asking specifically about sense of smell in the history is sufficient
- *Completion*: examination of the nose is not complete without looking into the mouth and pharynx
  - occasionally large nasal polyps, adenoids and tumours may be visible arising from behind the soft palate

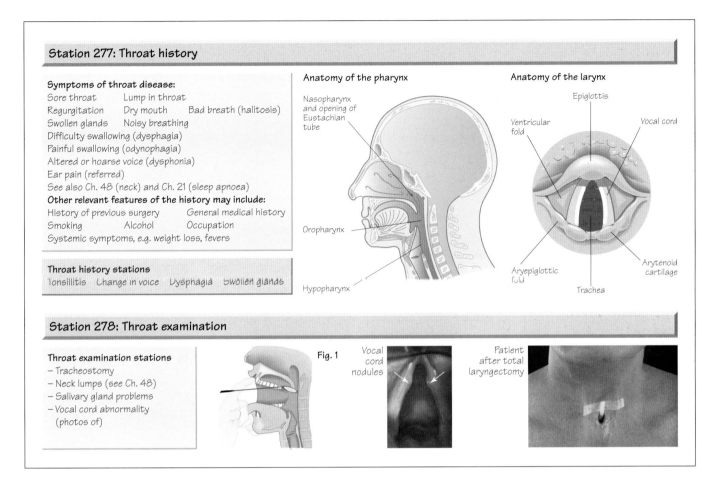

Station 277: Throat history

Symptoms of throat disease:
Sore throat   Lump in throat
Regurgitation   Dry mouth   Bad breath (halitosis)
Swollen glands   Noisy breathing
Difficulty swallowing (dysphagia)
Painful swallowing (odynophagia)
Altered or hoarse voice (dysphonia)
Ear pain (referred)
See also Ch. 48 (neck) and Ch. 21 (sleep apnoea)
Other relevant features of the history may include:
History of previous surgery   General medical history
Smoking   Alcohol   Occupation
Systemic symptoms, e.g. weight loss, fevers

Throat history stations
Tonsillitis   Change in voice   Dysphagia   Swollen glands

Anatomy of the pharynx
Nasopharynx and opening of Eustachian tube
Oropharynx
Hypopharynx

Anatomy of the larynx
Epiglottis
Ventricular fold
Vocal cord
Aryepiglottic fold
Arytenoid cartilage
Trachea

Station 278: Throat examination

Throat examination stations
– Tracheostomy
– Neck lumps (see Ch. 48)
– Salivary gland problems
– Vocal cord abnormality (photos of)

Fig. 1

Vocal cord nodules

Patient after total laryngectomy

Station 277: Throat history

• *A 72-year-old male smoker has been referred by his GP with a hoarse voice. Please take a structured history*

Hints and tips

• The key points you should aim to cover in your history are listed opposite
• Ascertain the patient's reason for attending and determine the main and associated symptoms
• Remember to assess impact of the symptoms on the patient's life and work
• Address any concerns the patient has

Station 278: Throat examination

Hints and tips

• See Chapter 48 for examination of the neck
• *Examine the oropharynx*: initially use a tongue depressor and pen torch to examine the oral cavity and oropharynx. You should assess:

• tongue
• hard and soft palate
• tonsillar fossa
• gingivolabial/gingivobuccal sulci
• floor of mouth/undersurface of tongue
• uvula and palatal movements
• teeth
• *Examine the larynx*:
  • initially listen to the patient speak to assess for dysphonia and noisy breathing
  • observe the breathing pattern
  • to examine the larynx it is necessary to perform indirect or fibre-optic laryngoscopy; these would not be assessed in an OSCE at undergraduate level
  • indirect laryngoscopy is demonstrated in Fig. 1 above
• *Completion*: a full neck examination including lymph nodes and salivary glands

Station 279: Ear cases

Otitis media

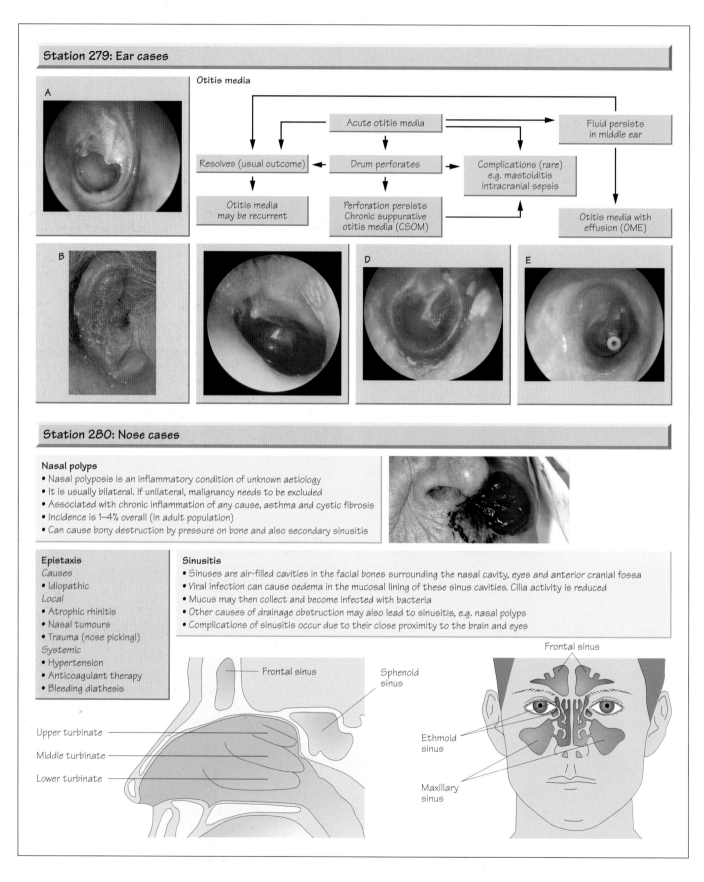

Acute otitis media

Resolves (usual outcome)

Drum perforates

Fluid persists in middle ear

Complications (rare) e.g. mastoiditis intracranial sepsis

Otitis media may be recurrent

Perforation persists Chronic suppurative otitis media (CSOM)

Otitis media with effusion (OME)

Station 280: Nose cases

Nasal polyps
- Nasal polyposis is an inflammatory condition of unknown aetiology
- It is usually bilateral. If unilateral, malignancy needs to be excluded
- Associated with chronic inflammation of any cause, asthma and cystic fibrosis
- Incidence is 1–4% overall (in adult population)
- Can cause bony destruction by pressure on bone and also secondary sinusitis

Epistaxis
Causes
- Idiopathic
Local
- Atrophic rhinitis
- Nasal tumours
- Trauma (nose picking!)
Systemic
- Hypertension
- Anticoagulant therapy
- Bleeding diathesis

Sinusitis
- Sinuses are air-filled cavities in the facial bones surrounding the nasal cavity, eyes and anterior cranial fossa
- Viral infection can cause oedema in the mucosal lining of these sinus cavities. Cilia activity is reduced
- Mucus may then collect and become infected with bacteria
- Other causes of drainage obstruction may also lead to sinusitis, e.g. nasal polyps
- Complications of sinusitis occur due to their close proximity to the brain and eyes

Frontal sinus

Sphenoid sinus

Frontal sinus

Upper turbinate

Middle turbinate

Lower turbinate

Ethmoid sinus

Maxillary sinus

Station 279: Ear cases

• *Please look at the pictures opposite and describe the lesions*

Station 279A: Squamous cell carcinoma of the pinna
Hints and tips

• The pinna is a common place for squamous cell carcinoma (SCC) to occur and is related to sun exposure
• Presents as an ulcerating, expanding keratotic nodule

Station 279B: Perforation of the ear drum
(Fig. A)
Hints and tips

• The cause may arise from either side of the tympanic membrane, e.g. external trauma or internal infection
• It may also be therapeutic or iatrogenic, e.g. immediately prior to placement of a grommet

Station 279C: Otitis externa (Fig. B)
Hints and tips

• Characterised by pain, discharge and itch
• Infected debris is visible within the ear canal and this must be removed under direct vision if possible, or aural toilet with cotton wool if too painful
• Ask about eczema, psoriasis and dermatitis

Station 279D: Myringosclerosis
Hints and tips

• White plaques on the ear drum
• Calcification from previous ear drum trauma, e.g. acute otitis media or following grommets
• No hearing loss

Station 279E: Otitis media

• These pictures show various sequelae of otitis media. Please discuss the presentation and complications of otitis media and describe the pictures shown

Acute otitis media (AOM) (Fig. C)

• Middle ear infection
• Painful
• Usually occurs in children following URTI
• Can lead to perforation of the ear drum

Chronic suppurative otitis media (CSOM)

• Persistent perforation of the ear drum with continuing infection
• With or without cholesteatoma (keratinised squamous epithelium in the middle ear)

Otitis media with effusion (OME, i.e. glue ear) (Fig. D)

• Fluid in the middle ear with intact tympanic membrane
• Commonest cause of hearing impairment in children
• Main feature on inspection is a dull tympanic membrane (occasionally an air–fluid level is seen)
• Often resolves spontaneously
• May need insertion of a ventilation tube (grommet; Fig. E) if OME persists beyond 3 months (or offer hearing aid)

Station 280: Nose cases

• *Please examine this patient's nose*

Station 280A: Nasal polyps

The box opposite outlines the aetiology and associations. Nasal polyps typically occur in male, middle-aged patients.

Sx   Blocked nose/nasal congestion
      Changes in sense of taste and smell
      Persistent postnasal drip
Rx   *Medical*   Intranasal topical steroid ± oral steroids
      Surgery   Polypectomy

Station 280B: Epistaxis
Hints and tips

• Nose bleeds are a common ENT problem
• It is important to remember that it may be life threatening, particularly in the elderly or those with co-morbid conditions
• The nasal septum has a rich blood supply (see figure in Ch. 100). A large anastomosis of arteries (Kiesselbach's plexus) occurs in the anterior septum (Little's area). Bleeding usually arises from here in young patients

Mx   ABCDE (see Ch. 11)
      Check FBC, clotting and G&S
      Sit patient upright and lean patient forward (to avoid
      swallowing or inhaling blood)
      Pinch cartilaginous nose for 15 minutes
      Pledgets soaked in lignocaine and adrenaline (1 : 10 000)
      Cauterise with silver nitrate (if bleeding point is seen)
      Insert special nasal tampons to tamponade bleeding (lubricate
      with gel and insert horizontally along nasal floor)
      Alternatively, ribbon packing can be used

Station 280C: Sinusitis
Hints and tips

• *Acute sinusitis*:
  • usually unilateral and after an URTI
  • symptoms usually last < 3 months
• *Chronic sinusitis*:
  • pain is less of a feature
  • symptoms last > 3 months
• Presentation is often non-specific
• Complications can be life threatening

Sx   Nasal congestion
      Purulent discharge
      Facial pain with headache
      Dental pain (maxillary sinus)
      Alteration in sense of smell
      Pain may be exacerbated by leaning forward or head movement

NB. Facial pain in the absence of nasal symptoms is unlikely to be sinusitis.

Rx   Cases are usually self-limiting
      Analgesia and decongestants
      Antibiotics
      Topical nasal steroids
Complications   Osteomyelitis
             Orbital cellulitis
             Intracranial involvement

Station 281: Hearing tests

Rinne's test

A

B

Weber's test

C

D

E

More complex

F

More complex

G

Station 282: Impedance audiometry (tympanogram)

Normal

Amount of sound absorbed by middle ear

Pressure in e.a.m. in da Pa

Glue ear

Amount of sound absorbed by middle ear

Pressure in e.a.m. in da Pa

Eustachian tube dysfunction

Amount of sound absorbed by middle ear

Pressure in e.a.m. in da Pa

Station 283: Pure tone audiometry (hearing test)

(a) Hearing loss in decibels

(b)

(c) Hearing loss in decibels

(d)

(e) Hearing loss in decibels

Air left ✗
Air right ●
Bone left]
Bone right [

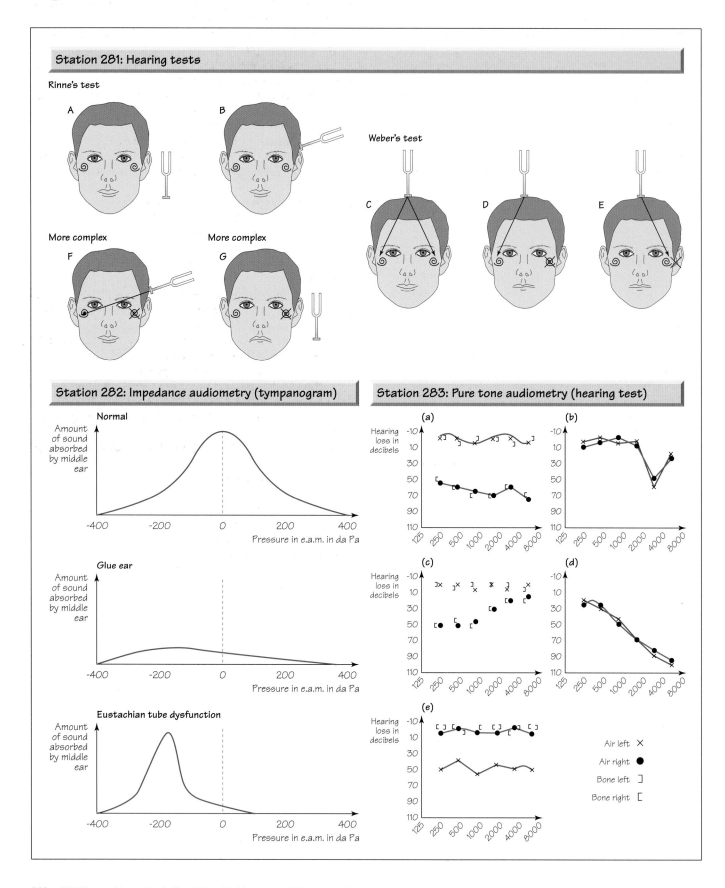

Station 281: Hearing tests

- *Use this tuning fork to assess this patient's hearing*
- *What methods of hearing assessment are you aware of?*
- *How could you assess whether a child has glue ear?*
- *This patient complains of hearing difficulties. How would you investigate the cause?*

Rinne's test

- Use a 512 Hz tuning fork as it has a slow decay in sound intensity
- The test compares the intensity of sound heard with air conduction (Fig. A opposite) and bone conduction (Fig. B)
- In patients with normal hearing, air conduction should be perceived as louder
- In conductive deafness (external auditory meatus blocked with wax or in a child with glue ear) bone conduction will be louder

Weber's test

- Place the tuning fork in the midline of the head/forehead
- In normal ears the sound should be of equal intensity in both ears (Fig. C)
- In unilateral nerve deafness (Fig. D) the sound should be louder in the 'good' ear
- In conductive deafness (Fig. E) the sound is perceived as being louder in the 'bad' ear because the 'good' ear is subject to ambient sound which decreases its sensitivity (i.e. raises its threshold)

False-negative Rinne

- This is the 'catch' with these tests
- It occurs in patients with unilateral nerve deafness
- The Weber's test is accurate and shows the sound heard in the 'good' ear (Fig. D); however in the Rinne's test, bone conduction (Fig. F) appears better than air (Fig. G)
- This is because the neural deafness means the patient cannot hear air conduction on that side but when bone conduction is tested the patient is actually detecting it on the other side

Station 282: Impedance audiometry

Hints and tips

- Impedance audiometry (tympanogram) allows the measurement of middle ear compliance and pressure
- It measures the amount of sound absorbed by the middle ear at different pressures in the external ear canal
- This is normally maximal when the pressures on both sides of the ear drum are equal (at atmospheric pressure)
- If the pressure in the middle ear falls then the ear drum is 'stiffened' and the maximum sound absorbance is when this is 'corrected' by reducing the pressure in the canal to match it
- This sort of picture is seen with eustachian tube dysfunction
- When the middle ear is filled with 'glue' very little sound is absorbed by the middle ear despite changes in the ear canal pressure

Discussion points

- How do grommets work?
- Why do your ears 'pop' on aeroplanes?

Station 283: Pure tone audiometry

Hints and tips

- The audiogram measures the loss of hearing (compared to normal) in decibels (y-axis) at various frequencies measured in cycles per second (cps = Hertz)
- Note that measurements of bone and air conductance are made for both sides and are given different symbols
- Five 'classic' audiograms are shown opposite:
  - unilateral nerve deafness (e.g. acoustic neuroma): Fig. a
  - noise injury (bilateral dip at one frequency): Fig. b
  - Ménière's disease (typically unilateral loss at lower frequencies): Fig. c
  - presbycousis (mainly high frequency loss, associated with ageing): Fig. d
  - left conductive deafness: Fig. e

Discussion points

- What is an acoustic neuroma?
- How may an acoustic neuroma present?
- What is Ménière's disease?

Station 284: Psychiatric history

Presenting complaint, history of presenting complaint
Past psychiatric history:
    Episodes, admissions, treatment, response
    Use of Mental Health Act (MHA)
Developmental history:
    Birth, early childhood, developmental milestones
    School - relationships with peers, academic ability
    Adolescence - sexual relationships, leaving home
    Adulthood - work, relationships, children
Forensic history:
    Age, penalty imposed, current conditions
Social history:
    Finances, current living arrangements
    Driving licence
    Illicit drug use - frequency, quantity
    Alcohol - units per week, binge pattern
    Symptoms of dependency
Family history
    Physical or mental illness, suicide
Pre-morbid personality

Station 285: Risk assessment

• Suicide, self-harm
• Self-neglect
• Harm to others
• Harm to children (emotional/physical/sexual abuse/neglect)
• Harm to property (including fire-setting)

Assessing suicide risk: Beck Suicide Scale [1]

1. Preparation	a. Planned in advance
	b. Suicide note
	c. Final acts (e.g. made a will)
2. Circumstances	a. Alone
	b. Intervention unlikely
	c. Precautions against discovery
3. After the act	a. Did not seek help
	b. Stated wish to die
	c. Believed act would be fatal
	d. Regrets its failure

Presence of five or more is considered significant risk

Station 286: Mental state examination

Appearance
Clothes: appropriateness
Hair/beard: well kempt or dishevelled
Facial expression

Behaviour
Non-verbal communication: eye contact, rapport, posture
Movement: agitation, involuntary movements (e.g. extrapyramidal side effects), psychomotor retardation

Speech (and form of thought)
Rate: e.g. pressure of speech
Volume
Prosody
Form of thought: flight of ideas, loosening of associations, thought block, neologisms

Mood (subjective and objective)
Depressed, anxious, irritable, perplexed, elated
Reactivity of affect: labile, blunt, flat

Thought content
Delusions (fixed, false beliefs out of context of cultural background – differentiate from over-valued ideas)
Themes: grandiose, persecutory, jealousy or self-referential (e.g. news reporter sending coded messages by way of his gestures)
Obsessional thoughts
Depressive thoughts
Suicidal thoughts

Perception
Hallucinations: visual, auditory, tactile, olfactory, somatic
Illusions

Cognition
Alertness   Memory
Concentration
Mini Mental State Examination (MMSE)

Insight
Into illness and treatment

Types of station

With an actor:
• History
• Mental state
• Risk assessment
• Explanation of medication
• Explanation of psychotherapy
• Explanation of prognosis/diagnosis

Types of station

Without an actor:
• Mental state: patient with psychotic symptoms on video
• Discussion of a vignette, e.g. differential diagnosis and management
• Discussion of the case you have just seen, e.g. discuss your assessment of risk with a consultant

Psychiatry OSCEs: introduction

In psychiatry OSCEs the examiners are likely to be assessing you in two ways:

• Your level of knowledge about diagnosis and management of common psychiatric disorders
• Your communication skills

You will be more likely to meet an actor than a patient and they may be instructed to behave as though they are anxious, angry or suspicious.

Station 284: Psychiatric history

Student info: *This young woman presented to A&E following an overdose of paracetamol yesterday. She is now medically fit for discharge. Please take a history*

Patient info: *You are a 25-year-old woman from a country in central Africa. You fled your home a year ago during a civil war in which several close members of your family were killed by men with machetes and you feared for your life. You have trouble sleeping and feel anxious a great deal of the time. You have to hide away your kitchen knives, because they remind you of what happened. You have requested asylum in the UK, but have to attend a hearing next week. You have been told that you are likely to be refused asylum. Today, you felt that you could no longer cope with life. You would rather die than face being tortured in your home country, so you took an overdose with the intention of ending your life*

Hints and tips

• Even if it is obvious that you do not need one for the OSCE, remember to say that you would arrange for an interpreter to be present if necessary
• Remember general communication skills and build a rapport carefully, the patient may be feeling distressed, anxious or suspicious
• The history you take should include a risk assessment
• To assess her symptoms you will need to ask about her current problems and go on to screen for other psychiatric disorders, particularly mood and anxiety disorders
• You should try to ask for some details about the reason why the patient fled or what exactly happened as she may need specific treatment or counselling (e.g. if she was raped or tortured)

ΔΔ   Post-traumatic stress disorder
     Adjustment disorder
     Depression

Further assessment/management

• Physical examination
• Collateral history: the patient may have workers within the asylum system who can provide further information on her asylum status and cultural factors that may be important

Station 285: Risk assessment

Student info: *This 25-year-old woman took an overdose of 30 paracetamol yesterday. Now she is medically fit to go home. Assess the risks for this patient*

Patient info: *You are a married, 25-year-old woman with twin 18-month-old daughters and a 4-year-old son. You previously worked as a chef but gave that up when you had children. You think you have been depressed since your father died unexpectedly of a heart attack 9 months ago. You have lost weight, wake up at 4 a.m. most days, have no energy and cannot remember the last time you enjoyed anything. You have been feeling quite isolated lately, but you are glad your husband works away because he sometimes hits you. Yesterday afternoon a friend came over to visit and you had a few glasses of wine. Afterwards you were feeling very low. You realised that your family would be better off without you, so you took the children to visit your mother and went home to take the overdose. You were certain that you wanted to die at that point. Your mother came round unexpectedly, realised what had happened and called an ambulance. Now you feel a bit embarrassed about the overdose, but you really cannot see any hope for the future, and do not know how you are going to cope. You have not told your husband anything yet, and the children are still with their grandmother. From the age of 15 until you were 18, you were treated for anorexia nervosa*

Hints and tips

• Be sensitive: suicide can be a difficult topic for patients to talk about, but broach the subject clearly and openly
• The Beck Suicide Scale can be used as a guide when asking about the presenting episode of self-harm
• Other factors in the history that should be elicited in this case are: previous recent suicidal thoughts (frequency and duration), past history of deliberate self-harm, and current depressive symptoms, particularly hopelessness and delusions or overvalued ideas of guilt or worthlessness
• Use of alcohol: continued alcohol use increases the risk of further impulsive deliberate self-harm
• Protective factors, e.g. sources of support
• Risk to others: has she thought about harming the children ('taking them with her')? Are the children at risk from neglect?

Discussion points

• What is your opinion about the level of risk in this patient?
• What is your differential diagnosis?
• How would you find out whether the patient currently has an eating disorder?
• How would you manage the risks in this patient?
• Could you use the Mental Health Act to treat this patient against her will? (Yes, if you are treating a psychiatric disorder, e.g. depression, and you believe that the treatment is necessary to protect the patient from serious harm, e.g. completed suicide)

Further assessment/management

• Collateral history, e.g. from mother
• Physical examination and investigations to rule out organic causes
• Risk management: in-patient versus out-patient; involve multidisciplinary team, GP, medication and social support
• Assess risk to children: it would be your duty to inform social services if you believed there was a serious risk of neglect or harm to the children, either physical or emotional
• Assess for other psychiatric disorders such as alcohol dependence and personality disorder (e.g. emotionally unstable, borderline type)
• Treat any underlying psychiatric disorder, e.g. depression

Station 286: Mental state examination

Student info: *You are a junior doctor on call for general surgery. A 44-year-old man has been admitted with appendicitis. The nurses on the ward say that he appears 'paranoid' and the anaesthetist has asked you to assess his mental state*

Patient info: *You are Mr G, a divorced 44-year-old mechanic. You have two teenage children who live with your ex-wife nearby. Your life has been pretty stressful for the past year. You have smoked* *amphetamines on and off for many years and last Christmas you bought large amounts from some dealers, hoping to sell it on. You ended up owing them a few hundred pounds, and only just managed to keep your job by promising your boss that you were 'clean'. Your girlfriend left you about a month ago. Now you are worried that the dealers are after you. They have been waiting outside your house and following you to work in a car. They have also been able to tap your phone. You have noticed people looking at you in the street. You have heard the dealers talking outside your house at night, but cannot make out what they are saying. You like watching Eastenders, but you think that one of the actors has been making threats to you personally through the story-line. You know this sounds a bit mad, and are not keen on telling the doctor. You are also worried that the doctor will turn you in to the police, so are very suspicious of him/her. You came in because you have excruciating abdominal pain, and you think this definitely has something to do with the dealers, perhaps they have poisoned your food . . .*

Hints and tips

- Set up will be important here. You may wish to have a nurse with you. A relative of the patient would also be likely to make your job easier, if the patient agreed. The patient is likely to be extremely suspicious of you, so ensure you have left your pager with a colleague and wait a while before you start writing things down
- Build a rapport with the patient/actor – find out what they are worried about early on, if you can, then explain that what they tell you is confidential (within the usual limitations)
- When you listen to the patient talk, check whether you are following his train of thought
- Have in mind introductory questions for parts of the assessment such as delusions and hallucinations, which the patient may not be keen to talk about, e.g. 'Sometimes people have experiences that they can't explain . . .'
- To assess abnormal experiences such as hallucinations, ask in detail about a recent time the patient experienced one. Ask about where they were, what they were doing at the time, how did they notice it, where was it coming from?
- Differentiate delusions from over-valued ideas. Ask about what evidence the patient has for these beliefs, without challenging them and losing their trust
- For the cognitive section, you can use the MMSE (mini mental state examination)

- When you ask about insight, find out the patient's explanation for what is wrong and what he thinks needs to be done about it

Discussion points

- What is your differential diagnosis?
- What are the risks in this patient (suicide, self-neglect, harm to others, medical risks (e.g. refusal to have the procedure), blood-borne infections if using IV drugs)
- How would you manage this patient? (Further history, examination and investigations, including urine toxicology screen. Consider drug-induced psychosis or delirium secondary to sepsis and treat these appropriately. Discuss with the anaesthetist and your consultant before the surgery (but do not delay the appendicectomy unnecessarily). Refer to a psychiatrist for further management of psychotic symptoms)
- How would you assess whether the patient has capacity to consent to an appendicectomy?
- Would you use the Mental Health Act to carry out the appendicectomy against the patient's will? (No, the Mental Health Act can only be used to treat mental disorders)

Capacity

If a patient has capacity to consent, then it must be obtained. Patients are deemed to have capacity until it is proven otherwise. The degree of understanding required to give or withhold consent varies depending on the procedure. In this case, the patient needs to be able to:

- Understand the medical condition (appendicitis)
- Understand the options for treatment (urgent appendicectomy is pretty much the only option)
- Understand the risks of the procedure and the likely consequences if he did not have it
- Remember and weigh up the information to come to a decision and communicate the decision

If the patient does not have capacity to give consent, then the procedure can go ahead without his consent only if it is deemed to be immediately necessary to prevent death or serious harm.

---

[1] Beck AT, Weissman A, Lester D, Trexler L. Classification of suicidal behaviours II: dimensions of suicidal intent. *Archives of General Psychiatry* 1976;**33**:835–7.

Station 287: Assessment of psychosis

Schneider's symptoms of first rank importance
The presence of just one of these symptoms suggests a diagnosis of schizophrenia

Delusions of thought alienation
An outside force is controlling the patient's thoughts in the following ways:
- Thought insertion
- Thought withdrawal
- Thought broadcast

Delusions of passivity
The patient is being made to do something, want to do something or feel something by an outside force, i.e.
- Made act
- Made will
- Made feeling

Somatic passivity
A delusional belief that an outside force is controlling a part of the body

Delusional perception
A normal percept (e.g. traffic lights changing) is interpreted in a delusional way (signals that his family are all dead). It comes as a fully formed delusion 'out of the blue' (autochthonous)

Auditory hallucinations
- Third person (talking about the patient as he/she/it)
- Running commentary
- Thought echo

Formal thought disorder is when the form of thought is disordered, i.e. the flow of thoughts and how they are linked together are abnormal. It is assessed by listening to how the patient talks (and can be seen in their writing). This is very difficult to act and the most likely way it could be included in an OSCE would be using a video of a patient. Examples you might see are:
- Loosening of associations - apparent loss of links between thoughts
- Flight of ideas - thoughts still have links between them, but flow of thoughts is too fast
- Thought block: - sudden loss of train of thought
- Neologisms - idiosyncratic use of words or made up words

Station 288: Biological management of psychosis

Subjects to include in an explanation about starting any drug (after ensuring it is safe to start treatment)
- Dose, timing, likely duration of treatment
- Usually start at low dose with gradual increase
- Delayed onset of action
- Side effects: common ones and rare but serious ones
- Frequency of blood tests/other monitoring, e.g. ECG
- Mechanism of action (in lay terms, e.g. correction of imbalance of chemicals in certain parts of the brain) and explanation that these are not drugs that cause addiction
- Stopping: medication should be gradually withdrawn under supervision of a doctor
- Special considerations, e.g. women of child-bearing age

All antipsychotics can cause almost all of the following side effects to some degree. Examples of the worst offenders are given:
- Extrapyramidal (typicals, e.g. haloperidol)
    Parkinsonism: rigidity, bradykinesia, tremor
    Akathisia: restlessness (motor/cognitive)
    Dystonia
    Tardive dyskinesia
- Weight gain
- Sedation
- Hyperprolactinaemia (risperidone)
- Sexual dysfunction
- Postural hypotension (clozapine)
- Diabetes, dyslipidaemia (olanzapine, clozapine)
- Reduced seizure threshold
- Cardiomyopathy (clozapine)
- QTc prolongation
- Neuroleptic malignant syndrome (haloperidol)
- Cholinergic, e.g. dry mouth (typical antipsychotics)
- Increased liver enzymes (olanzapine)

Station 289: Psychosocial management of psychosis

This is where the multidisciplinary team (MDT) becomes important. Know who would be in it and what each member would do

Formal psychological therapy
- Cognitive-behavioural therapy: targeted at the distress caused by psychotic symptoms, aiming to later challenge delusional beliefs or hallucinations
- Family therapy: based on the idea that levels of expressed emotion are high in some families of patients with schizophrenia ('hypercritical and over-involved').

Social
- Employment, finances, housing (social worker)
- Activities (occupational therapist)
- Social skills training

Station 287: Assessment of psychosis

Student info: *LK is a physics student. He has been brought to A&E by his housemate who says that he has been acting bizarrely for 3 weeks. He has been withdrawn and suspicious. Assess this patient's mental state*

Patient info: *You are a 19-year-old student. Your housemate has insisted on bringing you to hospital because he thinks you are unwell. You are angry that he thinks this because you are very worried that the students next door are plotting to kill you, and no-one seems to believe you. You owe them some money (£20) for some cannabis they gave you. You have been staying awake at night because you are too frightened to go to sleep. At night you hear them talking about you. You think they know where your parents and younger brother live, and are worried that if they do not kill you, it will not be long before they find your family. You are sure that the students are somehow listening in to your thoughts – you cannot say how – but this terrifies you*

Hints and tips

• Ascertain the patient's understanding of why he has come into hospital – this will allow you to gain an idea of his level of insight

• If the patient is distressed and anxious, it is important that you are empathic towards him, rather than challenging the truth of the experiences he is reporting

• Memorise a set of questions that you can use to ask about first rank symptoms

• Find out whether the patient needs to protect himself by carrying a weapon, whether he has any idea about who exactly poses a threat to him and whether he has considered harming this person. Also ask about whether he perceives any threat to his loved ones and ask about suicidal thoughts – he may be planning to commit suicide in order to protect his family

Discussion points

• Which of Schneider's first rank symptoms does this patient have? List the others

• What is the significance of having first rank symptoms?

• In a different scenario with a patient with delusions of persecution, you may be asked to carry out a risk assessment

ΔΔ   Drug-induced psychosis (amphetamines or cocaine are most likely to cause this picture)
Schizophrenia
Schizoaffective disorder
Acute and transient psychotic disorder
Organic illness, e.g. brain tumour

Ix   Collateral history from housemate and family (if the patient agrees, you can ask friends/family for further information, e.g. substance misuse, FH and to ascertain that the reported persecution is delusional)
Physical examination, including neurological with fundoscopy
Urine toxicology screen
FBC, U&Es, LFTs, TFTs, calcium, glucose, syphilis serology

Station 288: Biological management of psychosis

Management is likely to come up in a station where you are asked to explain something to the patient or a relative. In psychiatry this includes the psychological and social aspects of care in addition to medication. In general, for patients with an acute psychotic episode, you should assess the risks and consider in-patient management (or intensive home treatment from, for example, a crisis team) for further assessment before commencing antipsychotic medication.

Student info: *MS is a 21-year-old shop assistant. He has been on the psychiatric ward for 3 months. He was admitted this time with his second psychotic episode in 2 years and has been diagnosed as having schizophrenia. He stopped attending for his depot injections a few months before this episode began, and your consultant would like to start him back on an antipsychotic drug. You have arranged to speak to the patient about starting an antipsychotic medication. Choose one antipsychotic medication that you would like to talk about*

Patient info: *You have been told that you have schizophrenia. You know that this is because you were hearing voices, but you still do not really understand why it happened. You have stopped hearing voices now, but since you came back into hospital, you have lost your job, your girlfriend has left you and you have been evicted from your rented flat. The doctors have said that the depot antipsychotic worked well, but you disliked it. It was causing problems with your sex life, and you are quite embarrassed to talk about this. You say that you do not like taking it because it has made you put on weight, which is also true. It also made you feel stiff in your face and hands. You have no idea about what will happen in the future, but you really want to leave hospital*

Hints and tips

• Ensure that you remember all the usual points: find out how much the patient knows and whether he has any strong feelings about taking any medication for his symptoms; does he think he needs it, does he think the previous treatment worked?

• Ask about unwanted side effects he has experienced before. You may need to ask specifically about sensitive ones such as sexual side effects if you think it is appropriate/important

• Encourage the patient to weigh up the pros and cons of the previous treatment, so that you can find out what is important for him

• Know enough examples of antipsychotic drugs to choose one that would be appropriate for this patient

• If this was a female patient you would need to give appropriate advice about contraception, explain about the risks to the fetus and explain what to do if she were to become pregnant

Discussion points

• What is treatment-resistant schizophrenia? (Schizophrenia that has not fully responded to two trials of antipsychotic medication at an adequate dose for at least 6 weeks)

• How would you assess treatment-resistant schizophrenia? (Reconsider the diagnosis or co-morbid disorder such as drug misuse; assess whether the patient has been taking the medication as prescribed)

• How would you manage treatment-resistant schizophrenia?

• Explain how you would start a patient on clozapine (usually as an in-patient, with a baseline assessment to ensure it is safe to start, monitoring of BP, pulse, ECG, start at very low dose and gradually increase, weekly FBC initially)

Station 289: Psychosocial management of psychosis

Student info: *You are the junior doctor on a general adult psychiatric ward. Your patient JG is a 19-year-old man who was diagnosed with schizophrenia during an admission to an adolescent unit. He has had many different antipsychotic medications and has been on clozapine for the past 4 months. He has never responded well to medication and has severe negative symptoms. He still hears voices from time to time,* *but seems to have insight into these at least some of the time. He was admitted to your ward 6 months ago (before you started) and you have been told that he has made some progress since starting clozapine; for instance, he is now able to care for himself, occasionally visits the shops with a nurse and regularly goes to the gym or plays badminton with the occupational therapist. The plan is that he will be transferred to a rehabilitation unit. He would share a flat with other patients, and would be encouraged to be as independent as possible, but there would be nurses nearby 24 hours a day and check-ups with the psychiatric doctor whenever necessary. The patient has agreed for you to talk to his mother about his long-term management and prognosis. He did not want to be present for this discussion*

Relative info: *You are Mrs G. Your son is now 19 years old. You think he first became unwell at around 15 when he gradually became withdrawn and started to fall behind with his school work. He was not diagnosed with schizophrenia until he was 17, when he became frightened and started to act bizarrely. After he was discharged from the adolescent unit, you cared for him at home for a while, but you quickly realised you could not cope with him and you were worried that he might hurt your 8-year-old daughter. Since then, you have rarely seen the son you remember as a child, and you have been devastated that the doctors cannot do more for him. They have told you that this new medication he is on (clozapine) might help, but in general they do not seem very hopeful. Now he is going to be transferred to a rehabilitation unit. You are quite worried about this as you have been to visit and saw that he would have much less supervision than he has had in hospital*

Hints and tips

- Ascertain what Mrs G would like to talk about and what she knows about the outlook for her son and the proposed transfer
- Find out what her particular concerns are
- Explain the natural history of schizophrenia: some patients fully recover and have no further episodes, some fully or partially recover but have further episodes, some have little recovery and continue to have disabling symptoms in the long term
- Be realistic (negative symptoms are generally difficult to treat, and the prognosis for this patient is quite poor) but try to be hopeful where you can (his social functioning seems to have improved lately and patients may continue to improve on clozapine for many months)
- The general idea for rehabilitation in psychiatry is to enable the patient to live as full a life as possible, by optimising all aspects of their care, usually in the community. The long-term aims include a gradual move towards independent living and employment or education
- A key-worker usually coordinates the care of the patient and involvement from the MDT, and should be introduced to the patient when discharge planning begins

Discussion points

- What are the negative symptoms of schizophrenia? (Poverty of speech, blunted affect, loss of interest in social interaction)
- How can these be treated?
- What are good or bad prognostic indicators in schizophrenia?

Station 290: Assessment of mood disorders

Core symptoms of depression
Low mood, anhedonia, lack of energy

Additional symptoms
Low self-esteem, guilt, thoughts of suicide, poor concentration, psychomotor disturbance, sleep disturbance, change in appetite

Severity of a depressive episode (ICD-10)

	Number of symptoms	
	Core	Additional
Mild	2	2
Moderate	2	4
Severe	3	5

Somatic syndrome

Loss of mood reactivity	Loss of libido
Early morning wakening	Pervasive anhedonia
Loss of appetite	Diurnal mood variation
Loss of weight >5%	Psychomotor disturbance

Classification for differential diagnosis
A depressive episode can occur:
• With or without the somatic syndrome
• With or without psychosis
• As a single episode
• As part of a disorder, e.g. recurrent depressive disorder, bipolar affective disorder
• Secondary to other mental disorder, e.g. substance misuse, schizophrenia
• With co-morbid illness or disorder

Station 291: Biological management of mood disorders

Antidepressants
• Selective serotonin reuptake inhibitors
• Tricyclic antidepressants
• Selective noradrenaline reuptake inhibitors
• Monoamine oxidase inhibitors

Side effects

Hyponatraemia	Weight gain
Cardiac effects	Anti-cholinergic
Sexual dysfunction	Postural hypotension
Sedation	Discontinuation symptoms
Increase in impulsive behaviour, possible increase in suicidal behaviour in young people	

Mood stabilisers
Lithium, carbamazepine, sodium valproate
Used in:
• Mania
• Bipolar affective disorder
• Treatment resistant depression

Electroconvulsive therapy
Used in:
• Severe depression (life threatening)
• Intractable mania

Station 292: Psychosocial management of mood disorders

Social
• Housing
• Employment
• Finances
• Befriending scheme
• Leisure activities, education, social groups

Formal psychological therapy
• Cognitive-behavioural therapy
• Psychodynamic psychotherapy

Station 290: Assessment of mood disorders

Student info: *Take a history from this 35-year-old woman who gave birth 6 weeks ago*

Patient info: *You are a 35-year-old married secretary. You gave birth to your second daughter, Molly, 3 weeks ago. Your mother and husband have taken over most of the care. You think that Molly is a strange baby. She looks at you in an 'evil' way and you think she must be possessed by the devil. You are afraid that you might hurt her. Your husband does not seem to think there is anything wrong with Molly, but he is very worried about you. You have not been eating or sleeping much and struggle to get yourself washed and dressed each morning. You feel as though you have no stomach or heart and think that Molly has somehow taken your insides away. You were admitted to the mother and baby unit 2 years ago after the birth of your first daughter, when you had a manic episode. You stopped taking lithium 3 months before you conceived Molly*

Hints and tips
• In the history you will need to carry out an assessment of risk, including the risk of suicide and the risk of harm or neglect to Molly and her sister
• Assess whether the patient requires in-patient or out-patient management
• Assess the mood disorder and psychotic symptoms so that you can give a differential diagnosis
• Assess for co-morbid disorders such as anxiety and alcohol or drug misuse
• Investigations should include a physical examination to rule out organic causes and a collateral history from the husband or mother

Discussion points
• What is your differential diagnosis?
• How would you manage this patient?

- What medication would you use? (Antipsychotic and/or mood stabiliser; selective serotonin reuptake inhibitors (SSRIs) would be contraindicated due to the risk of precipitating mania)
- Can this woman continue breast-feeding?
- What advice would you give this woman about contraception if she is likely to continue using a mood stabiliser or antipsychotic medication long term?
- What are the organic causes of depression?

Station 291: Biological management of mood disorders

Student info: *Mrs Y is a 50-year-old primary school teacher who is depressed. You are her GP. You have given her advice and information over the past 6 weeks, but things have got worse and Mrs Y wishes to try an antidepressant. Choose a suitable drug and counsel her appropriately*

Patient info: *You have been depressed since your brother died unexpectedly in a car accident 1 year ago. You have trouble sleeping, your appetite is poor and you cannot enjoy anything. You previously enjoyed your job, but recently there have been some changes of staff and you are feeling a great deal of pressure at work now. Your two children are now teenagers and planning to go to university soon. Your husband works as a manager in a local factory. You have started to drink wine every night to help you sleep. You have tried the 'self-help' techniques that the doctor gave you last month, but it made little difference. You would now like to start an antidepressant, but have heard that they can be addictive. You take atenolol for high blood pressure*

Hints and tips
- See the box on starting medication in Chapter 105
- Find out what the patient knows
- Explain purpose of antidepressants (to relieve symptoms and shorten duration of episode)
- An important, serious side effect to include in the explanation is a possibility of increased suicidal behaviour soon after starting medication, which is most likely to occur in adolescents
- If starting an SSRI, explain the withdrawal phenomena and how to avoid them
- Emphasise the importance of other treatments, i.e. continue with life-style changes such as cutting down alcohol and taking regular exercise
- Offer continuing support: review every 1–2 weeks to check for response and side effects until stable
- Alcohol use may need further discussion and review – alcohol is thought to cause worsening of low mood and decrease effectiveness of antidepressant medication

Discussion points
- How would you ensure that Mrs Y is medically fit to have an antidepressant medication? (Ensure organic causes for depression have been ruled out; know contraindications and cautions)
- What advice would you give about the duration of treatment?
- Mrs Y would like to know what causes depression. How would you explain this?
- What factors in depression indicate a good or bad prognosis?

Station 292: Psychosocial management of mood disorders

Student info: *Assess this patient's depressive symptoms and explain to him the non-biological management of depression*

Patient info: *You are a 45-year-old widower. Your wife died 6 months ago from meningitis. You think she would not have died if the doctors at the A&E department had acted more quickly and you are suing the hospital. You have no children. You have a stressful job as a manager of a publishing company. Since your wife died, you have had several months off work with stress. You are taking Prozac and think it helps. Over the past month or so, you have hardly been to work at all, you have been drinking whisky every night to get to sleep and you are finding it difficult to get anything done around the house. You have been told that if you do not go back to work next month, you are likely to lose your job. You have booked an appointment with your GP because you have no idea how to manage any more*

Hints and tips
- Find out what are the most stressful tasks in the patient's life, and what he thinks are the most important things to deal with. Consider work, finances, self-care (including sleep), leisure activities and social life
- Find out what he thinks will help and what has already helped so far
- Support the patient in order to protect the things that are important to him, e.g. a letter of support to his manager or occupational health department would be likely to buy him some time with his job. He could aim for a graded return to work, rather than trying to return full time immediately
- Educate him about the benefits of lifestyle changes such as regular exercise and find out whether this is a plausible option for him
- Be hopeful. Depression is a treatable illness that the patient is likely to fully recover from
- Discuss his use of alcohol. Find out whether he has the dependence syndrome. If so, he is likely to need specific support to help him to cut down his alcohol intake
- Consider referring the patient for formal psychological therapy such as cognitive-behavioural therapy or psychodynamic psychotherapy

Discussion points
- What is treatment-resistant depression? How would you manage it?
- What is the dependence syndrome?
- How could cognitive-behavioural therapy be used with this patient? What factors would you consider if you were thinking of referring him? (Patient motivation, his understanding of the aetiology of depression, and his insight into the importance of psychological factors in the recovery process)
- What would be the contraindications for formal psychological therapy? (Current alcohol dependence would make it unlikely that the patient would be accepted if referred for formal psychological psychotherapy, but a referral could be considered if the patient's alcohol use was at a controlled level)

Dependence syndrome
This syndrome applies to drugs including alcohol.
- Narrowing of repertoire
- Tolerance (over time need more to have same effect)
- Salience (takes precedence over other activities)
- Withdrawal symptoms
- Avoidance of withdrawal symptoms by repeated use
- Subjective awareness of loss of control
- Reinstatement after abstinence

Station 293: Assessment of anxiety disorders

Anxiety disorders are characterised by marked fear or avoidance leading to poor social functioning

The diagnosis is not made on the anxiety symptoms, as these are common to all anxiety disorders, but on how the anxiety is provoked or experienced

Phobic anxiety disorders

Agoraphobia (with or without panic disorder): fear of crowds/public places, travelling alone/away from home

Social phobia: fear of social situations with risk of embarrassment

Specific phobia: highly specific fear, e.g. spiders

Other anxiety disorders

Generalised anxiety disorder: constant anxiety

Panic disorder: discrete intense short-lived episodes, no trigger

Obsessive compulsive disorder (OCD)

Obsessive thoughts are:
- Repetitive
- Intrusive
- Unpleasant
- Recognised as patient's own thoughts
- Resisted by the patient

Compulsions are unnecessary behaviours that the patient cannot resist performing

Station 294: Psychological management of anxiety disorders

Cognitive-behavioural therapy (CBT)

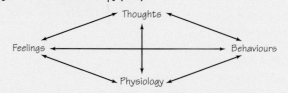

CBT assumes that a person's thoughts, feelings, behaviours and physiological state constantly interact. When an anxiety disorder develops, the interactions become distorted in such a way that a vicious circle becomes set up, e.g. a panic attack in a public place leads to avoidance of going out, distorted beliefs reinforce the fear of going out. CBT aims to identify and challenge these patterns

Techniques include thought diaries and activity scheduling. The process must be collaborative ('guided self-help') and is carried out at a pace that suits the patient. It is usually brief and problem focused, taking place over about 12-18 weekly sessions

CBT model	Condition
Graded exposure	Social phobia Specific phobia Generalised anxiety disorder
Systematic desensitisation	Agoraphobia
Exposure and response prevention	Obsessive compulsive disorder

Station 295: Biological management of anxiety disorders

Drug treatment for anxiety disorders other than OCD should usually be used second line after/with psychological therapy

Long-term management: SSRIs or serotonergic tricyclic antidepressants, e.g. clomipramine

Short-term management: benzodiazepines, but there is a risk of dependence if used for more than 4 weeks

Station 293: Assessment of anxiety disorders

Student info: *You are a GP. Take a psychiatric history from this 40-year-old woman*

Patient info: *You are a housewife with two young children. You have had 'attacks' since you were about 20. They have been getting more frequent lately and you have stopped going out. Occasionally you have a glass of wine before you go out, to settle your nerves. Otherwise, you tend to avoid going out and you feel isolated. It is a huge effort to get out of the house and your husband has insisted on bringing you today. He is in the waiting room and you are already feeling very anxious. The 'attacks' were diagnosed as panic attacks by another GP last year but you think that these episodes are heart attacks. You are extremely worried about your heart and would like the GP to check it is okay. The attacks come out of the blue, beginning with your heart racing, you feel sweaty and short of breath and then feel as though you are going to pass out and die. Your father died of a heart attack aged 45 years*

Hints and tips

- Take a history of the presenting symptoms to find out whether these are panic attacks (sudden onset, rapid build up, typical symptoms and thoughts of impending doom, death, fainting or embarrassment)
- Identify any situations that provoke anxiety: panic disorder is commonly co-morbid with agoraphobia
- Take a sufficient history to rule out organic causes (such as ischaemic heart disease), and say what examination and investigations you would like to do
- Assess for co-morbid depressive or obsessional symptoms
- Past psychiatric history: discuss other anxiety disorders and previous treatment (drugs or psychotherapy)
- Drug and alcohol use: is the patient self-medicating? Has she got the dependence syndrome?
- Assess impact on social circumstances – employment, children, relationships
- Premorbid personality: differentiate anxiety disorder from anxious/avoidant personality traits
- Differentiate from hypochondriasis

Discussion points

- What investigations would you use to exclude cardiac causes?
- Do you know of any other causes of these symptoms? (Classically phaeochromocytoma causes sudden episodes of palpitations and sweating)
- Explain to the patient what happens physiologically during a panic attack
- Please explain cognitive-behavioural therapy (CBT) to this patient
- What difficulties with engagement could you foresee for this patient?
- What roles could other members of the psychiatry MDT play in the management of this patient?

Station 294: Psychological management of anxiety disorders

Student info: *You have referred this 25-year-old man with social phobia to your local psychotherapy unit for CBT and he has been accepted. The patient has come to see you so that you can explain what will be involved*

Patient info: *You are a single, 25-year-old software engineer who works from home. You live with your parents. You have always found it difficult to mix socially. At school you were often bullied. You still blush easily and constantly think you are about to embarrass yourself if you are with your friends. You only go out socially after you have had a few drinks to calm your nerves. You would like to do something about your symptoms as you have become socially isolated*

Hints and tips

- Find out what the patient understands about his condition and the problems it causes so that you can fit your explanation around that
- Explain the process, e.g. setting, frequency and number of sessions
- Briefly explain CBT as it would apply to this patient (graded exposure) in terms that he understands
- Provide information without overwhelming
- The patient's alcohol use would need to be maintained at a controlled, non-harmful level. There would be a risk that if he is facing difficult situations as part of his therapy, the patient may become more dependent on alcohol

Discussion points

- Can the patient continue taking medication while he is attending CBT?
- What is the prognosis for this patient?
- What role can the patient's family play in the use of CBT?

Station 295: Biological management of anxiety disorders

Student info: *You are a junior doctor in the psychiatry general out-patients clinic. Mr F has come to see you because he has been diagnosed with obsessive compulsive disorder (OCD). He has tried CBT but his symptoms have worsened and the consultant has advised that he should commence medication. Choose a suitable drug and advise Mr F appropriately*

Patient info: *You are Mr F, a 42-year-old accounts manager for a small company. You have always been quite fastidious, but for the past 8 years or so this has gradually got much worse. At work you always stay behind for several hours to check over everything you have done during the day. You have to check and re-check every task you do. At home you have to stay up until 2 or 3 a.m. every morning so that you can go through a checking routine to make sure everything is safe before you go to bed. If you try not to check things you become extremely anxious. You have frequent intrusive thoughts about people in your family coming to harm in gruesome ways. You tried CBT last year. It helped a little but you want to start medication in order to try to keep your job*

Hints and tips

- See the box in Chapter 105 about starting medication
- Discuss the rationale for starting medication – the patient is at risk of losing his job and may be pinning his hopes on a tablet. He may also need to find additional ways of coping and/or may wish to combine medication with CBT
- Selective serotonin reuptake inhibitors (SSRIs) for OCD are used at higher doses than when used for depression
- Explain that these medications are not addictive, but that the patient may well experience withdrawal symptoms if he suddenly stops taking them

Index of OSCE stations